PAIN CONTROL *with* EMDR

TREATMENT MANUAL

8TH REVISED EDITION

MARK GRANT, MA, MAPs.

First published in 1998
By Mark Grant
1 Holroyd St
Kew VIC 3101
Australia

All enquiries to markgra@ozemail.com.au

Publisher's note

This publication is designed to provide accurate and authoritative information in regard to the subject matter covered. It is sold with the understanding that the publisher is not engaged in rendering psychological, financial, legal or other professional services.

A Catalogue In Publication is available from the National Library of Australia.

ISBN 978-1-925457-44-5

Cover: Cherryart
www.cherryart.com.au
Typeset by BookPOD

Dedicated to my family

I am grateful to Bruce Eimer whose seminal EMDR pain protocol helped me get started with this application of EMDR. Ray & Zbik's 2001 chapter on CBT therapies and beyond, in Tollison et al. (Eds.) *Practical pain management* (3rd edition), gave me an early theoretical basis for this application of EMDR and has stood the test of time. I'd also like to thank my father for the gift of ADHD—a somewhat challenging inheritance incorporating a mix of sensitivity and focus vs. distractibility and a lack of a sense of limitations (to name a few). A reminder that we are all different, we do not come into this life as "blank slates," and the Greeks were right about the need to "know thyself."

My thanks to Francine Shapiro who edited the first edition of this manual many years ago, Sylvie Blair and Dalida Boustead for their patience and attention to detail in producing and editing over the years, Esta Porter and Phil Harford for collegial review, and my wife Ana for her unfailing support and encouragement.

Last but by no means least I'd like to thank my patients whose courage, resilience, and compassion have been a constant source of inspiration and wisdom.

"When a patient comes to you tremendously handicapped, how handicapped is he really? What brain cells does he have unused?"

—Milton Erickson

Contents

Introduction

Chronic pain/MUS (medically unexplained symptoms) is one of the oldest, most complex human problems, involving a combination of disabling mental and physical symptoms, mysterious etiological factors, and devastating effects on all aspects of human functioning. Saint Augustine (354–430 AD) described physical pain as "the greatest evil." Arguably, chronic pain/MUS stimulated the birth of modern psychiatry/psychology through Jean Martin Charcot's employment of hypnosis with hysteria in the late 19th century. All subsequent approaches, including psychoanalysis, behaviorism, and cognitive behavior therapy have grappled with the challenge of this problem, with mixed results. Remarkably, given the advances in the healing sciences of the last century, chronic pain/MUS remains one of the most common human afflictions, affecting one in four people.

EMDR (eye movement desnsitization and reprocessing) therapy, which originated as a treatment for post-traumatic stress disorder (PTSD), presents as a natural alternative because of its efficacy with trauma, which is often a contributing factor to chronic pain/MUS, and its ability to stimulate physiological changes.[1] Depending on how you look at it, the method also either stimulated or caught a wave of increased recognition of the traumatic antecedents of a wide range of psychological and physical problems. Trauma is here defined not only as sexual abuse, but also the effects of emotional abuse, neglect, and adversity. Some will argue correctly that the latter are not traumatic in the true sense of the word, yet their effects are actually more profound for the trajectory of a person's life and health. We also know that no matter how much denial, repression, or dissociation the individual employs, their body will keep replaying those learned survival responses, which either include pain or lead to pain through their long-term effects on the central nervous system. These understandings have also stimulated what could only be called a revolution in our approach to psychotherapy, toward body-based, bottom-up approaches and practices which are increasingly informed by neuroscience.

This manual represents an attempt to operationalize these discoveries based on an EMDR framework. A growing body of research (there are currently over six randomized controlled trials, or RCTs) supports the method's potential as a treatment for pain.[2] I have been refining this application of EMDR for over 20 years via a combination of clinical work and peer-reviewed research, hence the need to continuously revise it.

This manual is divided into three parts addressing the theoretical, practical, and adjunctive therapeutic demands associated with treating sufferers of chronic pain/MUS.

Part One reviews our understanding of pain as a psychological problem from hysteria through to current trauma-informed models. It will be seen how pain can be, and often is, a product of multiple etiological factors including attachment deficits, trauma, complex health problems, and even medical procedures. Dissociative processes, ranging from everyday changes in consciousness to structural dissociation, are inevitably present. Chapter 3 reviews recent discoveries regarding the structure and functioning of the brain, the effects of severe stress on the brain, and its implications for psychotherapy. It will be shown that EMDR fulfills many of the criteria for a neurobiologically informed psychotherapy.

Part Two describes a protocol for the treatment of chronic pain using EMDR. EMDR was developed with the aim of being adopted and used according to a manualized protocol, enabling accurate dissemination of the method and facilitating research testing. The protocol section includes extensive information about the history taking, assessment, and preparation phases of EMDR treatment of chronic pain, including what to look out for when assessing chronic pain sufferers, how to develop workable EMDR "targets," how to deal with "blockages," how to use bilateral stimulation to reduce pain, and how to install resources and future templates. Reflecting the unique demands of chronic pain/MUS, eight key differences between the standard trauma protocol and the pain protocol are identified and summarized. It will be seen that EMDR often has to be supplemented with adjunctive strategies such as hypnosis, ego state work and somatically focused interventions.

Part Three consists of treatment resources for the therapist and the client. The first section consists of Therapist Resources for assessment, treatment planning, and applying the pain protocol, including an abbreviated working version of the pain protocol.

The Client Resources section contains many handouts and worksheets designed to help clients understand their pain, increase their self-care, sleep better, and better manage the physical and emotional aspects of their pain. The "Chronic pain fact sheet" and "Pain management recipe" are vital client information resources for every new client.

All of the therapist and client resources are available as separate PDFs from the self-help pages of www.overcomingpain.com. Clients are referred to as patients and clients alternately throughout this text. Although the term "client" was adopted to address the power imbalance in medicine, its commercial connotations do not reflect the nature of the therapeutic relationship. The therapeutic relationship is a healing one, based on care, trust, intimacy, the provision of safety (so the patient can be vulnerable/regressed), and responsibility (on both sides).[3]

I hope that this manual will extend your work as an EMDR clinician and that it will also stimulate more research and wider acceptance regarding this application of EMDR.

Mark Grant

Melbourne
December, 2023

PART ONE

RESEARCH AND THEORY

1

The Problem of Pain

Any approach to the treatment of chronic pain/MUS begins with the challenge of defining pain—is it physical, mental, or a combination of both? Why is this even an issue? More than any other "psychological" problem, our understanding of pain is shaped by historical and cultural factors which influence how our patients experience pain, and how we engage with them, in ways which we may not be conscious of. Before Descartes there was little distinction between physical, mental, and spiritual pain. Now we view pain in terms of chronic vs. acute, functional vs. organic, nociceptive vs. neuropathic. Something has been lost. How can we understand, let alone treat, patients who have developed crippling pain following a minor injury or sometimes no injury at all? What is the relationship between present physical pain and past emotional pain? What unmet needs might pain be signaling? How can we bridge the gap between past and present, mind and body, in the most healing way?

What is pain?

The word "pain" comes from the Latin *poena*, meaning punishment, torment, hardship, suffering. In our modern post-Enlightenment era, after much conflict about the nature and origins of pain (see below), the term has a more mechanistic connotation (pain as a signal of injury). Despite belated attempts by organizations such as the IASP (International Association for the Study of Pain) to reintroduce emotion into our understanding of pain, the biological view continues to dominate. The disbelief, fatigue, and frustration that this condition evokes in many (though not all) treatment professionals, let alone family and friends, attests to this. It's not a bad thing that we understand pain as something other than a curse from the gods, but when that understanding is not associated with effective treatment, then it (pain) might as well be. We need to recharge this word with its original emotional power—it would better reflect the subjective experience of pain. Ironically, one trend which may help in this regard is the discovery that most of the brain circuitry associated with chronic pain/MUS involves affective functioning (see Chapter 3). Perhaps our science-based world, where concepts such as neuroplasticity are part of the zeitgeist, will help us reconnect with this older, more phenomenological understanding of pain.

Ostensibly, physical pain begins with injury—a fracture, a ruptured disk, a torn muscle, and so on. Physical pain arises out of nerve signals stimulated by tissue damage, which travel from the body to the brain. The brain responds by signaling the muscles to tighten and protect the injured part of the body. It also guides us to "rest and protect" the injured area. Over time the damaged tissue heals, the central nervous system ceases to send out signals, and the pain goes away. This kind of pain, which is how most of us think about pain, is known as acute pain. Acute pain is time-limited, consistent with the injury which caused it, and generally manageable.

There can also be many non-medical precipitants of medically unexplained pain, as we will see shortly. Experientially chronic pain looks and feels different to acute pain (although the two often occur together). Subjectively it may be more diffuse, described by qualities like dull, throbbing, aching (although there's often a vagueness about it). Chronic pain often affects multiple bodily sites, and tends to be unpredictable and fluctuating in nature. Other health problems, fatigue, and emotional distress are typical. Where there is injury or physical pathology, it is generally insufficient to account for the level of pain and distress that is being experienced. Ronald Melzack, one of the fathers of modern pain management, famously described chronic pain as a "challenge" and a "puzzle."

Early theories of pain

From a psychological perspective, modern psychological pain management could be said to have begun with Pierre Janet in the late 19th century. Janet believed that unexplained physical symptoms were a way of preserving and reproducing trauma or severe stress via dissociation.

Janet defined dissociation as a separation between the conscious and the subconscious which only occurred when the central nervous system was overwhelmed:

> *"The memory traces of the trauma linger as subconscious fixed ideas that cannot be 'liquidated' as long as they have not been translated into a personal narrative and instead continue to intrude as terrifying perceptions, obsessional preoccupations, and somatic reexperiences. The capacity to adapt breaks down and the patient ends in a state of chronic helplessness expressed through both psychological and somatic symptoms."*

Janet was not the first psychiatrist to talk about dissociative reactions (Briquet and even Descartes talked about dissociation), but he was the first to systematically study dissociation and identify it as the crucial psychological process with which the organism reacts to overwhelming trauma and which results in the wide variety of symptoms then classified as hysteria.[1] Before Janet, pain theories reflected evolving attempts to explain pain in terms of discernible physiological pathology. Pain that did not fit what they knew about disease processes at the time was thrown into the diagnostic bins of hysteria or neurosis.[2] We will return to dissociation and its involvement in chronic pain/MUS in Chapter 2.

Note that not all chronic pain sufferers' symptoms are a result of dissociation due to big "T" trauma (e.g., sexual abuse)—Janet said it is the emotionality of the event that is the key to whether it becomes traumatic or not. Janet was right about emotionality, but wrong about linking trauma-related pain primarily to a single overwhelming event. It does happen, but other less dramatic forms of adversity are now known to play a much greater role in predisposing individuals to the onset of chronic pain/MUS. Insecure attachment has been found to be associated with two times the prevalence of chronic pain.[3] Bowlby's theory of attachment traces its origins as far back as at least the psychoanalytic era and concepts such as object relations theory. Freud also had a theory of attachment—that infants' attempts to stay near a familiar person were driven by survival needs such as food and also were part of attempts to satisfy libidinal desires.[4]

Efforts to understand pain in biological terms began with Descartes who described pain in terms of a disturbance in the body which got communicated to the brain via nerve fibers. This understanding of pain as a product of physical injury is the basis for our understanding of acute pain, also known as specificity theory. Before Descartes, pain was thought to emanate from outside the body (e.g., a curse from the gods, malevolent spirits, fairies, etc.). After Descartes there was a quest to understand pathological anatomy—where does pain originate and how does it get transmitted?

An early successor of Descartes was Robert Whytt (1715–1769) who thought that every disorder was based on nerves. By nerves I don't mean emotions but actual nerves, the neural pathways that transmit sensations through the body. Whytt thought that nervous disorders were caused by too great a delicacy of the nervous system—or irritable spine. For example, Whytt believed that irritated nerves of the uterus produced the symptoms of hysteria in pregnant women. He did demonstrate that the spinal cord was the center of nerve communication in the body. After Whytt, William Cullen (1710–1790) took a more either-or approach and tried to distinguish between nervous conditions and conditions with a more organic origin. Cullen viewed hysterical and hypochondriacal disorders in terms of nerves. While Whytt would have been content to define neurosis in physiological terms (oversensitive nerves), Cullen looked at disease in broader terms—considering the role of both action and feelings in disease. He believed that if no biological explanation could be found, then any disease must be considered to be the product of a nervous disorder.

This either-or approach is arguably driven by the left hemisphere of the human brain, which dislikes ambiguity. Human beings have the option of seeing reality through two alternate lenses, that of the left hemisphere and that of the right. Ideally they work in tandem, with primacy assigned to the right body-centered sensing hemisphere, followed by interpretation by the analytical left. We will talk more about how the brain mediates reality in Chapter 3, but for now hold the idea that the left hemisphere likes to win and will push its view, even in the face of disconfirming information. Understanding this tension between the two different takes of reality of the left and right hemispheres will make the endless see-sawing between mind and body in pain theories more understandable.

Cullen did not view nervous disorders in purely physiological terms. Cullen considered that nervous ailments involved the mind and the body—including the disease and how it affected the organism's intellectual functioning. He was the first person to refer to an imbalance in a person's emotional stability, or mind-body connection, as a neurosis. And he was the first to use the terms "hysteria" and "hyperchondriasis." His recognition of the importance of a patient's mental state led to him introducing placebos (another first), which could be active or inert substances, to address a patient's psychological needs, such as comfort and hope. Cullen's ideas were eventually replaced by a return to focusing on pathological anatomy as a basis for understanding disease in the 1820s.[5]

As a result of this return to focusing on the nervous system, reflex theory emerged. Reflex theory was developed by Marshall Hall (1790–1857)—a Scottish gynecologist who saw the spine as a central control board of a vast network of reflex actions. Reflex theory was based on the idea that nervous connections running down the spine constituted a second nervous system that regulated all bodily organs, and that any body organ can influence any other organ in the body. Reflex theory combined elements of previous theories, the idea of spinal irritation, and reflexes. For example, according to this theory the cramps of pregnancy were a product of reflexes and spinal excitation. Hysteria (e.g., lump in throat, paralysis) was thought to be caused by convulsions in the uterus. Reflex theory led to the use of surgery on the uterus to cure hysteria (as wrong-headed as it was, this trend to base treatments on theories is evident throughout the history of pain and any disease really). Reflex theory was part of attempts to make medicine more scientific by distinguishing between conditions for which there was discernible biological basis and conditions which were medically inexplicable. The aim was to develop a more precise description of conditions based on observable physiological phenomena. But it led to just about everything for which there was no discernible physiological basis being labeled as neurosis.

Jean Martin Charcot (1824–1893), the famous neurologist, based his theory of hysteria on reflex theory. Charcot believed that hysteria was inherited and that it had a physical basis (like Descartes and Whytt). He performed autopsies on deceased patients in an attempt to find the physiological bases for medical conditions. He once hired an elderly man who had a bad tremor to work in the kitchen at the Salpêtrière Hospital with a view to performing an autopsy when he died (you can imagine that the head of catering was not keen on his new hire). Indeed, after many broken plates the man eventually died, and Charcot was able to perform his autopsy—leading to the uncovering of the physiological symptoms of multiple sclerosis (MS). He also mapped the symptoms of Lou Gehrig's disease. Charcot hoped he could do the same with hysteria—an impossible task. Reflex theory disappeared fairly rapidly after Charcot's death due to four things:

1. The discovery of the endocrine system in 1870. The endocrine system is, of course, the collection of glands that produce hormones that regulate metabolism, growth and development, tissue function, sexual function, reproduction, sleep, and mood, among other things. Hormones enable one part of the body to influence what happens in another part of the body, even though there is no connection (think of it as being like Wi-Fi). For example, the pituitary gland regulates the thyroid through thyroid-stimulating hormone (TSH). The adrenal glands are regulated via the release of cortisol.

2. The rise of research methods—researchers performed a procedure on the uteruses of 20 hysterical women. Only one got better—and it was found she had visited a sanitarium while recovering from the procedure!
3. A physician by the name of James Israel found that patients suffering from hysteria got better after pseudo surgery, which rather disproved the notion that these patients had anything physically wrong.
4. The rise of psychological explanations, especially recognition that trauma could lead to physical symptoms, as described by Janet.

Sigmund Freud also believed that physical pain could be a manifestation of psychological hurt.[6] Freud thought there were three kinds of pain: pain from the body (which he regarded as transitory), pain from the world around us, and pain from our relations with others (which he regarded as the most challenging). Freud initially shared Janet's ideas about the role of early trauma but later abandoned them in favor of his theory of sexual repression. It's thought he was intimidated by the reaction from society at the time to the idea that sexual abuse could be happening. The psychoanalytic view of pain posits that unconscious conflicts between the Id (your instinctive self) and Superego (conscience) are resolved by the unconscious production of physical symptoms. The resolution of such conflict is termed "primary gain." "Secondary gain" refers to the social benefits which may accrue from having pain, e.g., support and attention, and relief from responsibility.

Theories of pain then took another swing back toward purely biological explanations—as Bessel van der Kolk notes, from the beginning of the 20th century, for the next 60 years, attention to the psychological effects of trauma was relegated to a few studies of the "war neuroses" and psychological sequelae of the Holocaust. After Charcot's death, French psychiatry gradually fell in step with the prevailing medical attitudes, and the exploration of psychopathology continued along increasingly divergent paths, with little communication between the biological, cognitive, and psychodynamic points of view.[7] The advances in the natural sciences fostered study of organs and organic functions at the expense of such psychological phenomena as consciousness, emotions, and motivation, for which the only tool of exploration was clinical observation. Janet pursued his studies in increasing isolation.

However, by the mid 20th century the limitations of the medical model could no longer be ignored (e.g., its inability to explain problems such as phantom limb pain—PLP), which stimulated the development of Melzack and Wall's gate control theory (GCT). In a way that

Cullen would have approved of, GCT proposed that pain was maintained by both physical injury AND mental factors such as attention, which mediated the experience of pain via a "gate" in the spinal cord. Melzack developed this theory after observing than animals who had undergone sensory deprivation reacted differently to painful stimuli than animals (dogs or mice) who had been reared normally. Melzack attempted to describe the neurological underpinnings of the gate in terms of large and small nerve fibers. Downward impulses (from the brain) on large fibers were said to close the gate while upward impulses (from the body) through small fibers were believed to open the gate.

Although well accepted now, GCT was quite controversial when it was first proposed and was met with vicious resistance.[8] Even now, over 50 years since the GCT was proposed, there are still medical professionals whose preference is to consider chronic medically unexplained pain in hysterical terms—as a sign of malingering, weakness, or maladjustment. Interestingly, over 100 years ago Pierre Janet rejected the Descartian division of mind and body outright—he thought it a tired debate.

GCT coincided with the development of behaviorism and then cognitive therapy and cognitive behavior therapy (CBT). CBT fitted well with GCT to explain how cognitive inputs (for example) might moderate the experience of pain.

The cognitive behavioral approach

Fordyce's operant conditioning model, based on principles of behaviorism, followed the GCT. Behaviorism was an early psychological approach which posited that all human behavior can be understood in terms of animal learning. Namely, that the repeated pairing of a particular stimulus with a particular response leads to the development of a learned behavioral response. For example, as the pain sufferer seeks to avoid aggravation of their pain through avoiding activity, the relief obtained represents a kind of reward, which encourages the sufferer to further avoid activity (as described in the discussion regarding secondary gain above). Excessive inactivity is thought to increase pain through lost muscle tone and reduced circulation. The process by which behavioral responses are learned is called operant conditioning. In contrast to psychodynamic or client-centered approaches, behaviorism represented a kind of "black box" approach to understanding human behavior, wherein all behavior can be understood as a response to either "rewards" or "punishments."

However, problems with a strictly behaviorist approach (people did not always respond in a predictable fashion) led to the introduction of cognitive factors in understanding the experience of pain. CBT, as the approach became known, viewed chronic pain as being primarily a product of negative thoughts, feelings, and behaviors rather than physical pathology. In chronic pain, the patient's suffering and disability are thought to be maintained by the patient's thoughts and beliefs about their condition. For example, chronic pain sufferers' disability is increased by their avoiding activity because of misinterpreting pain signals as meaning there is something wrong with them or that they will hurt themselves. Treatment was based on the premise that pain could be reduced by changing negative thoughts and beliefs thought to exacerbate pain perceptions.[9] The IASP's definition of pain as "... an unpleasant sensory and emotional experience" added emotion to the list of psychological factors thought to be involved in pain.

Collectively, these theories represent what's known as the biopsychosocial model of pain. In contrast to the traditional view of physical disease, the biopsychosocial model is concerned with illness, which refers to the physical discomfort, emotional distress, and behavioral limitations associated with pain and disability. The biopsychosocial model also posits that whatever their pathophysiological status, chronic pain sufferers have certain psychological characteristics in common, to explain the development of "maladaptive chronic pain behaviors" beyond what would be expected for a given injury or illness.[10]

For example, pain is thought to be increased by avoidance of activity, which causes physical deconditioning. By incorporating people's reactions to disease or injury, as well as biological processes, the biopsychosocial model provides a better framework for understanding the often disparate levels of pain and disability in relation to specific conditions and/or pain where the physical cause is unknown. However, the biopsychosocial model has largely failed to acknowledge the contribution of traumatic stress to chronic pain and it has overextended psychoanalytic concepts such as secondary gain.

The notion of secondary gain was picked up by the behaviorists who saw it as a reinforcing factor for pain behaviors. Nicholas (1996) writes: "a person seeking help for chronic pain could be said to be inactive with secondary physical deconditioning, to hold unhelpful beliefs, to be overly passive or reliant on others for resolution of his/her problems." Secondary gain has traditionally been used to explain the actions of pain sufferers. In a recent study where women chronic pain sufferers were found to have greater levels of disability than men, it was speculated that perhaps they were using the pain as an excuse to stay at home, something the author described as "a powerful secondary gain." (Gatchel 1995). But secondary gain has been overused with harmful effects for chronic pain sufferers. Pilowsky (1996) warned of the danger of an approach which emphasizes patients "taking responsibility" for their pain becoming a basis for patients being blamed for poor treatment outcomes. Eccleston et al. (1997) noted that many pain patients were confused and angry at treatment which seemed to focus on their own behavior and at being blamed for their own suffering and misery. May et al. (1999) has observed that the disparity between expressed symptoms, pathological signs, and perceived disability in chronic low back pain (CLBP) has led to the moral character of the sufferer forming a constant subtext to medical discourse about the condition. Obviously, unquestioning application of the secondary gain concept is unhelpful and only a careful, individualized assessment can ascertain the presence and nature of secondary gain in any given case. (See Fishbain D.L., Rosomoff, H.L., Cutler, R.B., & Rosomoff, R.S. (1995). Secondary gain concept: a review of the scientific evidence. *Clin J Pain, Mar, 11*(1), 6–21).

Despite hundreds of controlled studies over a period of three decades, CBT can only claim small overall effects in treating pain and "weak effects" in terms of pain relief. A Cochrane review also found that there was no clear theory regarding the mechanisms of change in CBT trials and a lack of clarity regarding specific and non-specific effects of therapy.[11] The authors also noted that central assumptions such as deconditioning and poor physical status in chronic pain remain unsubstantiated. The reviewers concluded that better theories are needed to generate hypotheses about processes and mechanisms of change.

In recent years there has been a return to acknowledging trauma as a causal factor of pain/MUS, thanks to the work of pioneers such as Charles Engel, Peter Levine, Robert Scaer and Babette Rothschild. Although trauma is generally understood as exposure to a life-threatening event, such as rape or combat, both of which can precipitate medical and medically unexplained pain, one of the most common and damaging types of chronic stress is physical and/or emotional abuse and neglect in childhood. Emotional abuse means being subject to criticism or ridicule by one's parents, being manipulated and/or being held responsible for things which are outside a person's control. Emotional neglect means not receiving adequate love and affection either because one's parents were not around or because they were unable to show love. Emotional abuse and neglect tend to occur in families where there was mental illness, alcoholism or drug abuse, intergenerational abuse or neglect, violence, and instability. However, they can also occur in apparently normal families where everything may appear happy on the surface, but there is no real intimacy.

Another type of stress comes from experiencing (or witnessing) life-threatening situations such as a motor vehicle accident, physical or sexual abuse during childhood, rape, assault, war combat, and even being diagnosed with a life-threatening illness. The event must also have involved feelings of intense fear, helplessness, or horror, although sometimes these feelings may not have occurred until sometime later. PTSD involves more severe symptoms than those of normal stress, including nightmares and flashbacks, avoidance, numbness, trembling, and catatonia. PTSD can also involve re-experiencing symptoms, wherein the sufferer actually relives the traumatic event in their body. These reliving symptoms can incorporate physical pain, making PTSD the most potent form of stress in terms of causing pain. PTSD-like symptoms can also result from non life-threatening stressors such as emotional abuse and neglect, workplace bullying, the unexpected death of a loved one, and being sued. Of course, these effects are increased when traumatic stress is combined with emotional neglect.[12]

Ronald Melzack (1999) recognized how the effects of severe stress could cause, maintain, and exacerbate pain:

> *"Stressors have destructive effects on muscle, skeletal and hippocampal tissue which may become the immediate basis of pain or provide a basis for the devastating effects of later minor injuries in which the severity of pain is disproportionately far greater than would be expected from the injury."*

Severe stress is also more common than is generally thought; emotional stress such as anxiety and depression affects 20% of people in many countries. Even traumatic stressors, which used to be considered unusual, have been found to occur in over 50% of people, with problems such as child abuse and neglect affecting as much as 25% of children in developed nations.[13] Chronic pain is also stressful; it impairs physical functioning and mental health and adjustment. The stress from chronic pain can take various forms including negative feelings (anxiety, depression), memories (of past pain), and thoughts ("I can't stand this anymore"). The stress caused by chronic pain has long been thought to explain the additional suffering associated with this problem. We will explore the relationship between trauma, adversity, and pain more fully in the following chapter.

Nosology of pain

There are three broad categories of pain: nociceptive (related to tissue damage), neuropathic (combination of tissue and nerve damage), and functional (no organic pathology). Nociceptors are nerve cells that carry the pain to the spinal cord, where it gets relayed to the brain. It is called somatic pain if it results from injury to muscles, tendons, and ligaments. Somatic pain is usually well localized. It is called visceral pain if it results from injury to the internal organs like stomach, gall bladder, and urinary bladder. Visceral pain is usually diffuse and non-localizing. Somatic pain in turn is classified into cutaneous somatic pain if the pain arises from the skin, and deep somatic pain if it is from deeper musculoskeletal tissues. The various causes of joint pain are grouped under musculoskeletal pain.[14]

Nociceptive pain starts out as acute pain, at least in the early stages, whereas neuropathic pain is always chronic. Nociceptive pain is called central pain if the lesion is in the central nervous system. It is called peripheral neuropathic pain if the lesion is in the peripheral nervous system. Neuropathic pain is often described as severe, sharp, lancinating, lightning-like, stabbing, burning, cold, numbness, tingling, or weakness. It may be felt traveling along the nerve path from the spine down to the arms/hands or legs/feet. It does not respond to routine analgesics.

- Hyperpathia—increased sensitivity to nociceptive pain
- Allodynia—increased sensitivity to non-painful stimuli
- Hyperalgesia—increased sensitivity to painful stimuli
- Myofascial pain—pain associated with multiple trigger points

Nociceptive pain and neuropathic pain are not exclusive—nociceptive pain often leads to neuropathic pain. Another key difference between the two is that neuropathic pain is usually less explicable in terms of physical pathology/injury. But the classic psychological pain is functional pain. Functional pain is medically unexplained pain which exists to satisfy some usually unconscious (dissociated) psychological need. For example, a woman who was sexually abused as a child, but is amnesiac of that abuse, might develop vaginal pain when tired or stressed as a way of expressing her needs without actually having to verbalize them. Abused children often grow up with a fear of being seen and heard since any attention can lead to further victimization. This is not done consciously or deliberately. Similarly, a woman who grew up not being allowed to express her needs might develop headaches as a way of holding the tension caused by inner conflict between expressing her needs and causing problems in the family (for example) vs. not expressing her needs and denying herself. Functional abdominal pain (e.g., irritable bowel syndrome) is one of the most common pain complaints in children and adolescents.

Below is a summary of the types of pain most commonly associated with these three categories.

Different types of pain		
NOCICEPTIVE	**NEUROPATHIC**	**FUNCTIONAL**
Mechanical low back pain	Hyperpathia	Tremors
Postoperative	Hyperalgesia	Convulsions
Arthritis	Allodynia	Fatigue
Myofascial pain	Neuralgia	Paralysis
Cancer pain	CRPS	Gastrointestinal pain
Inflammation	Fibromyalgia	IBS
Burn pain	Phantom limb	Headaches

Figure 1.1 Nosology of pain

Pain classification systems

Classification systems such as the DSM and the ICD offer a way of defining chronic pain/MUS for purposes of diagnosis and case formulation, as well as communicating with third parties such as insurance companies. Classification systems also provide a kind of objective validation of the patient's suffering—as van der Linden et al. (2022) note, "If it can't be coded, it doesn't exist."[15] Despite their limited clinical utility (no diagnostic code can hope to capture the reality of a patient's suffering), classification systems are important for communicating with and accessing treatment funding from third party providers, but care needs to be exercised when using them for forensic purposes. At the same time, the complex, overlapping physical and mental phenomena that constitute pain/MUS have proven difficult to neatly conceptualize.

In the DSM-IV pain was categorized according to whether it was considered to originate primarily from psychological or medical factors. Namely,

- Pain disorder associated with psychological factors (i.e., PTSD, depression)
- Pain disorder associated with a medical condition only (i.e., cancer pain, arthritis)
- Pain disorder associated with both psychological factors and a medical condition (e.g., some types of headache pain, vaginismus)

The term "somatoform disorders" referred to symptoms suggesting physical illness or injury, but which may not be fully explained by a medical condition. In the DSM-5 this category has been replaced with somatic symptom disorder (SSD) which is based on excessive worry or preoccupation about somatic symptoms. This change is meant to be in recognition of the fact that psychological factors can play a role in pain whether or not a person has a medical diagnosis. This de-emphasis on the presence of a medical diagnosis is consistent with increased understanding that somatic symptoms can arise because of other factors than objective physical pathology (e.g., perception, emotion).

Unfortunately, the DSM-5 categorization does not easily capture people who are suffering from pain as a result of past trauma, who may present as indifferent regarding their somatic symptoms or fluctuate between indifference and worry. In patients with developmental abuse, it also misses the dissociation and/or lack of self-care that precedes and maintains their somatic symptoms. Despite mountains of evidence that they overlap, dissociative disorders, trauma and stress-related disorders, and somatic disorders are all filed in separate sections of the DSM. Other than acknowledging that problems such as PTSD or DID (dissociative identity disorder) have a somatic component, no space is given to pain which has its roots in early developmental trauma. With its classification of chronic pain as a disease in its own right, the ICD-11 offers a more clinically useful classification than the DSM in this regard.

Criticism has been leveled at the DSM-5 that the SSD categorization may lead to overdiagnosis of mental disorders in people suffering from unexplained pain. In the ICD-11 the authors have attempted to redefine pain from simply being understood as a response to injury, which has had the unintended effect of delegitimizing medically unexplained pain. Chronic pain is now categorized as either primary (the pain is the main problem) or secondary (the pain is a symptom of a medical injury or illness). Chronic primary pain refers to pain that is not consistent with an identifiable pathology (e.g., chronic regional pain syndrome, fibromyalgia, irritable bowel syndrome, non-specific low back pain), whereas chronic secondary pain refers to pain as a symptom of another disease (e.g., work accident, rheumatoid arthritis, diabetic neuropathy). Chronic primary pain is roughly equivalent to what might previously have been called idiopathic pain. Terms such as "somatization" and "functional pain" have been dropped on the grounds that they are potentially laden, but some critics have argued that the new categorization unreasonably de-emphasizes psychiatric processes.

Regardless of how pain is officially categorized, it seems likely that sufferers of medically unexplained pain will continue to struggle with being believed by others and even believing in the reality of their own experience. Hopefully some of the information about the processes underlying chronic pain presented here will help sufferers feel more validated and clearer about how to address the contribution of unresolved trauma to chronic pain.

2

Trauma and Pain

Trauma, particularly early childhood adversity, is now recognized as the primary causal factor of chronic pain/MUS. As the history of pain demonstrates, this is not a new idea, but given the trends and preferred treatments of the 20th century, it is a paradigm-altering development with radical implications for wide swaths of our profession which still frame chronic pain in cognitive-behavioral terms. What are the effects of trauma and how do they lead to ill-health and pain? How are these effects best addressed and neutralized? How important is connecting present symptoms with past learnings for healing? It's more than just knowing how to connect past trauma with present pain (as hard as that is)—we also must address the problem of dissociation, one of the most important mediating factors between trauma and chronic pain/MUS.

PTSD and pain

Trauma is caused by life-threatening events such as physical or sexual abuse in childhood, assault, rape, accidents, disasters, combat exposure, torture, medical mishaps, and even being diagnosed with a life-threatening illness.[1] This kind of simple trauma is most commonly associated with a diagnosis of PTSD. The symptoms of PTSD are well known and include:

1. Increased physiological arousal

   Increased physiological arousal in PTSD often involves intense levels of physical tension including feeling jumpy or "edgy," sleeping problems, and uncontrollable physical trembling. The main symptoms of increased physiological arousal are:

   - Insomnia: difficulty falling or staying asleep
   - Emotional dysregulation: including mood swings, irritability, etc.
   - Hypervigilance: feeling anxious and "on edge"
   - Exaggerated startle response: feeling "jumpy"
   - Concentration problems

2. Avoidance

   Avoidance associated with PTSD means avoiding thinking, talking about, or visiting places that remind you of the trauma. This can also mean avoiding thinking or talking about what happened. PTSD-related avoidance can also involve involuntary physical, emotional, and mental responses which are outside of conscious awareness. The main symptoms of avoidance:

   - Physical avoidance: avoiding situations which remind you of the trauma
   - Anesthesia: numbness or loss of sensation to parts of the body
   - Emotional: alexithymia and dissociation—decreased ability to recognize and express emotions, feeling "split off" from what you're feeling and what you're thinking or experiencing
   - Mental: avoiding thinking about the trauma
   - Amnesia: inability to remember part or all of what happened

3. Re-experiencing symptoms

   Re-experiencing symptoms is unique to PTSD and involves reliving the traumatic event through recurring thoughts, memories, and feelings associated with the original experience. Re-experiencing symptoms includes:

- Recurring and intrusive thoughts, memories, and dreams (including nightmares)
- Acting or feeling as if the traumatic event were happening again (including a sense of reliving the traumatic experience, "freezing up," hallucinations, and dissociative flashback episodes)
- Experiencing intense physical and emotional distress when exposed to situations that symbolize or resemble the traumatic event (including heart palpitations, indigestion, feelings of intense fear, terror, and anxiety)

For PTSD to be diagnosed, the initial reaction to the event must involve intense fear, helplessness, or horror. Children tend to display disorganized or agitated behavior.[2] PTSD can also involve "body memories" wherein sufferers re-experience the pain, helplessness, and/or terror of the original trauma. Body memories are physical sensations that were felt at the time of the original trauma. Body memories can incorporate a range of physical sensations including nausea, aches and pain, fatigue, heart palpitations, dizziness, etc. A classic example of this is the paralyzing back pain author and WWII soldier James A. Michener experienced after stumbling into a small ditch hours after he had walked away from a plane crash (see below).

Between 10% and 80% of chronic pain sufferers also have PTSD.[3] The types of trauma most commonly associated with pain include:

- Early childhood adversity (e.g., physical or sexual abuse, witnessing domestic violence, having a parent with a mental illness, emotional neglect, etc.)
- Serious accidents
- Surgery
- Diagnosis of a life-threatening illness
- Abortion
- Combat trauma
- Exposure to political violence

Another type of trauma which is often overlooked is medical trauma. For example, 77% of women who lost a child in childbirth were found to have PTSD. Up to 59% of ICU patients have been found to develop PTSD.[4] Bill developed PTSD after being told his foot would have to be amputated after a botched medical procedure. Five surgeries later the doctors told him his foot would be okay. But by then he had already spent two weeks preparing himself for having his foot amputated (including being measured for a prosthesis) and he was suffering intrusive thoughts, nightmares, and episodes of deep sadness and crying that would persist for years after leaving the hospital.

The types of pain most commonly associated with PTSD include nausea, muscle aches, headaches, back pain, stomachache, genital pain, and chronic widespread pain.[5] PTSD has been linked to several chronic pain syndromes including fibromyalgia, reflex sympathetic dystrophy, chronic fatigue syndrome and temporomandibular disorders.[6] PTSD seems to exacerbate pain following injury: injured people with PTSD complain of greater levels of pain than injured people without PTSD and require higher amounts of medication than non-PTSD pain patients.[7] PTSD sufferers also respond less well to medical treatment and are more likely to have complications.[8] PTSD has also been linked to health problems, including diabetes, recurring headaches, heart disease, bladder problems, immune disorders, digestive and genitourinary disorders, irritable bowel syndrome, skin problems, and increased risk of fractures.[9]

Complex trauma (CPTSD) and pain

Most people with chronic pain/MUS have suffered from more than one trauma, as well as childhood adversity in the form of emotional abuse and neglect. In one of the largest investigations of its kind, a study of 9,508 adult members of a health plan in the USA found that people who had suffered severe stress were more than twice as likely to have health problems (e.g., heart disease, diabetes, fractures, and occupational health problems) compared with people who had not.[10] These researchers also found that the most common form of severe stress came in the form of interpersonal violence (family violence, abuse, growing up in a family with mental health problems, or substance abuse). They also found that the more stressful events a person had experienced, the greater their risk of pain and illness.[11]

People who have experienced multiple traumas, particularly interpersonal abuse and neglect in childhood, develop a more severe version of PTSD known as Complex PTSD (CPTSD). Interpersonal violence typically begins in the family and can include criticism, threats, conflict, neglect, betrayal by parental figures, abandonment by parental figures, or assigning a child "adult" responsibility.

Note that the individual stressors in CPTSD may not constitute what are generally considered big "T" trauma, but cumulatively, over time, they create a chronic sense of threat and isolation that is sufficient to generate the symptoms of CPTSD. Complex trauma is also seen among people who have survived persecution, false imprisonment, torture, or sex trafficking. Although not as widely recognized as PTSD, CPTSD is actually more common.

In addition to the symptoms of normal PTSD, CPTSD involves damaged sense of self, emotional dysregulation, and relationship difficulties (see Figure 2.1). Because it involves repetitive assaults on the nervous system over prolonged periods, CPTSD involves much more "wear and tear" on the body than normal PTSD. CPTSD is associated with a greater range of illness and pain, including fatigue, headaches, back pain, gastrointestinal pain, tremors, and paralysis. Sufferers of CPTSD are also more likely to dissociate, a key link between trauma and chronic pain/MUS.

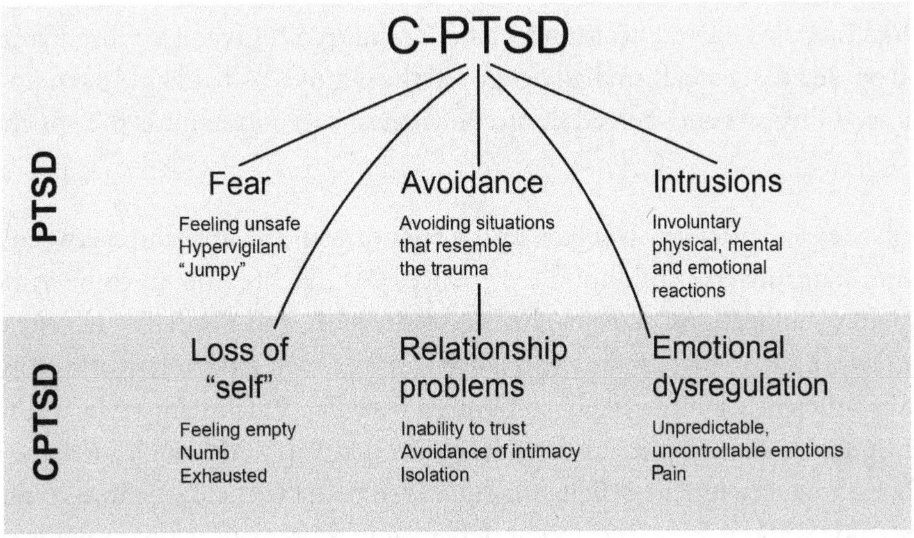

Figure 2.1 PTSD vs. CPTSD

Attachment problems are a primary etiological factor in the development of CPTSD. A secure attachment is where we learn how to manage physical and emotional pain. A secure attachment tells the child that their needs matter and that it is safe to express them. An anxious or insecure attachment tells the child that it is not safe to have needs, leading to the development of defense mechanisms such as dissociation (see below) and substitutes. For example, the child might learn not to show its needs to avoid the pain of rejection (Knipe's "shame is my safe place"). Or the child might develop perfectionistic tendencies to "earn" the right to have needs.

Attachment problems, abuse, and neglect typically occur in the family—a place which in modern times is ideally regarded as a bastion of safety but historically was anything but. For most of human history, depending on where they lived, children were regarded as chattels, slaves, or mini-adults with no rights. In Roman society the father had complete control over the family, to the extent that he could kill his children for disobedience.[12] Sexual abuse of children was common, with children often sold into prostitution. During the Industrial Revolution orphaned children as young as five were forced to work in factories, often chained to their workstations and whipped to ensure productivity. As recently as WWII, children were regarded as capable of making sexual choices and unlikely to be harmed by unwanted sexual experiences.[13] Despite advances in attitudes toward children, challenges persist. In the modern era, advanced capitalism has been linked to greater instability in intimacy and family life, and increased likelihood of mental health problems in children.[14] Over a hundred years ago, G.K. Chesterton opined that capitalism had destroyed the family: "What has broken up households and encouraged divorces and treated domestic virtues with contempt is the epoch and power of capitalism."

Although there has not been a lot of research regarding the relationship between attachment problems and pain, adverse childhood experiences (ACEs) are known to be associated with increased pain complications, catastrophizing, depression, and poorer treatment outcomes.[15] One of the few studies to investigate the relationship between attachment and pain found that chronic pain sufferers are more likely to have an insecure attachment style and report more fear, hypervigilance, catastrophizing, and less pain control.[16] Although we have some good theories about how attachment deficits might lead to pain (see below), more research is needed to support ideas about how attachment deficits might predispose the individual to chronic pain/MUS.

People with anxious attachments tend to be more hypervigilant, ever fearful of judgment and rejection. As can be imagined, this heightens the physiological response to physical and emotional pain. Individuals with avoidant attachment tend to respond to injury and pain with deactivating strategies—they downplay their experience. Individuals with avoidant attachment also tend to be more self-reliant and have difficulties with intimacy.

Mary Owen, a famous Australian women's liberationist, was raised by a stepmother after her mother died when she was a baby. Although Mary's stepmother provided adequately in a material sense, there was little emotional affection displayed. When Mary had children of her own, she adopted the same style of mothering. Reflecting on this toward the end of her life she concluded, "I never learned to love people ... I think I worry more than love."

Goodwin & Attia (1999) have described an attachment-based model for chronic pain wherein emotional pain may be misapprehended as physical pain and/or they dissociate from their body as a way of coping.[17] With the former there is a focus on physical pain to avoid emotional pain ("I am my pain"). With the latter there is distancing from the pain as a numbing strategy ("the pain is not me"). In both cases there is a distorted relationship between mind and body and denial or amnesia of childhood adversity.

Dissociative phenomena in chronic pain and MUS

Dissociation is the key process that connects traumatic stress and pain/MUS—"the engine rather than the caboose" as Sandra Paulsen describes it. Dissociation is generally understood as a process of separation between normally integrated elements of conscious experience, specifically as a defense against overwhelming distress. Kluft describes it as a splitting of awareness from consciousness as a way of dealing with overwhelming events.[18] This process-driven view of dissociation is a modern post DSM-III conceptualization. Before the 1980s, dissociation was more commonly understood as a division in the personality or consciousness—compartmentalization.[19] This conceptualization is a legacy of Pierre Janet who viewed dissociation structurally, wherein an alternate part of the personality gets created, comprising the unintegrated psychological and behavioral elements of the trauma.[20] The contemporary view of structural dissociation is that compartmentalization involves the separation of the psyche into two or more separate ego states. The structural model of dissociation identifies two key ego states: the EP, or Emotional Part, is responsible for animal defense survival responses (e.g., fight-flight/freeze), and the ANP, or Apparently Normal Part, which is responsible for actions necessary for everyday survival (e.g., working, socializing).[21]

Dissociation also affects the mind (psychoform) and body (somatoform) functioning. As the terms suggest, somatoform dissociation involves physical symptoms such as loss of motor control and reliving symptoms such as whiplash pain or pelvic pain, while psychoform dissociation involves mental phenomena such as depersonalization, amnesia, changes in identity, and idée fixe ("the world is a dangerous place").[22] Both types of symptoms are involved in the production and maintenance of pain and other medically unexplained symptoms.

Some take the view that dissociative phenomena occur along a spectrum between everyday compartmentalization, while others separate dissociation between normal and pathological (for taxonomic purposes—not in any pejorative sense). For example, inner conflict about choices can be a product of normal separation of consciousness, but when personality is organized around psychic entities which may not even be aware of each other, a pathological threshold is reached. Pathological dissociation may involve the identity diffusion of DID, maladaptive levels of absorption, and excessive ability to numb survival-related pain and emotional distress.[23] It's also characterized by unintegrated ego states which transition spontaneously and discontinuously between each other.

Some individuals are more prone to dissociation than others, a quality that has been linked to hypnotizability.[24] Janet also wrote about this—he felt that some individuals dissociated because of decreased integrative capacity due to illness, exhaustion, personality factors, and exposure to overwhelming stress.[25] Dell notes that about 15% of people are highly hypnotizable and that such individuals tend to be more reactive to stress (or any environmental stimuli). However, they are not necessarily dissociative unless they have also experienced adversity, such as early childhood neglect or abuse. Dell feels that such individuals employ dissociation as a default coping mechanism for stress, ranging from subclinical levels of emotional avoidance to more clinical manifestations. This high hypnotizability is associated with PTSD, somatization, conversion disorders, and more severe forms of dissociation such as DID.[26] The more trauma a person has suffered, the more likely they are to develop symptoms of somatoform dissociation.[27]

The purpose of dissociation is to protect the individual from pain/overwhelming distress. In the short term, dissociation may afford good protection against the pain of abuse, trauma, or neglect. The physically abused child can separate themselves from the affective reality of what happened. The victim of neglect can develop a separate self that seems unaffected by the love that was missing. Unfortunately, overuse of dissociation ultimately leads to a feedback loop wherein dissociative processes such as avoidance of feelings and compartmentalization can maintain pain (see Figure 2.2).

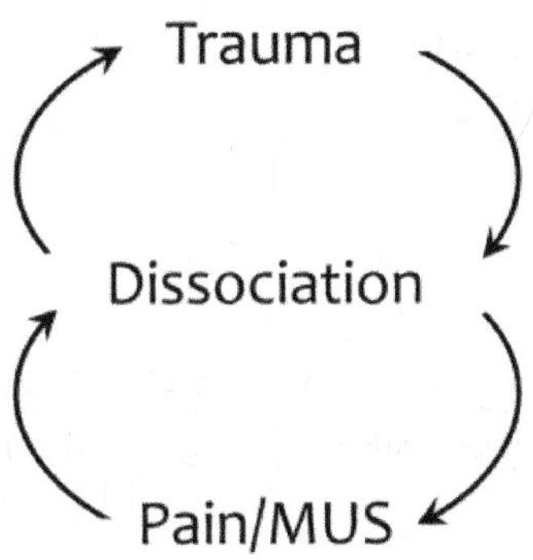

Figure 2.2 Trauma, dissociation, and pain

This places dissociative processes at the center of case conceptualization and treatment. While dissociation is not the only cause of medically unexplained symptoms (e.g., genetic factors, suggestibility, or physiological effects of chronic stress), it is certainly the central one when treating trauma survivors, i.e., most chronic pain sufferers. It also presents a challenge because of the inherent invisibleness of dissociative processes. Addressing dissociative processes requires having a clear understanding of what dissociation is and how it manifests in sufferers of chronic pain/MUS.

Dissociation is a complex, multi-faceted phenomenon—understanding of which begins with two core processes, "detachment" and "compartmentalization." As outlined above, detachment refers to the active separation of mental and sensory elements of experience in the moment. It involves a decoupling of sensory and mental responses to stressful experiences. For example, not feeling pain when hurt, not taking protective action when threatened, etc. In contrast, compartmentalization refers to a longer-term structural division of mental processes, a division between functioning elements of personality (or "parts") that operate autonomously and independently.[28]

Detachment and compartmentalization involve a range of distinct but overlapping processes, including:

1. Avoidance
2. Depersonalization
3. Amnesia
4. Ego states
5. Somatization

These five dissociative processes are the hidden link between trauma and pain. Understanding and being able to recognize them is the key to the effective treatment of trauma-related pain.

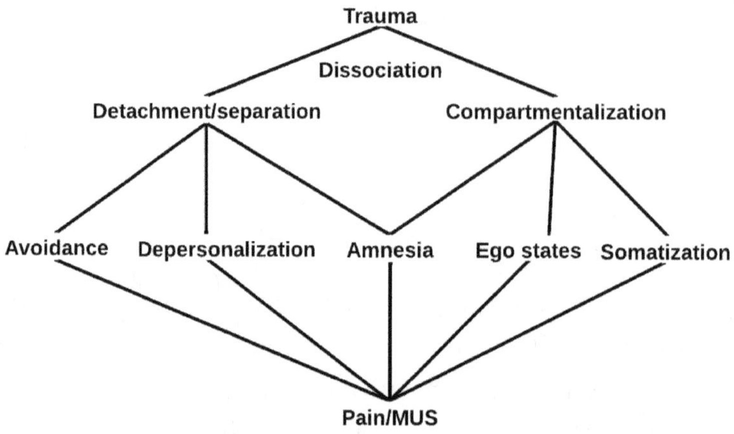

Figure 2.3 Dissociative phenomena in chronic pain/MUS

Dell emphasizes that the chronic, dissociative symptoms of an adult always originate as active, intentional mental efforts to escape from pain or distress, the unexpected success of which leads to their becoming habitual. Dell also notes that: 1) dissociative phenomena are sustained by negative reinforcement, and 2) by the time a dissociative person encounters a therapist, the defensive origins of their dissociative symptoms are long obscured. The people-pleaser does not remember why they chose to deny their own needs. The workaholic does not remember why they decided that continually pushing their body to its limit was necessary to survive.

Below is a brief description of each phenomenon and how it relates to chronic pain/MUS.

Avoidance involves a narrowing of the field of consciousness to exclude material that is too aversive or intolerable—avoidance of one thing in order to focus on another. It might be avoidance of unpleasant feelings or memories, or people or places, or feelings that are unsafe to show or shameful—anything that threatens the self. Generally speaking, avoidance leads to decreased ability to recognize and attend to deeper emotional (and physical) needs. For example, ignoring feelings of fatigue to maintain a sense of being strong, without needs. When employed consciously, avoidance is not dissociative. But in dissociation, this avoidance is involuntary and habitual. The comfort that it brings comes at the price of being effectively able to fully engage with the present. Dissociative detachment, as it's known, also comes at the cost of decreased mental functioning, such as disorganization, forgetfulness, spaciness, and undue drowsiness, which impairs one's ability to respond adaptively to environmental stimuli.[29] For example, Samantha was conversing with a colleague about problems she had been having with her manager, when she failed to notice a chair that a workman had left in the hallway and tripped and fell. The fall resulted in a back injury which soon developed into chronic pain and disability. While this accident could be attributed to inattention or bad luck, Samantha was normally very situationally aware and would usually have been able to detect the chair while holding a conversation, but in the months prior to the fall, she had noticed increasing anxiety, fatigue, concentration problems and impaired decision-making. At the time of the fall, Samantha was suffering from undiagnosed PTSD after 10 years of workplace bullying which she had endured in the naive (survivor part) belief that if she didn't "give up," she could win.

Samantha's story illustrates how an exhausted, mentally impaired individual has decreased capacity to learn from experience, is less able to cope with situational demands, more prone to accidents or injuries, more likely to experience pain more intensely, and less able to cope with pain. Dissociative avoidance is also a feature of depersonalization/derealization, amnesia, and compartmentalization.

Depersonalization is characterized by a sense of separation (or detachment) from oneself and one's body (body alienation)—it's a more intense form of internal avoidance. Individuals affected by depersonalization may describe feeling numb, unreal, and like they are just "going through the motions" of life. They also often describe feeling spaced out or disconnected from what's going on around them, including other people (derealization). In chronic pain/MUS sufferers, depersonalization can be a response to stress, illness, fatigue, and medication. Even Milton Erickson, who used his finely honed hypnotic skills to cope with his lifelong post-polio pain, once told a friend, "Sometimes my body feels like a stranger to me."[30] Depersonalization is not restricted to dissociative disorders but is a feature of many psychiatric diagnoses, including depression, substance abuse disorders, borderline personality disorder, and seizure disorders.

As a short-term coping mechanism for stress, depersonalization is adaptive and common. However, chronic depersonalization, which is usually autonomous of the original stressful trigger, is associated with structural dissociation and tends to be more maladaptive in terms of emotional processing, body awareness, cognitive functioning, and effects on relationships.[31] Depersonalization, which is distinguished by a total absence of emotional immediacy, is associated with elevated baseline cortisol levels, decreased cognitive functioning, amnesia, decreased coping, impaired ability to engage in relationships, and increased disability.[32] Like many dissociative phenomena, the short-term benefits of depersonalization are outweighed by its long-term consequences for emotional regulation and life-functioning. Despite these effects, its contribution to disability is less than that of dissociative amnesia and structural dissociation/identity effects.[33]

Amnesia is another dissociative phenomenon associated with detachment/separation and is common in chronic pain sufferers.[34] Dissociative amnesia involves pushing of uncomfortable information out of awareness. Amnesia can range from an inability to remember recent events (e.g., conversations, where one left car keys) to an inability to recall autobiographical material. Amnesia can arise from feeling spacey and tired as a result of detachment.[35] This causes material not to be encoded whereas amnesia associated with compartmentalization involves the storage of material in separate ego states, making it unavailable to normal consciousness. Amnesia can contribute to chronic pain through intrusions and as part of the compulsion to re-enact. The dissociated trauma survivor may experience physical reactions (including pain) in response to current stressors that seem out of proportion to what is happening but are not connected with any memory. Or somehow keep putting themselves in harm's way even though they are consciously aware they shouldn't engage in risky behaviors.

An example of dissociative amnesia comes from the life of Stephen King, the famous horror writer who also suffers from chronic pain after a hit-and-run accident. King had a traumatic childhood involving loss, abandonment, and instability. King was raised by his single mother, who was addicted to painkillers after his father walked out on her when he was about five years old. Although his mother did her best, the family moved around a lot and King was often left in the care of relatives. This period so alienated King, he remembers feeling "evicted from life." Recalling his childhood as an adult, he described his memories as "a fogged-out landscape from which occasional memories appear, like isolated trees."[36]

Amnesia contributes to chronic pain by separating past experiences from present consciousness, leading to decreased ability to learn from past experiences. This, along with post-traumatic re-enactment, explains why the abuse survivor keeps "missing the signs" when they start dating yet another abusive guy, or why they choose to continue working in an unsafe workplace. Of course, disadvantaged individuals don't always have much of a choice about where they work, or what risks they might have to take to provide for their families. But there are also often many choice points where the safer option was not taken. When detachment becomes enshrined in personality structure in the form of dissociative parts, it's known as compartmentalization.

Compartmentalization refers to the development of ego states or parts due to habitually having to separate elements of consciousness to survive. Note that dissociative experts distinguish between ego states and parts in the sense that parts can sometimes function autonomously, with separate knowledge and memories, while ego states are always an aspect of the self. Basically, all dissociative parts in DID are ego states, but not all ego states are dissociative parts or alters. For the purposes of this text these terms are used interchangeably since we are not discussing DID. Compartmentalization generally involves at least two prototypical ego states, a child and an adult. As mentioned earlier, in structural dissociation these are labeled as the Apparently Normal Part (ANP), responsible for daily life, and the Emotional Part (EP), responsible for defense.[37] The ANP engages in avoidance of the EP (and its traumatic contents) that might intrude upon the ANP's ability to maintain normal life functioning. These intrusions can include images, feelings, thoughts, and sensations. This is a Janetian view wherein hysterical symptoms (i.e., conversion disorders) arise from the separation or dissociation of traumatic material from consciousness. In structural dissociation the parts are not aware of each other and function separately albeit normally. Compartmentalization is characterized by a deficit in the ability to deliberately control processes or actions that would normally be amenable to conscious control.[38] Compartmentalization enables quite traumatized individuals to maintain an appearance of normal and sometimes very successful living.

Individuals with this personality structure can be recognized through statements like "I don't know why I did that" or "a part of me always ..." These parts together constitute the whole personality, but even if not full-blown DID, it's a divided personality. Symptoms are due to the actions of the EP *and/or* the ANP. For example, an EP may intrude upon an ANP with images (flashbacks) that the ANP then tries to avoid by drinking alcohol. Symptoms can also arise as a result of conflict between the parts—a "damned if you do, damned if you don't" aspect to life choices. For example, Mary experienced headaches whenever she visited her narcissistic mother, due to inner conflict, and felt that she was unable to ever express her needs. As long as she kept quiet about her true feelings, she was able to maintain some sort of connection with her mother. But at the same time, she was losing her connection with herself, which she found increasingly intolerable.

Gregory Bateson called this a double bind, and it is something every chronic pain sufferer faces, even without trauma and dissociation. *"Do the benefits of this medication outweigh the side effects?" "Is the pain that performing this activity will trigger worth the satisfaction that it will bring?" "How do I maintain a relationship with my loved ones without burdening them with my problems?"* Double binds, or at least ego state conflict, is inevitable. The question is how does the individual live with the conflict between their parts and how well are they able to balance their competing needs? Maybe the side effects of that medication are a lesser evil than the consequences of not taking it. Maybe the exacerbation of pain caused by attending a daughter's graduation is worth the satisfaction of fulfilling a parental role.

Another useful way of categorizing these ego states comes from Internal Family Systems or IFS. As with structural dissociation theories in IFS, the parts are categorized according to their roles. So, the EP becomes an exile, the ANP might take the form of a manager or protector, and there might be another part that deals with emergencies called a firefighter.[39] When an ANP or protector part is working very hard to maintain normal functioning, typically without any regard for the needs of the EP or exiled parts, it entails a way of being that is energy-intensive and dismissive of need for rest and support, which ultimately results in exhaustion and dorsal vagal shutdown. Uniquely, the IFS approach also acknowledges the existence of the self which, unlike parts, does not have a separate purpose (defending or carrying emotional wounds) but exists for the joy of living, loving, and learning. The self is defined by qualities such as connectedness, curiosity, compassion, creativity, and courage. The self is generally calm and confident.

Compartmentalization can involve unexplained neurological symptoms (e.g., paralysis), conversion symptoms, and amnesia.[40] As discussed above, amnesia involves an inability to bring normally accessible information into consciousness, necessary for adaptive decision-making. Dell believes that individuals with increased hypnotic capabilities are more able to do this and in fact do this automatically. When the desire to escape an uncomfortable reality is accompanied by hypnotic capacity, there occurs a "full-blown" splitting off, resulting in amnesia regarding the traumatic event. This is generally associated with structural dissociation.

Somatization is the physical expression of mental distress. In trauma survivors, it involves pain as a somatic memory of unprocessed trauma (e.g., pelvic pain in an abuse survivor, whiplash pain in a motor vehicle accident survivor).[41] Scaer has theorized how this might occur in whiplash, which he views as one of the purest examples of trauma-related pain. He describes whiplash as a somatic manifestation of an undischarged freeze/immobility response, which may be triggered by external cues and enhanced by endorphinergic mechanisms inherent to the initial response to threat.[42]

Somatization may also be understood as a product of variations in vagal responses. Porges' polyvagal theory posits that the human nervous system cycles between three states according to its capacity to respond to environmental demands: 1) fight-flight/freeze (hypervigilance, exaggerated startle), 2) ventral vagal (normal social engagement), and 3) dorsal vagal shutdown (deadness, disconnection, lethargy). For example, a baby ideally enjoys a state of engaged, joyous attunement with the mother (ventral vagal), but it cries when its mother leaves (fight-flight response). If the mother doesn't return within a reasonable time, the baby eventually transitions into a state of blank numbness (dorsal vagal shutdown).[43]

In trauma survivors, somatic symptoms may arise because of either an overactive fight-flight response or dorsal vagal shutdown. The formerly sustained hyperarousal enhances somatic distress associated with organic pathology or generates somatic symptoms independently. For example, the paralysis that author and WWII veteran James A. Michener describes suffering following a plane crash.

As a soldier in WWII, Michener, who had suffered from his childhood adversity, had to make regular trips to American Samoa. These trips involved traveling in the back of a military aircraft and landing at a dangerous mountain-ringed airstrip. On one occasion, as the aircraft was making its final approach, Michener realized that the pilot had failed to execute a tight turn correctly and that they were almost certainly going to crash. He glanced across the fuselage at the only other passenger, a fellow officer, who said nothing but twirled his fingers to indicate that yes, the plane was "going over." Neither man showed any trace of the dread they must have felt, as they were officers in the U.S. Army. Michener's plane spun out of control when the wing tip contact ed the runway, and Michener and his fellow passenger were thrown violently around the cargo hold of the aircraft. Miraculously, the fuselage remained relatively intact, and no lives were lost. Once Michener and his fellow passenger had untangled themselves from each other, they gathered their belongings and exited the wrecked aircraft. As they walked to the nearby officers' club, neither man spoke, but both were quietly pleased with their "coolness under stress" and the fact that they had acted "rather well" in the emergency compared with some of the younger men from the crew.

After dinner, Michener walked across the base back to his hut. In the dark, he fell into a ditch left by a crew digging a service line. Overcome with shock and the emotion of the day, Michener felt frozen with fear, so much so that he couldn't even call out for help. Michener lay paralyzed in the ditch for what seemed like an eternity. He was only rescued when someone from the club happened by, saw his predicament, and summoned help to haul him out.

The next morning, after a Valium and a good night's sleep, Michener went to inspect the ditch he had fallen into. He was shocked to find that what had felt like an 8-foot-deep trench was in fact no more than 18 inches deep! Michener realized with a deep sense of humility that perhaps he was not as impervious to battle fatigue, nervous exhaustion, and back pain seizures as he'd previously thought (this was his third plane crash!).[44]

Conversely, when the sympathetic system becomes exhausted due to severe chronic stress, it shuts down, leading to fatigue, mood, and biochemical changes. While dorsal vagal shutdown involves decreased sensitivity to bodily signals, its overall effect is to increase pain sensitivity. The vagus nerve has anti-inflammatory properties—the low vagal tone has been noted in painful and inflammatory diseases, including fibromyalgia.[45] Low vagal tone is also associated with social disconnection and impaired ability to recognize and express feelings (alexithymia). Long-term inability to express emotional needs is associated with a variety of somatic symptoms including headaches, gastrointestinal problems, muscle pain, and fatigue.[46] See Chapter 3 and Figure 3.5 for more information about the relationship between the polyvagal theory and chronic pain.

It is also likely that survivors of complex PTSD are not in a state of shutdown permanently, but cycle between fight-flight and shutdown. For example, during the fight-flight response, they may relive the pain they felt during the trauma, or experience pain more intensely due to increased affective distress. During shutdown they may experience pain more intensely due to decreased energy levels.

As will been seen later, the polyvagal lens helps determine the nature and order of treatment inputs. A simple PTSD sufferer with good underlying health might be able to benefit from EMDR immediately and might not need much else. A CPTSD sufferer with a complex medical history, fatigue, and shutdown, might be more likely to benefit from a slower, less intense therapeutic approach incorporating hypnosis, affect regulation skills training, and somatic strategies, interspersed with EMDR. The recognition that states of arousal can be moderated by interpersonal connection is another vital implication of this theory—it's not just what you do, it's the quality of the relationship within which you do it (see Chapter 5).

The somatic and emotional changes associated with somatization have been linked with a wide range of conditions or "diseases of stress" that defy medical explanations. Diseases of stress can affect any bodily system, including the heart and lungs, the gastrointestinal system, the musculoskeletal system, the skin, and so on.[47] Not surprisingly, diseases of stress rarely occur in isolation. For example, fibromyalgia is often associated with headaches and irritable bowel syndrome.[48] Hypertension is often associated with obesity, diabetes, and COPD.[49] Diseases of stress often represent the "tip of the iceberg" in terms of systems collapse.

Gastrointestinal Disorders:
- Diarrhea
- Ulcer
- IBS
- Obesity

Respiratory Disorders:
- Asthma
- Hay fever
- Tuberculosis

Skin Disorders:
- Pruitus
- Eczema
- Urticaria

Musculoskeletal Disorders:
- Rheumatoid arthritis
- Low back pain
- Migraine headache
- Fibromyalgia

Metabolic Disorders:
- Hyper/hypothyroidism
- Diabetes
- Long COVID

Cardiovascular Disorders
- Coronary artery disease
- Essential hypertension
- Congestive heart failure

Figure 2.4 Diseases of stress

Diseases of stress are often accompanied by diagnosable medical conditions (e.g., back injury, hyperthyroidism, stroke), making the task of distinguishing between what's organic and what's "psychological" even more challenging. Any chronic illness will trigger emotional distress reduction which may alleviate pain and suffering. The degree of pain relief achievable would seem to be dependent upon the extent to which the pain is organically based.

Assessing dissociation in pain/MUS

There are various instruments for assessing dissociation, including the DES, the SDQ, and MID (see Therapist Resources section). In addition to the phenomena described above, here are some other signs and symptoms that may be indicative of dissociative processes:

- Changes in voice tone and apparent age
- Overlapping or discrepant facial expressions
- Persistent eye closure, blinking, fluttering eye-rolls
- Avoidance of eye contact

- Rocking, rhythmic leg or foot tapping
- Amnesia
- Out of body experiences
- Trance phenomena (spaciness, time distortion, unexplained physical sensations)
- Compartmentalization

Remember, the function of dissociation is to conceal something. Recognizing dissociation depends upon being able to detect what Chefetz calls "little curls": subtle mismatches or shifts in a client's presentation. Often these will trigger a sense of confusion or disconnect in the therapist, a brief sense of something having shifted, easily lost in the attempt to stay with the dominant narrative. An alexithymic woman I was treating recently started tearing up as she talked about the recent death of a friend (the only emotion I had ever seen her display). Almost immediately she changed her gaze and started talking about something else. I felt a visceral sense of disjuncture and thought "What just happened?" When she came to a pause in her talk, I gently shared my reaction with her, and expressed curiosity about what was happening for her during the switch from talking about her deceased friend to talking about something else (which is rather less intrusive than saying "Hey, you seemed pretty upset about the loss of your friend"). She took the opportunity to share more about why emotions didn't feel safe for her, and it became a therapeutic opportunity.

Summary

In summary, chronic pain/MUS is often associated with PTSD, particularly CPTSD, which involves more profound physical and mental effects. Dissociation is often present. Dissociation is a defense mechanism triggered by trauma, ranging from big "T" trauma to small "t" trauma such as emotional neglect and abuse, and attachment deficits. Dissociative processes (as defined here) can range from alterations in consciousness associated with normal avoidance to full-blown dissociative identity disorder. Dissociation is a multi-faceted process comprising two key processes (detachment and compartmentalization) and five overlapping sub-phenomena: avoidance/distancing, depersonalization, amnesia, compartmentalization, and somatization. These phenomena constitute an incremental process that may begin with a non-pathological alteration in consciousness but culminates in structural dissociation and somatization. While dissociation is initially helpful in containing unpleasant affect, over the long term it may preserve it through hyper/hypo-arousal, decreased ability to process memories, decreased ability to cope with stress, unintegrated ego states, and biochemical changes. The net effect is the creation of a negative feedback loop between the mind and the body wherein the initial pain-ameliorating effects of dissociation come at the cost of an ever-decreasing capacity to manage sensory experience.

Most chronic pain sufferers are not affected by "pathological" dissociation, but are experiencing anxiety, memory problems, some degree of depersonalization, compartmentalization and exacerbation of somatic complaints as a result. Being able to distinguish between PTSD and CPTSD, and knowing how to identify the different dissociative phenomena associated with chronic pain/MUS, is essential for EMDR targeting and knowing when to supplement EMDR with adjunctive strategies such as hypnosis. We will examine the implications of this in treatment planning in Chapter 4.

3

Pain and the Brain

In addition to increased recognition of the role of traumatic stress in chronic pain/MUS pain theories have always reflected the scientific and cultural zeitgeist, which currently includes an appreciation of the role of neurological factors. While we are far from fully understanding the role of the brain in producing chronic pain/MUS, we know enough to start applying what we do know to the kinds of treatments we use. In this chapter we will attempt to answer some of the following questions: What is the differing role of brain areas responsible for sensory processing vs. emotion, memory, and motivation in acute vs. chronic pain/MUS? What is memory and to what degree can chronic pain be considered a memory? What relevance do evolutionary, threat-related autonomic responses have? What implications might the fact that the brain is divided into left and right, each side responsible for processing different elements of experience, have? To what degree might EMDR align with the kind of treatment approaches implied by such understandings?

Pain in the brain

Since the turn of the 21st century there has been an explosion in our understanding of the role of the brain in trauma, pain, and dissociation. The brain is the center of the nervous system and integral to all experience. The brain consists of a mixture of software and hardware, with some parts responsible for specific functions ("point to point") and other parts more flexible in their functioning ("random access"). Roughly speaking, the brain is designed in a hierarchical way wherein sensory information (feelings, sensations) follow an "upward" direction and mental information (thoughts, attitudes, and beliefs) follow a "downward" direction.

The involvement of the brain in pain is implied in the IASP definition of pain as subjective and not involving actual injury. Aristotle defined pain as an affect, to separate it from the primary senses. Descartes, of course, viewed pain in much more physiological terms, what we would equate with acute pain. The areas of the brain responsible for acute pain are well established: the thalamus, the ACC (anterior cingulate cortex), the somatosensory cortices, the insula, the PAG (periaqueductal gray), and the prefrontal cortex.[1] Collectively these areas are known as the pain matrix. While not completely mutually exclusive, the areas of the brain responsible for sensory-affective processing (blue) are most active with chronic pain while acute pain is more reliant on pain regions responsible for sensory processing (red)—see Figure 3.1.

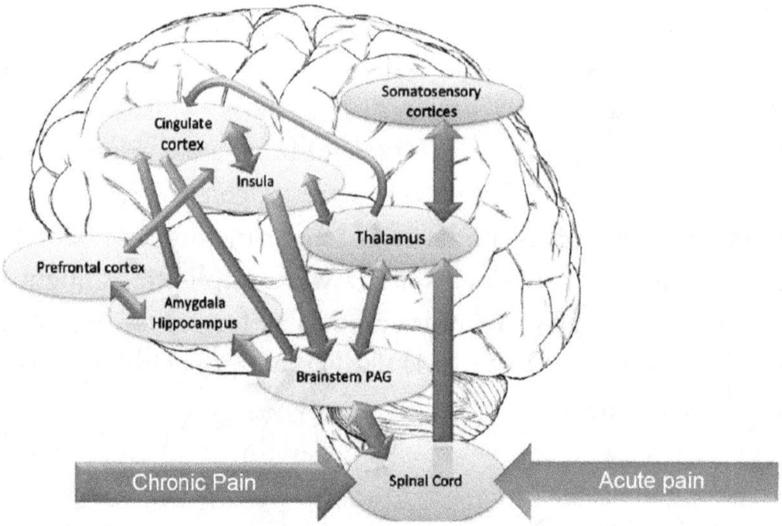

Figure 3.1 The pain matrix

The thalamus

The thalamus is a kind of relay station which reroutes incoming information (affect, bodily sensations). Sensory information enters the CNS (central nervous system) via the thalamus, from whence it is passed on to the amygdala and the prefrontal cortex. More than just a relay station, the thalamus is also involved in the sensory-discriminative and affective motivational components of pain. The thalamus also plays a role in modulating incoming pain signals from the body. Decreased gray matter has been found in the right thalamus (and prefrontal cortex) of chronic back pain sufferers equivalent to 10–20 years of normal aging.[2]

The thalamus has connections to the periaqueductal gray (PAG) which mediates pain perception and regulation, as well as risk assessment and defensive responses to traumatic stimuli. The PAG is also responsible for the development of learned emotional and behavioral responses to noxious stimuli including anxiety, panic attacks, and depression.[3] The PAG also mediates the orienting response, along with the superior colliculus (SC) and the locus coeruleus (LC). Stimulation of the PAG produces analgesia, leading to its incorporation in the Gate Control Theory.[4] The PAG also communicates with the anterior cingulate and mPFC (see below), and constitutes the medial network of the prefrontal cortex, which is responsible for processing sensory information.[5]

The amygdala

The amygdala interprets the emotional meaning of information. The amygdala connects strong emotions (e.g., fear, panic) to experiences, people, and things. Information evaluated by the amygdala is passed on to areas in the brain stem that control behavioral, autonomic, and neurohormonal response systems. Amygdaloid processing happens prior to higher order (frontal cortex) processing. The right amygdala (along with other regions of the cingulate cortex and medial prefrontal cortex) has been implicated in the production of spontaneous pain, a feature of chronic pain/MUS.[6] It's thought that this is part of the "survival/defense valence" function of chronic pain, which some novel research involving squid seems to confirm (more details below).[7]

The frontal cortex

The frontal cortex is divided into the prefrontal cortex, the medial prefrontal cortex, and the orbito prefrontal cortex. The prefrontal cortex (PFC) is where higher level thinking, planning, and goal formulation take place. The PFC is also involved in attention and mindfulness, and the downregulation of negative affect. Scientists have found that people who are able to recover from negative emotional events have more active PFCs. Damage to the PFC leads to reduced ability to override feelings and make rational, socially appropriate decisions.

The medial prefrontal cortex (mPFC) links the body and the brain, and balances the sympathetic and parasympathetic nervous systems. The sympathetic and parasympathetic nervous systems are like the accelerator and brakes of the nervous system. The mPFC is also important for self-awareness, intuition, and the ability to have attuned communication with others. The orbito prefrontal cortex is involved in self-discipline, setting plans and priorities, and is highly connected to reward and punishment feedback loops.

The anterior cingulate cortex

The anterior cingulate cortex (ACC) is responsible for emotional processing, attention, and correcting mistakes. It also seems to allow for monitoring of results, especially in terms of how they relate to emotional goals. The ACC and the amygdala are thought to be involved in the experience of pain and fear induced negative emotion, as well as the sensory component of pain. The ACC is also involved in the expression of negative emotions associated with physical pain. It also has a full body map, unlike the amygdala and the orbito prefrontal cortex.

The insula

The insula has mapped to it sensations from the body's interior and surface that are related to homeostasis, such as itch, pain, burning, cold, hot, etc. The right insula is activated when a person experiences pain and/or emotion. The insula thus connects the state of the body with the state of the brain. The insula is said to be where the mind and body unite; it gives rise to an individual's sense of emotional self—it is the foundation for emotional intelligence. The insula also has strong connections to the amygdala, the ACC and the orbito prefrontal cortex.

The insula is the part of the brain where all the internal sensory input comes together, including heart, lungs, stomach, intestines, and so on. Signals such as thirst, hunger, and the need to breathe. The insula also gets input from a separate set of receptors on the skin and mouth: temperature, pain, itch, ache, and touch. Many inputs, such as being pinched, will signal both the insula and body touch maps.

The insula plays a key role in pain management. Pain is handled in the same way as an emotion, both of which result in elevated activity in the insula. This is why meditation and biofeedback can both be effective ways to deal with chronic pain. By helping someone learn to turn down the activity in their insula, they can learn to reduce the ongoing sensation and stress from pain. The same kind of learning can help people who are anxious and have a generally high level of arousal in their insula to be less anxious and stressed.

The hippocampus

While not traditionally regarded as part of the pain matrix, the hippocampus is important because of its role in cognition and memory and in modulating the overall pain experience. The prefontal cortex, amygdala, and hippocampus are areas of the brain known to be most sensitive to damage following early childhood adversity.[8] Changes in hippocampal volume have also been noted in chronic pain (and PTSD) sufferers.[9] Rauch posits that PTSD patients exhibit hypersensitivity within the amygdala and a failure of the mPFC to exert governance over the amygdala. He asserts that hippocampal damage results in amnesia, learning problems, and memory.[10] Alterations in amygdala and limbic irritability are thought to underly an enhanced fight-flight response. Hippocampal abnormalities are also thought to foster the employment of dissociation as a defense mechanism.[11]

The hippocampus facilitates long-term learning from experience. The hippocampus, along with the amygdala, is involved in the laying down of fear memories associated with pain. Overlapping molecular processes have also led to the hippocampus being implicated in the depressive aspect of chronic pain.

Precisely how the elements of the pain matrix interact to produce pain is still not completely understood, with widely varying neural responses to noxious stimuli reported between and within individuals. Brain activity also varies between different pain conditions.[12] So the application of neuroscience to the understanding and treatment of chronic pain/MUS, though promising, is somewhat in its infancy.

Brain hemispheres and pain

The brain is also divided into left and right, again with each side being responsible for different aspects of information processing. In very simple terms, the right hemisphere is responsible for receiving information about bodily states and emotions. The left hemisphere is responsible for rational abstract thought (e.g., maths and problem-solving), planning, and language. The left hemisphere mediates focused attention; the right mediates open attention. The left hemisphere tends to see the "small picture" ("I had a car accident and almost died") while the right hemisphere sees the "big picture" ("I had a car accident and almost died, but I survived"). Not surprisingly, anything which disrupts communication between the hemispheres disrupts a person's ability to "read" what is going on in their body, practice self-care, and integrate experience. It's also thought that the right hemisphere deals with novelty and the left with routine. The right hemisphere is responsible for much of the emotional distress associated with physical or emotional pain. This is because of its close connections with some parts of the limbic system such as the amygdala and the anterior cingulate cortex.

The most in-depth analysis of the differences between the left and right hemispheres is Iain McGilchrist's *The Master and His Emissary* (Yale University Press, 2009). One of the most important differences McGilchrist highlights is that the left hemisphere prefers the known world and has a narrow focus of attention while the right hemisphere has a wider focus of attention and attends to the external world in a more open way. New information enters the brain via the right hemisphere, in a raw unprocessed state, gets transferred to the left hemisphere (via the corpus callosum), is analyzed, and then returned to the right hemisphere. Problems such as trauma and pain, which have a significant affective component, disrupt normal information processing in the brain, resulting in imbalances in hemispheric functioning. For example, decreased left hemisphere and increased right hemisphere functioning has been noted in sufferers of these conditions. Conversely, disorders which involve disconnection from the body and sensory deficits (e.g., schizophrenia, DID) are related to overactivity of the left hemisphere and decreased activity of the right. Figure 3.2 shows the left–right division of the brain and the different tasks that the two hemispheres are responsible for.

Although the left and right hemispheres perform different tasks, they also work closely together to process information. For example, when listening to music the right hemisphere notices the melody, but the left hemisphere notices the tune. Musicians have been found to rely on their right hemisphere early in their careers when they start learning to play, but their left hemisphere later in their careers when they become proficient. For this reason, one has to be cautious about making gross generalizations on the basis of differences between the brain hemispheres.

The relevance of the hemispheres to understanding chronic pain/MUS relates to the effects of trauma on the brain, dissociation, and the experience of pain. We know that trauma causes hemisphere-related changes to the amygdala, the anterior cingulate cortex, the hippocampus, the prefrontal cortex, and the insula. These changes are associated with increased brain activity in the right hemisphere.[13] The left PFC is normally responsible for downregulating the brain's fear circuits, but because of the intensity of activity in the right hemisphere when traumatized, the PFC can't do this.[14] The brain of the traumatized individual is essentially in a state of hypervigilance with little ability to put the brakes on. Other mental functions, such as concentration, memory, and decision-making, also suffer. Increased activity in the right brain is also thought to be associated with less integrated functioning between the left and right hemispheres.[15]

When trauma is associated with dissociation, an asymmetry can occur wherein right hemisphere functioning is suppressed in favor of the left. As Fisher (2017) notes, "The left brain generally stays positive, task-oriented, and logical under stress, while the right brain panics, searching for where to run, freezing in fear, praying for rescue ... or being too overwhelmed to do anything but submit. This dissociative split allows us to separate the trauma-related parts of ourselves and to *function* in daily life without awareness of having been traumatized."[16] The left brain also drives coping strategies such as amnesia, avoidance, and keeping busy as a way of coping, all in service of managing what's happening in the right. In pain sufferers this preserves the ability to maintain an appearance of normal functioning, which can bolster self-esteem and identity, but at the cost of freezing out positive social and other life experiences necessary for unlearning right-hemisphere pain maintaining affective patterns.[17] Finally, in survivors of early childhood adversity, dissociation effectively "primes" the brain for pain by blocking experiences of positive affect necessary for a comfortable sense of self physically and mentally. See Chapter 2 for a more detailed review of how dissociative phenomena contribute to chronic pain/MUS.

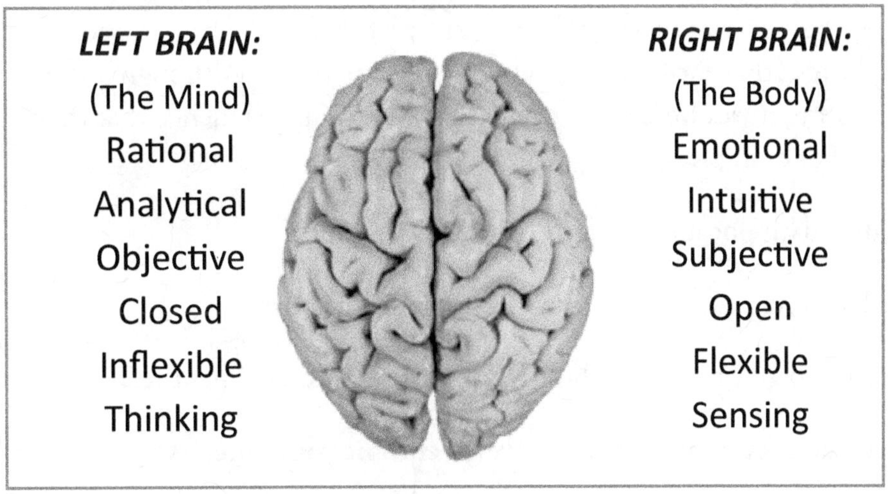

Figure 3.2 Left and right view of brain functioning

Body schemas and maps

The brain exists to serve the body, but the body is also there to serve the brain—brain development is dependent upon embodiment (how else is it going to learn stuff?). The brain is a kind of virtual reality machine which contains within it various representations of the body including body schema and body image. Body schema refers to an individual's felt sense of the body based on its physical properties. Body image refers to how an individual perceives their physical self. Body image is based on learned attitudes about the body (including beliefs and memories). Body image can persist despite physical changes. For example, a person who loses a leg might still see themselves as a two-legged person. A person with a bad back might still see themselves as physically capable of lifting heavy weights. This may be why it's so hard to get some chronic pain sufferers to alter their physical routines: their brain still thinks they can do everything they could prior to being in pain.

In a revealing experiment, Schwoebel et al. (2001) found that when chronic pain sufferers with bilateral arm pain had to select images based on their good and bad arm, by pressing a button with their good arm, they took fractionally longer when selecting the images that corresponded to their injured arm, even though they did not have to move that arm.[6]

Neuroplasticity and pain

The brain communicates and functions via neurons, which fire weak bioelectrical impulses across synaptic gaps. Memories are formed by strengthening of synaptic connections ("Neurons that fire together wire together") and lost by weakening of synaptic connections. Neuroplasticity is the idea that the brain is modifiable by experience. Although it used to be thought that the brain's structures were fixed, there is now too much evidence that they can be altered by experience. For example:

- Reduced hippocampal volume in PTSD sufferers[18]
- Reduced corpus callosum in adult survivors of abuse[19]
- Decreased gray matter in fibromyalgia sufferers (three times the loss in normal aging)[20]
- Hyperactivity in prefrontal cortex (in chronic pain sufferers)[21]
- Alterations in the functional connectivity of cortical regions (in chronic pain sufferers)[22]

Just understanding one aspect of neuroplasticity (brain chemistry) illuminates the pathways between psychological stress and physical pain. Severe stress causes biochemical changes, including decreased GABA (gamma-aminobutyric acid), serotonin, and norepenephrine, which affect mood, sleep, energy levels, and pain sensitivity. Victims of severe stress have been found to have increased levels of substance P, a neurotransmitter that increases sensitivity to pain.[23] Severe stress also causes reduced BDNF (brain-derived neurotrophic factor), a protein necessary for cell repair and regrowth. Because of decreased GABA (which balances the system), these changes tend to become self-perpetuating over time. This is why people with chronic pain and/or PTSD experience such dramatic fluctuations in mood, energy levels, and mental functioning, even though nothing much externally seems to have changed.

Pain as a memory

Increased understanding of the effects of adversity on the brain, particularly in relation to areas involved in emotional memory (e.g., the amygdala and the hippocampus), have led to pain being viewed as a memory.[24] Borsook et al. (2007) have defined pain as "an altered brain state in which there may be altered functional connections and systems and ... degenerative aspects of the CNS."[25] Apkarian (2011) defines pain as "a product of functional and morphological reorganization of the brain constituting memories, reinforced by long-term learning mechanisms."[26]Memory is a two-dimensional phenomenon—declarative and/or procedural. Declarative memory involves the memory of events, the who, what, and when. Procedural memory involves learned emotional responses, bodily reactions, and skills. Affective memories are associative, meaning that events involving similar emotional responses are stored in the same area of the brain. This explains how traumatic memories are triggered by unrelated events which involve similar emotional responses.[27] Rome and Rome postulate that a sensitization occurs in vulnerable individuals which results in an augmented pain response to later stimuli, which may not even be nociceptive in nature.[28] Remember Michener's paralysis after he fell into a ditch following that plane crash (Chapter 2)? In addition, individuals who have experienced a relatively minor physical injury can develop pain which is much greater than would be expected. And then there are all the traumatic things that can go wrong in the medical treatment of injury and disease.

There is a groundswell of interest in developing brain-based psychological therapies for chronic pain/MUS. In a recent review of the neurobiological mechanisms underlying chronic pain, Borsook (2018) concludes "there is an urgent need for neurobiologically informed psychotherapy."[29] Apkarian (2011) feels that neurological discoveries have more to offer the treatment of chronic pain/MUS than acute pain because it is so poorly understood and, "Anatomical and functional specificity of the brain in distinct chronic pain conditions ... suggests the possibility of unique therapies by targeting the underlying specific pathways for each type of chronic pain."[30] There is already a growing literature regarding what a neurobiologically informed psychotherapy might look like.[31] Based on a review of the current literature regarding the implications of brain science, the following four conditions (by no means a complete list) have been identified as necessary for neurobiologically informed psychotherapy. It should:

1. Emphasize the therapeutic relationship and repair of attachment deficits.
2. Be congruent with brain processes associated with learning and memory.
3. Involve "top-down" (cognitive) and "bottom-up" (experiential) inputs in a way that capitalizes on the brain's capacity to learn from experience.
4. Emphasize awareness of bodily experience in the here and now.

While the specifics and operational details of each of these elements will require years of research to attain the status of "evidence based", the theoretical and clinical literature regarding the role of the brain in attachment, memory processing, and bottom-up processing is likely to be sufficient for clinicians who base their therapeutic choices on broader parameters.

Although not conceived as a neurobiologically informed psychotherapy, let alone a pain therapy, EMDR has been found to fulfill many of the conditions that would satisfy such an approach. The AIP (adaptive information processing) model references the nervous system in its account of memory and learning. Initially it simply posited that human beings have an innate capacity for processing experience in an adaptive way, and that traumatic stress thwarted this. The term "information" as used in EMDR therapy refers to affect, cognition, sensory, and somatosensory or other internal or external input as perceived at the time of the event leading to memory formation. Later attempts to explain the mechanisms of EMDR resulted in more detailed accounts of the neurological bases of the AIP and the brain processes that likely underpin EMDR.[32] These include stimulation of areas of the brain known to be involved in formation of traumatic memories (the mPFC, the amygdala, and the hippocampus). These are largely the same areas of the brain associated with chronic pain/MUS.[33] Electroencephalogram (EEG) and functional magnetic resonance imaging (fMRI) scans have shown decreased activity in the mPFC and the amygdala following EMDR.[34] One study found changes in hippocampal volume following EMDR.[35] A similar study found increased volume in the left amygdala following EMDR, but no change in hippocampal volume.[36] Bilateral stimulation has been found to promote the attenuation of fear via a pathway mediated exclusively by the superior colliculus.[37] Bilateral stimulation has also been found to stimulate increased access to positive memories via, or at least associated with, increased activation of the right STS (superior temporal sulcus) and decreased activity of the PFC.[38]

There have also been attempts to explain EMDR in terms of physiological and psychological processes. For example, EMDR has been found to stimulate psychophysiological changes associated with inhibited sympathetic arousal and decreased pain.[39] Baek et al. (2019) reported that fear conditioning in rats was more fully extinguished when they engaged in EMDR type eye movements than with other extinction learning interventions. The Baek et al. results also found a psychophysiological path involving the colliculus, thalamus, and amygdala which appeared to account for the effects of the bilateral eye movement.[40] In addition to the method's efficacy with PTSD, it was EMDR's unique ability to stimulate physiological changes that stimulated research as a treatment for chronic pain.[41] Psychological models reference the orienting reflex (OR) and working memory effects.[42] The OR model posits that EMDR stimulates activation/deactivation of the OR reflex, an evolutionary response involving decreased physiological arousal. Working memory models posit that EMDR works by taxing working memory. This popular EMDR theory posits that the method derives its effects from the competing stimulus of bilateral stimulation and focused attention. This theory makes intuitive sense when applied to EMDR treatment of traumatic memories. Reflecting the general trend toward integration in mind-body medicine, it seems likely that any overarching theory regarding the mechanisms of EMDR will consist of a combination of neurobiological and psychophysiological theories.

The therapeutic relationship was not emphasized in early iterations of EMDR, but as with neurological aspects, it has gained in prominence.[43] It is recognized that unconscious emotional processes (transference and counter-transference) are an important dimension of the therapeutic process.[44] The therapist is not just a detached technician who makes a diagnosis and applies the appropriate treatment, but a person with their own history, including possible trauma and neglect, which can get activated by the client's sharing of theirs. Being able to be aware of and manage their own emotional responses is vital for attunement and repairing therapeutic ruptures. At the same time the therapist needs to provide sufficient structure for the therapeutic process. Hase (2022) also states that the therapist's ability to provide emotional security in the therapeutic relationship is an important condition for the activation of the adaptive information processing system in a way that is supportive but unintrusive.[45] There needs to be a sense of congruence between therapist and patient, something Shore (2022) describes as "right brain to right brain communication."[46] According to Shore, the sense of safety and connectedness generated by an attuned therapeutic relationship can also help ameliorate stress-related physiological arousal and promote long-term emotional growth. Given the significant percentage of patients who are survivors of attachment problems in addition to their trauma and/or pain, the provision of a reparative emotional bonding experience as a core element of treatment seems both intuitive and essential.

Top-down vs. bottom-up interventions seek to take advantage of brain structures and functioning associated with sensory vs. analytical functioning. The top part of the brain is the thinking, analytic part (i.e., the PFC). The bottom part of the brain refers to the sensing, feeling regions, such as the amygdala and cingulate gyrus. Bottom-up approaches zero in on a client's raw emotions and defense systems by working with clients to modulate their bodies. Meanwhile, top-down approaches look to shift the way a client thinks—whether it's veering them away from unhelpful rumination or encouraging curiosity for their reactions.[47] In trauma survivors, the brain's ability to regulate arousal through cognition is decreased. Researchers like Dr. Joseph LeDoux have theorized that information entering the brain through its primary cognitive processing center—the dorsolateral prefrontal cortex—typically remains stuck in the prefrontal cortex and cannot reach the emotion regulating centers of the brain. Otherwise helpful cognitive capacities like perspective taking, reason, problem-solving and decision-making, and the capacity for impulse control routinely falter in the face of trauma.[48] As van der Kolk notes, "No matter how much insight and understanding we develop, the rational brain is basically impotent to talk the emotional brain out of its own reality."[49] Under these circumstances, the brain is more receptive to somatically driven bottom-up interventions (e.g., bilateral stimulation, body scan/somatic tracking, yoga) which afford more direct access to the limbic system.[50] See Figure 3.4 for examples of top-down and bottom-up interventions. See Chapter 6 for more information about the role of the therapeutic relationship in treating sufferers of chronic pain/MUS.

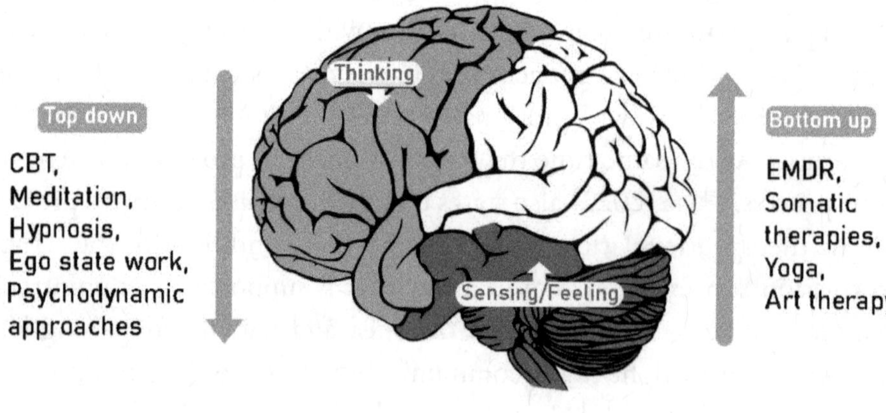

Figure 3.4 Top-down and bottom-up therapies

Some trauma experts believe that accessing the limbic system via interoceptive awareness, mediated by the mPFC represents a third pathway—what Dr. Joseph Spinazzola refers to as the brain's secret *side door*.[51] Interoceptive awareness is a person's awareness and perception of internal experience (bodily sensations, feelings, and thoughts). Van der Kolk believes that mind-body interventions such as interoceptive awareness, EMDR, and yoga (to name a few) engineer change by forging communication and restoring balance between the rational and emotional systems through the mPFC.[52]

These theories are beginning to filter through to mainstream pain literature. In *The Migraine Brain*, neurologist Carolyn Bernstein proposes that the brain cells of migraine sufferers are more easily aroused by stimuli such as fatigue, stress, temperature changes, and certain foods. Bernstein bases her model on research wherein migraine sufferers were found to have brain abnormalities including thickening of the somatosensory cortex—the area of the brain that relays pain and sensation. Other research has found structural impairments in the brains of chronic pain sufferers which affect their brain's ability to maintain itself in a balanced state while they are performing mentally demanding tasks. Bernstein concludes that one of the causes of migraines is that the brains of people who have migraines are different and function differently.

One of the most useful perspectives in terms of understanding chronic pain/MUS comes from Porges' polyvagal theory, which describes traumatic stress and its effects in terms of evolutionary, threat-related autonomic responses.[53] Given the correlation between trauma and adversity and chronic pain/MUS, this theory is also particularly relevant. The polyvagal theory posits that rather than binary fight-flight vs. normal states, the human nervous system is actually capable of a third state which occurs when the fight-flight response is thwarted or exhausted: shutdown. The theory derives its name from the vagus nerve which serves the parasympathetic nervous system (the "brakes"). As is commonly known, the fight-flight response is generated by the sympathetic nervous system to deal with threat. The fight-flight response involves a range of biological responses which can be both pain ameliorating and pain exacerbating. For example, increased cortisol (together with other immune-inflammatory and hypothalamic-pituitary-adrenal, or HPA, axis biomarkers). Cortisol is produced in the adrenal glands and the human body contains millions of receptors for this chemical in every organ and muscle. It is cortisol which increases heart rate and blood pressure in the fight-flight response. Cortisol can also have the effect of reducing inflammation and boosting immunity in the initial stages of stress.[54] However, cortisol and adrenalin can also sensitize peripheral nerves, leading to pain in the absence of injury. Individual cortisol responses are genetically determined: motor vehicle accident survivors with a rare gene variant were found to be more prone to developing chronic pain as a result of an increased cortisol response than individuals without this variant.[55] A prolonged stress response can also lead to fatigue, increased inflammation, emotional distress, and catastrophizing.[56]

When the fight-flight response is not available or exhausted, the parasympathetic nervous system shuts down. An example of this would be a child who is trapped in a sexually abusive parental relationship—they cannot fight back, nor can they escape. The only way to survive is to not feel. This state is called dorsal vagal shutdown. The term "dorsal" refers to the location of this part of the nerve toward the back part of the brain, an area which is associated with sensation and perception. Dorsal vagal shutdown is associated with decreased heart rate variability (HRV), a proxy measure for vagal activity thought to involve a disturbance in the descending inhibitory pathway.[57] HRV refers to the variation in time between each heartbeat—higher HRV is associated with greater cardiovascular fitness, well-being, and resilience. Decreased HRV has been linked to a variety of problems, including increased inflammation, gastrointestinal pain (GI), and fibromyalgia.[58] Dorsal vagal shutdown typically involves fatigue and exhaustion, which also exacerbate pain.[59] Both the fight-flight response and dorsal vagal shutdown are associated with social withdrawal, which is another exacerbating factor for pain and illness. Social interaction is an important activity for calming the fight-flight response and stimulating positive emotions. Decreased capacity for social engagement also creates a need for defensive strategies such as dissociation.[60]

Normal (ventral vagal) arousal refers to when a person feels safe and able to engage socially and energetically with the world.[61] The ventral vagal state constitutes a state of relaxed engagement, open-heartedness, curiosity, capacity for joy, ability to live life to the full. When a person is in a ventral vagal state they feel connected to their body in an okay way—able to "smell the roses" and experience their present reality appropriately and viscerally. Because of how it involves sensory engagement with the world, the ventral vagal state is vital for new emotional learning and growth. Unlike the survival-oriented view of life associated with the fight-flight response, ventral vagal states involve feelings of confidence and well-being and the perspective that while not perfect, on the whole life represents endless opportunities to learn about oneself and one's potential. Survivors of early childhood adversity may have no memories of what this feels like. Survivors of later adversity may have become so accustomed to living in a fight or flight state that they have forgotten. Josie, a 58-year-old survivor of chronic emotional abuse in childhood, had always wanted to learn how to dance. But she lived in a state of fear about trying anything new (going on holiday, joining clubs), in case something bad might happen, as had in her childhood whenever she asked for anything. For most of her adult life she had lived a very routine, vanilla kind of life, involving no close friends and very few novel activities. Following EMDR reprocessing and some somatic work, she began to feel calmer and safer in her body which gave her the confidence to finally enroll in those dancing lessons. Josie's story illustrates another point about psychological treatment of chronic pain/MUS—it doesn't necessarily involve spending a lot of time talking about pain!

In terms of PTSD and CPTSD diagnoses, the fight-flight response is more typically associated with PTSD while dorsal vagal shutdown is more typical of CPTSD. However, many sufferers of complex trauma cycle between fight-flight and shutdown (see Figure 3.5).

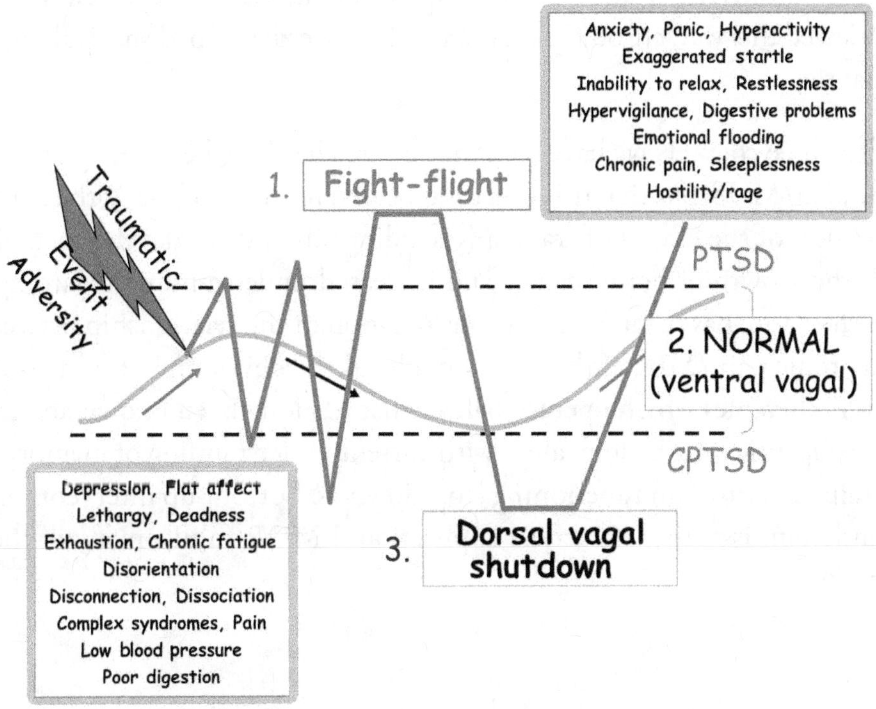

Figure 3.5 The polyvagal theory, PTSD, and pain

The connection between trauma and pain and chronic pain being a product of neuro-physiological survival responses is also supported by some novel research involving squid. In 2014 researchers from the University of Texas decided to test this popular view of acute vs. chronic pain by inducing central sensitization in squid and seeing what happened. They did this by cutting the ends off some of the squid. They then anesthetized some of the injured squid and then compared how normal (healthy, uninjured), injured no-pain (anesthetized), and injured/not anesthetized (chronic pain) squid reacted when faced with predators. The researchers found that the squid in the chronic pain condition were better at avoiding predators than both the healthy and injured no-pain squid. One of the researchers, Robyn Crook, speculated that the hyperaware state in the injured non-anesthetized squid must be serving to protect them from the increased risk of death associated with their injury.[62] The researchers concluded that "the propensity to develop chronic pain is an evolutionarily encoded feature of complex neural systems."

The research findings regarding central sensitization in squid indicate that far from lacking survival value (as per traditional models of chronic pain), chronic pain is just another manifestation of the well-known hyper-alertness that survivors of abuse and neglect develop to protect themselves. Viewed this way, chronic pain is part of an overdeveloped survival response that is essentially adaptive.

In these first three chapters we have seen that trauma has long been recognized as a precursor to chronic pain/MUS, but that this link disappeared for most of the 20th century. A resurgence in awareness of the effects of trauma (including all kinds of developmental adversity), coupled with the growth of brain science and increased understanding regarding the effects of trauma on the brain, has stimulated a reconsideration of the relationship between traumatic stress and chronic pain/MUS. It has also stimulated the development of neurobiologically informed psychotherapies which operationalize what has long been known about the importance of the therapeutic relationship, align with current understanding of memory processing, and reflect brain structure and functioning (top-down vs. bottom-up interventions). From its theoretical underpinnings to its practical application, EMDR fulfills many of the criteria of such an approach.

4

EMDR as a Treatment for Pain

EMDR can be defined both in terms of what it does (memory processing) and how it does it (the eight stages). Any definition involves certain assumptions about, for example, the nature of memory, the human nervous system, its inherent capacities and limitations, and the nature of psychotherapy. If we assume psychotherapy is an attempt to assist the patient to overcome the effects of aversive experience in a way that best takes advantage of those innate capacities, including enhancing them when needed, how should this be operationalized? What are the unique demands associated with chronic pain/MUS? What adaptations to standard practices might be necessary? What exactly is EMDR therapy and how does it answer these challenges?

As is well known, EMDR emerged in the late 1980s, following Francine Shapiro's fortuitous experience of feeling better following spontaneous eye movements. Shapiro discovered that traumatic memories could be resolved rapidly through concentrating on the memory while simultaneously concentrating on a bilateral stimulation—a procedure known as dual attention stimulus. In her groundbreaking initial scientific study of EMDR, Shapiro found that the method could stimulate significant reduction in physical and emotional distress associated with PTSD in just a few sessions.[1] Since then, dozens more studies led to the general acceptance of EMDR as an effective treatment for PTSD.[2]

Scelles (2021) found that EMDR has also been reported to have positive effects on a range of conditions including somatoform disorders, pain, sleep, mood disorders, anxiety disorder, and neurodegenerative disorders.[3] A recent review by Matthijssen et al. (2020) identified a total of eight RCTs that examined the efficacy of EMDR in the treatment of chronic pain.[4] Good efficacy was also found here for secondary forms of pain such as rheumatoid arthritis pain (Nia et al., 2018),[5] back and musculoskeletal pain (Estergard, 2008; Suarez, 2020; Gerhardt et al., 2016),[6] as well as neuropathic pain disorders and phantom limb pain (Brennstuhl et al., 2016;[7] Rostaminejad et al., 2017).[8] EMDR was also found to significantly ameliorate pain and associated distress,[9] in contrast to traditional approaches which have little effect on these aspects.[10] The effects of EMDR were found to be maintained over time and sometimes even increased post intervention.[11] Tesarz (2023) concludes that while the small number of cases and monocentric nature of the studies do not yet allow conclusive statements to be made about the efficacy of EMDR for chronic pain, the research results are promising.

More recently a growing number of studies indicate that EMDR can also be effective in the treatment of chronic pain.[12] Pain experts are excited by the promise of this method.[13]

Pain and the AIP model

Shapiro posits that human beings possess an adaptive information processing capacity. This gives us the capacity to transform even painful memories into useful learning and an increased ability to thrive and survive. According to this view, PTSD represents a failure of adaptive information processing since the painful feelings continue to dominate the person's existence long after the traumatic trigger has ended. Shapiro and others have suggested that the intense nature of traumatic anxiety simply overwhelms the nervous system's ability to process this material. Instead of analyzing and integrating the memory of what happened, avoidance and fragmentation occurs. Regardless of the mechanisms, the result is that the person continues to suffer physical or emotional pain well after the circumstances that triggered the injury have ended.

Chronic pain can also be understood in terms of this model. Physical pain is a response to injury or disease. It is signaling a problem, and that action needs to be taken (rest, seek medical help)—remember Goodwin's "natural sequence" from Chapter 2. Once appropriate action has been taken, healing is supposed to occur and the pain is supposed to fade away. Every adult human being has experienced this adaptive resolution of injury and understands pain this way. When pain persists beyond normal healing time frames, there appears to have been a failure in adaptive information processing, similar to what occurs with PTSD. The exception is where there are biological processes (possibly unknown) maintaining the pain. EMDR is founded on the role of memory networks in the brain that store information which can be both adaptive and maladaptive depending on the degree to which they have been processed. Non-organic pathology is thought to be a manifestation of inadequately processed memories. So, an example might be a highly stressed female executive with unresolved childhood sexual and emotional trauma who develops vaginismus and a urinary tract infection (UTI) at a time when she feels overwhelmed by current stressors. Although a UTI is an organic condition, people with PTSD, for example, are more prone to such infections. Other overlapping organic-psychological conditions include "diseases of stress" such as irritable bowel syndrome, headaches, vaginismus, etc. As discussed in Chapter 2, diseases of stress can affect all bodily systems and rarely occur in isolation. Dysfunctionally stored memories are normally the primary focus of treatment, but with chronic pain associated with a non-traumatic injury, the "memory" could be purely visceral (or at least experienced as such) based on the physical discomfort associated with the precipitating injury or illness.

Central sensitization is the process wherein acute pain becomes chronic. As the name suggests, it involves a process of increasing sensitization of the central nervous system to pain, leading to a lower threshold, also known as nociplastic pain. Examples would be hyperalgesia, which involves increased sensitivity to pain, and allodynia, which involves pain from non-painful stimuli such as a light touch. Models involving the brain are increasingly sophisticated. Apkarian (2018) has described how continuous nociceptive input reorganizes memories and their associations within the cortex via projections from the spinothalamic system to the amygdala, hippocampus, and prefrontal cortex (see previous chapter).[14]

Where the pain started spontaneously, it could be a product of the cumulative physiological effects of long-term fight-flight and/or dorsal vagal shutdown. In other words, learned psychobiological patterns of responding that ultimately exhaust and damage the body in the absence of or in combination with organic injury or disease. In a review of the relationship between childhood adversity and gastrointestinal disorders, Kolacz and Porges (2018) describe how stress-related physiological changes (e.g., heart rate variability associated with respiratory sinus arrhythmia) might produce non-organic pain.[15] Viewed through the lens of overactive evolutionary survival responses and associated learned psychophysiological responses, chronic pain/

MUS constitutes a procedural memory, regardless of what declarative memories the individual might have regarding their childhood adversity.

Regardless of prior trauma or adversity, the experience and effects of chronic pain can be quite traumatic in and of themselves. Chronic pain sufferers are beset by persistent physical discomfort, sometimes quite severe, sleeping problems and fatigue, loss of physical capabilities, loss of vocational possibilities, economic losses, strained relationships, social stigma, health fears, and identity effects.[16] In Chapter 2 we reviewed dissociative phenomena commonly found in trauma and pain sufferers. While we are used to thinking of dissociation in relation to trauma, it is also often part of the pain experience. As Marlene Hunter notes, "Pain is a dissociative experience, it separates us from what's going on around us."[17] Kleinman et al. (2011) noted that chronic pain involves various traumatic-like stress reactions, including intrusive thoughts, avoidance, and arousal. They postulated that symptoms of emotional numbing in chronic pain sufferers (i.e., pain-related emotional detachment) were reflective of post-traumatic symptomatology which occurs in response to pain.[18]

EMDR treatment model

EMDR is indicated as a treatment for pain because of its efficacy with trauma, which is highly correlated with chronic pain/MUS, its physiological effects, the trend to view chronic pain/MUS as a memory, and the method's coherence with neurologically informed psychotherapy.

As originally developed for PTSD, EMDR is an eight-phase treatment process incorporating History, Assessment, Preparation, Desensitization, Installation, Body scan, Closure, and Re-evaluation. These eight phases are designed to support the "desensitization" procedure which lies at the heart of EMDR (stages 3 and 4). The relaxation and distancing which follows bilateral stimulation enables sufferers of physical and emotional pain to see their pain in a different, transformative way. The rest of the stages are about preparing the client for the dual attention stimulus (DAS)/bilateral stimulation (BLS) (stages 1–2) and then stabilizing them and integrating whatever changes they have experienced (stages 5–8). Over the years, additional elements have been added to the EMDR treatment mix (e.g., safe place, past, present, and future approach to targeting, and resource development).

In an attempt to define EMDR, Hase (2021) has identified seven core elements or levels: 1) the AIP model, 2) The eight phases of EMDR therapy, 3) The different protocols, 4) The procedures, 5) Dual attention bilateral stimulation, 6) Clinical interventions, 7) The therapeutic relationship.[19]

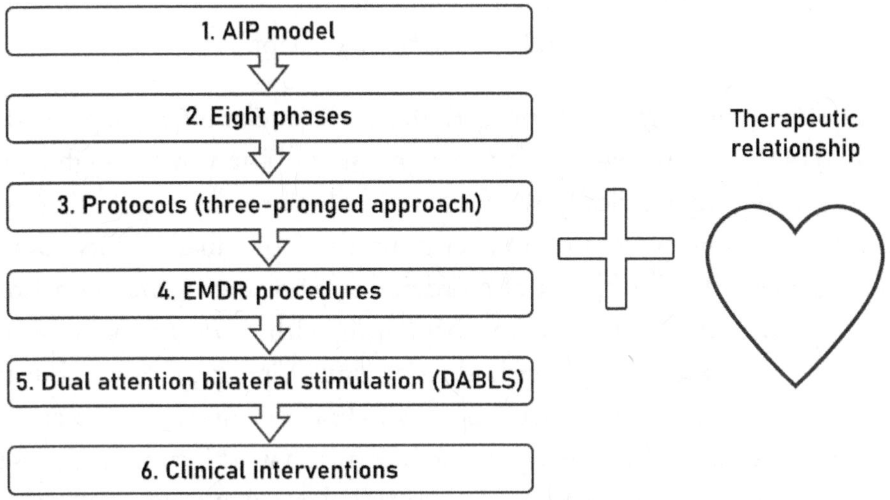

Figure 4.1 Structure of EMDR

This definition identifies the elements that distinguish EMDR from other treatment approaches (e.g., AIP model, dual attention bilateral stimulation, etc.) whilst recognizing that EMDR also incorporates elements that are common to all (e.g., the therapeutic relationship). We have already described the AIP model (above). The remaining elements will be described in Part Two. Before describing how to apply this to chronic pain/MUS, let's review some of the challenges and aims of psychological treatment of pain.

The 7 tasks of pain management

As we have seen, pain can be both a symptom (of much more than tissue damage) and a problem in its own right. Every new pain patient presents with an unspoken menu of competing needs, including unresolved trauma/effects of adversity, inadequately managed pain, affect management, coping with the effects of injury/illness, and existential and identity issues. As Tesarz (2014) notes, "EMDR in the treatment of chronic pain requires a greater variety of targets and more flexibility in the protocol application compared with the treatment of PTSD. Targets for desensitization and reprocessing should neither be restricted to the pain nor to traumatic life events but should be adapted to the individual as required."[20] Based on 30 years of research and clinical experience I have identified seven common tasks common to most treatment situations: 1) Tame the pain, 2) Emotional regulation, 3) Trauma processing, 4) Uncovering the meaning of pain, 5) Dealing with present stressors, 6) Self-care, and 7) Integration. As this is a list of potential therapeutic targets, it does not include the history and case conceptualization phase of treatment (these are described in the following chapters).

Awareness of these tasks gives the practitioner a comprehensive "map" of the treatment needs associated with chronic pain from the pain itself all the way through to its effects on identity. Conceptually and practically, the focus moves between pain and other problems with an awareness that other problems may impact upon the individual's ability to make progress with pain management. These tasks are also ordered in a bottom-up way, consistent with Janet's sequenced approach to trauma therapy, beginning with more sensory emotional aspects of pain ("tame the pain") and ending with identity issues ("reintegration"). But they are only a road map and not meant to suggest treatment is so linear or neat; some clients may need to start with trauma processing, others may need to begin with working on their present pain, still others might need to learn how to self-care (and to believe that they are worth it). You may work on several tasks in a parallel fashion, going backward and forward in the course of treatment. As you can imagine, each task involves different aims, strategies, and skills, including EMDR but also other interventions such as hypnosis, somatic interventions, ego state/parts work, etc.

1. Tame the pain

   Often, though not always, one of the most urgent needs of most chronic pain sufferers is to develop some degree of control over their pain. Unpredictable, uncontrolled pain keeps an individual in a state of anxiety and vulnerability, similar to that experienced by victims of trauma (except that with chronic pain the enemy is within). Chronic pain also keeps a person disabled, helpless, and unable to feel safe or comfortable in their own body. Developing some control and relief from the physical discomfort helps restore a person to a more normal and in control state. In terms of the eight phases of EMDR, this task is part of the stabilization phase. Taming the pain can be achieved through EMDR, particularly when there is a significant, treatable emotional component. If the client's pain levels are intolerable, they may not be able to engage in EMDR until the pain is brought under control using other methods. Pain management skills may be divided into short-term first aid strategies such as soothing activities or distraction, to more long-term strategies such as imagery and meditation.

2. Emotional regulation

Emotional regulation refers to the ability to experience and express emotions in a stable and effective way and is a core element of normal social and vocational functioning, as well as providing a foundation for identity. Emotional dysregulation problems are a feature of CPTSD and chronic pain, in addition to many other psychiatric conditions.[21] In addition to its unpredictability and negative effects on executive functioning, emotional dysregulation is also associated with identity disturbance, which is also a feature of CPTSD and chronic pain.[22] Emotional dysregulation is thought to exacerbate chronic pain (and disability) through increased negative affect, effects on sensory inputs into the CNS, increased catastrophizing, expressive suppression, and decreased coping.[23]

While emotional dysregulation (ED) may have been present in CPTSD sufferers prior to the onset of pain, it is likely exacerbated by the onset of pain, particularly when of sufficient intensity to affect physical functioning and well-being. This stems from the fact that trauma survivors have often developed body-dependent strategies to compensate for emotional regulation deficits, such as workaholism, achieving goals, distraction, and dissociation. These strategies depend upon maintaining a certain level of mental and, particularly, physical health. Chronic pain/MUS undermine these coping strategies, promoting a crisis in terms of ability to survive and identity. As Robert, a hard-working coal miner now disabled due to a work injury, declared, "Without my job I can't support my family; without my job I am nothing."

ED problems may present as fluctuations in mood, inability to contain negative emotions, feeling overwhelmed by negative emotions, and having feelings that are "not me." In polyvagal terms ED should be viewed as an indicator of lack of safety and extreme vulnerability. The patient is essentially cycling between fight-flight and dorsal vagal shutdown. Kolacz and Porges' (2018) review of the relationship between stress and heart rate variability in fibromyalgia sufferers describes how this might occur.[24] Some overcontrolled individuals may do quite a good job of concealing how vulnerable they really feel, but non-verbal signs such as sleeping problems, fatigue, flat mood, lack of motivation, concentration and memory problems, and relationship difficulties tell another story.

3. Trauma processing

   As we have seen, chronic pain is often preceded by some sort of traumatic stress. Trauma processing requires identifying the primary trauma that is maintaining the pain and processing it with EMDR. Where the pain was precipitated by a discrete trauma such as an assault or motor vehicle accident (MVA), this is relatively simple. Where the client has suffered multiple traumas, including before and after the incident that triggered their pain and/or other adversity, it is more complicated. For example, a simple case of mild whiplash following an MVA in an otherwise healthy, relatively well-adjusted person can be easily treated using the normal trauma protocol. But the same case with the addition of early childhood trauma or adversity, other health problems, other adult trauma, including medical complications, etc., would require a much more integrated approach (see Chapter 6).

4. Uncovering the meaning of the pain

   Whether as a symptom of injury, a dissociated traumatic memory, an impediment to living a full life, or an expression of the long-term effects of severe stress, pain can mean many things. The key to treating pain from a psychological standpoint is to both address its more obvious significance (health issues, vulnerability, loss) and uncover its hidden significance (dissociated trauma/effects of adversity). There is always a dissociated component. Irrespective of whether or not the patient experienced childhood adversity, most chronic pain sufferers will have learned to hide their pain to avoid feeling stigmatized by family, friends, and even treating professionals.[25] Denying feelings of helplessness may also be part of an attempt to cling to their pre-pain identity. Despite the stereotypical view of chronic pain sufferers playing up their pain to attract sympathy and other benefits, most chronic pain sufferers are regularly pushing themselves beyond their physical limits to avoid facing the negative emotional and social consequences of their weakened self.[26] Denial is also a common coping strategy for chronic illness.[27]

   Survivors of trauma and childhood adversity are generally used to hiding their feelings as a coping strategy and may be particularly adept at portraying themselves as more okay than they really feel. Peeling back the layers requires time and compassion. Geoff, a young man in his late teens, developed debilitating chronic leg pain following a motor vehicle accident where his father was the at-fault driver. The doctors could find nothing wrong with his leg, causing him to feel confused and ashamed. He tried to pretend that he was okay and relied on painkillers to function normally. In therapy he anxiously confessed that he was angry at his father for mistreating him for most of his childhood (Geoff was different to his siblings due to undiagnosed autism) and terrified that if he expressed his feelings, it would break his parents' marriage. Once he'd made that connection, Geoff was able to separate his sense of responsibility for himself from his family and express his repressed feelings. After that his leg pain slowly diminished.

Geoff's story illustrates three important points. 1) That chronic pain/MUS can often be a symptom of unexpressed trauma. 2) That bringing this to consciousness and addressing it can facilitate healing. 3) That the type of illness or pain is often diagnostic regarding the nature of the emotional issues that underly it. For example, in traditional medicine leg pain is ascribed to an inflexible personality, unexpressed anger, and fatigue from feeling responsible for the family.[28] These qualities characterized Geoff perfectly. The notion that emotional problems can lead to physical pain dates back to the 19th century (as discussed in Chapter 1), however it's a much older idea in Chinese medicine.[29] Self-help books such as Louise Hay's *You Can Heal Your Life* and Evette Rose's *Metaphysical Anatomy* offer diagnostic maps based on Chinese medicine (see Figure 4.2). These can be useful guides when searching for possible emotional issues underlying pain/MUS.

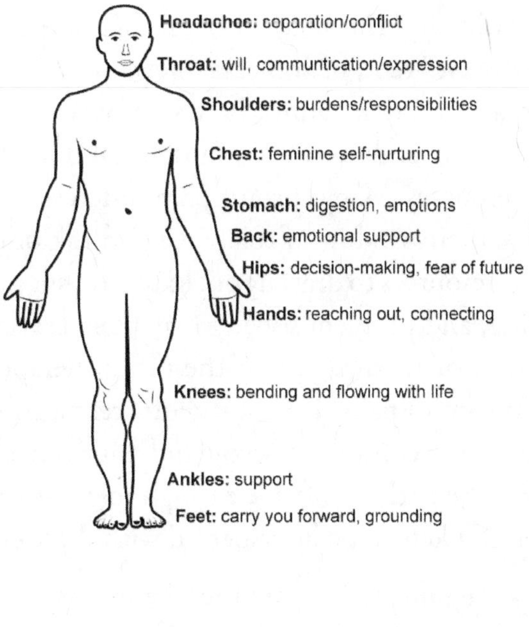

Figure 4.2 Body organs and diseases of stress

Scientifically minded readers may find such a categorization fanciful and wonder "where is the evidence?" The answer lies in the growing literature regarding the relationship between trauma and pain and the recognition of diseases of stress (as reviewed in Chapter 2). There is also a growing rapprochement between what the ancients knew and recent discoveries about the relationship between stress and specific organs. For example, emotional suppression has been linked to fibromyalgia.[30] Unresolved traumatic stress has been linked to gastrointestinal problems in fibromyalgia sufferers.[31] Low emotional intelligence and anger have been linked to migraine headache.[32]

A knowledge of the bodily organs most vulnerable to different types of stress can be helpful in guiding the direction of therapeutic inquiry, validating connections and guiding treatment (e.g., encouraging emotional expression, defining more appropriate levels of responsibility, becoming more flexible, etc.). These ideas should be taken as a guide. They should rarely be used to tell patients what their pain means—other than when a patient needs help articulating a connection they have already made. Everyone is unique and needs to be treated as such.

5. Dealing with current stressors

A significant proportion of chronic pain sufferers enter therapy in a state of crisis because of the sudden loss of their physical functioning, health, livelihood, financial security, future plans, and identity. They may have lost their job and not know how they are going to make next week's rent, or sometimes even put food on the table. These are real world existential issues that cannot be waved away with EMDR, unless the patient is lucky enough to be endowed with substantial untapped, easily accessible, mental and emotional resources. Many chronic pain sufferers are exhausted as a result of years of living outside their window of tolerance (I think of it as an "energy envelope") and have very few resources to draw upon. Extensive supportive psychotherapy, resourcing, skill-building, and problem-solving may be necessary to create sufficient safety and stabilization prior to engaging in the other therapeutic tasks associated with psychological treatment of pain. The therapeutic relationship is frequently a key aspect of therapy under these conditions—you and your office may be the patient's one safe place. Even after the patient is stable enough to commence psychotherapy of a deeper kind, treatment is likely to be interspersed with these elements.

Although the seven tasks (Figure 4.3) of pain therapy are presented in a linear fashion, clearly the course of therapy is dictated by the needs of each individual patient. Many will need crisis counseling and/or help with emotional regulation, or better pain control. A rare few will be strong enough to proceed directly to addressing the trauma or adversity that underlies their pain.

6. Self-care

   One of the defining characteristics of trauma survivors (and most chronic pain sufferers) is poor self-care. As van der Kolk (2001) notes, "Many people who were traumatized in their own families have great difficulty taking care of their own basic needs: hygiene, rest, and protection, even as they may be exquisitely responsive to other people's needs."[33] A person's capacity for self-care is a reflection of how they feel about themselves. If a person feels worthless or unlovable, they will believe they are not worth being cared for, or that they have to earn it, or that others' needs are more important than theirs. They will put the job ahead of their own health. Even Elon Musk, the billionaire entrepreneur who seems to have the world at his feet, struggles with self-care. Musk is the son of a harsh and abusive father, who was also bullied at school to the point of needing hospitalization.[34] As he grew into adulthood, Musk developed an almost inhuman work ethic. He once said, "Work like hell. I mean you just have to put in 80 to 100 hour weeks every week. [This] improves the odds of success." He has been known to sleep on the factory floor at Tesla. While this has clearly resulted in great success for Musk, it has come at a physical (and mental) cost. He has experienced weight fluctuations and sleeping problems and had struggles with anxiety and depression.

   Self-care means looking after one's physical and emotional well-being—making sure that they get the requisite amount of love, joy, rest, and nutrition. Self-care involves much more than exercise and diet. It requires a belief than one is worthwhile, something which is missing in most sufferers of trauma and pain. While self-care can be taught, it's far more effective when it evolves naturally as a result of emotional and attitudinal changes. Maria, a CPTSD/chronic pain sufferer, could never say no to her family. Because of her condition she found she could only perform physical and mental tasks in the morning. By the afternoon even preparing a meal, which she had done for years, was just more than her mind could manage. One day, after some months of therapy in which Maria had become more self-aware of the cost of her other-centeredness, her mother called and asked her to do something for her late in the day. Quite spontaneously Maria replied that she couldn't do it then but would do it the following morning. This small, almost trivial interaction symbolized a seismic shift in Maria's attitude toward herself and her capacity for self-care. It also represented a step toward learning to make healthier decisions for herself and reversing the behavioral patterns that were maintaining her stress and pain. Maria's therapist invited her to be curious about what this incident meant and what it might mean for her well-being if she was to do this more often.

7. Integration

The aim of therapy is integration. In EMDR integration refers to a state wherein traumatic memories have been processed and are now stored in an adaptive way, meaning they are integrated healthily with existing knowledge and identity. Things are linked up. The trauma survivor can know that they nearly died but that they didn't, both cognitively and emotionally. The adult survivor of childhood adversity can know that the mistreatment they experienced wasn't their fault and that they can ask for what they need without guilt or shame. The amputee can know that although something has been lost, they are still a whole person, still capable of engaging in life joyfully and productively. These changes are deeply felt and believed, rather than a product of forced positivity.

Dan Siegel, the famous Harvard neuropsychiatrist, says, "Health comes from integration. It's that simple, and that important. A system that is integrated is in a flow of harmony. Just as in a choir, with each singer's voice both differentiated from the other singers' voices but also linked, harmony emerges with integration."[35] Although he's talking about ego states/parts, Siegel's quote also implies the mind-body integration that is necessary for a person to live in the world as someone through whom experience can flow, shape, and grow adaptively. So, integration means more than just the reunification of dissociated sensory and mental elements of experience—but rather a whole person mind-body reconnection involving an embodied sense of self.

In survivors of trauma and pain, integration is not generally attained without what Jung called a "hero's journey" involving being willing to be vulnerable, facing the unknown, grappling with physical and mental pain, letting go of defenses, and, ultimately, transformation. Although EMDR is often seen as a rapid form of treatment, the complexity and chronic traumatization that these patients have endured, including dissociative defenses, means that this journey can take anywhere from a few months to many years of treatment. It is the therapist's job to act as guide and mentor on this journey, a journey where s/he will undoubtedly have to face their own fears and limitations. At the end of it all the patient has grown from and transcended their trauma and pain. From feeling overwhelmed by their trauma and pain they can look back and value painful "lessons learned." From living in the past, they can experience themselves fully in the present.

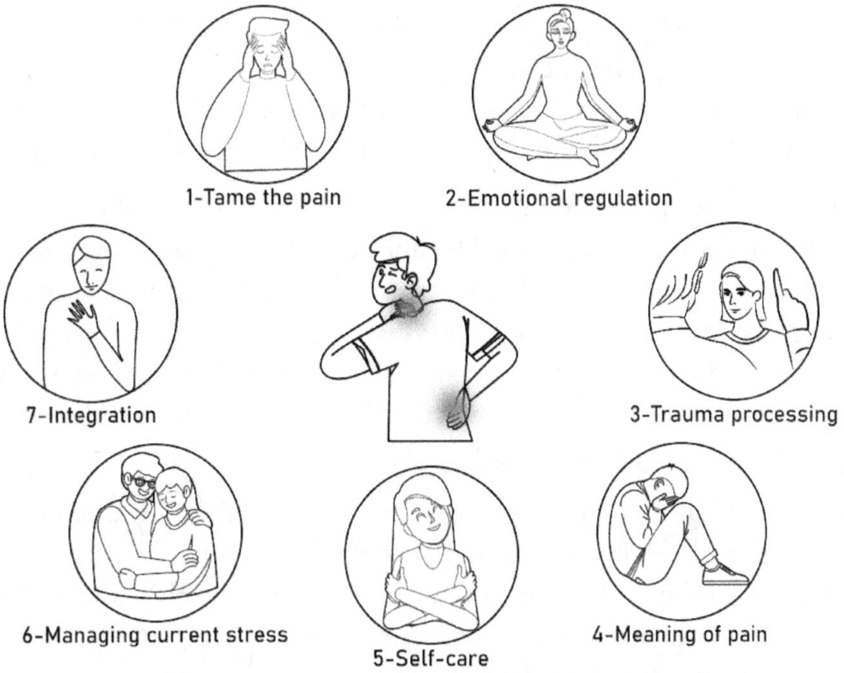

Figure 4.3 The 7 tasks of psychotherapy for pain

Harvey developed chronic pain after he fell off the back of a truck and suffered a ruptured disk at L-4, S-5 18 months prior to his first session with me. An operation some six months earlier had partially alleviated the pain (in his lower back and right leg) but the pain returned after he went back to work. Harvey said that he was not the sort of person who quit easily, but this made him feel defeated. Harvey's pain was more or less constant, but he could control it to some degree if he avoided activities which aggravated it. This was hard because Harvey's occupation as a truck driver entailed him sitting in one position for long hours, which aggravated his pain considerably.

About five years earlier he'd suffered another back injury, which entailed six months of rehabilitation. Although to all appearances Harvey had recovered from his first injury, he had found the six months of disability deeply traumatizing in the sense that it took away his previously strong confidence in his health and well-being. After that he was more careful but worked extra hard to prove to his employer that he was not a liability in what was a cutthroat business. When he got injured a second time, Harvey felt shocked, angry, and depressed. This time there would be no going back to truck driving and Harvey was faced with an uncertain future. Harvey's employer offered him less strenuous duties in an office, but with his poor schooling and limited literacy skills this terrified Harvey—as he put it, "If I can't drive a truck, there is no job for me." The whole situation made Harvey feel lost and out of control. Harvey's marriage and relationships with his three children were also suffering because of his moodiness.

At his first session Harvey recounted his story in a flat, matter-of-fact voice. Since neither medical professionals or physical rehabilitation experts had any effect on his condition, it was clear that he didn't have much hope that a psychologist could do much. Nevertheless, because of the way he'd been feeling, and behaving toward his wife and children, Harvey did accept that he needed some help. In order to help Harvey, I needed to know more about the forces that had shaped him and who he was or used to be, behind the tragic face he was currently presenting.

Harvey was a middle child of three, raised on a farm. He had wanted to join the air force, but he stayed on the farm to help his elderly parents run it. His brothers had moved away and did not maintain contact with the family. He was a dutiful son who put others first. There was a history of mental illness in the family—he admitted his father suffered from depression. Harvey felt his childhood was normal and although vague about details, denied any history of physical or sexual abuse. He admitted his father was distant because of his depression and that he got most of his affection from his mother, when she wasn't too busy or tired from working. When his parents went bankrupt and had to sell the farm, Harvey moved from the country to the edge of a major city, where he found work as a truck driver and married. Life had not been easy. Harvey had no qualifications or trade, but prior to the accident he had been able to support his family and pay the bills.

Harvey had a distinct personality. He was the sort of person who liked to know where he was going in life; he abhorred uncertainty. He had a high need for control and was self-reliant. He was also a goal-oriented person, who could adapt to changing circumstances. He was an emotionally stable man with no history of mental illness prior to his health problems. He was also a very private person who avoided showing his feelings, but especially emotional vulnerability. Harvey had high expectations of himself, and he could not accept the limitations imposed by his pain. It made him feel out of control, vulnerable, and inadequate. He struggled against the reality of the pain; he tried to avoid excessive physical activity but eventually he would get frustrated and throw himself into a physically demanding task such as mowing the lawn, after which his pain would flare up for several days and he would be more or less forced to rest until the pain subsided. Suitably chastened, he would take a more cautious approach to activity for a while, until his frustration escalated again.

As a result of the history and my own impressions about Harvey's personality, I summarized the main targets for treatment, in order of priority, as:

1. Tame the pain
2. Emotional regulation (Harvey's depression and irritability)
3. Self-care
4. Uncovering the meaning of the pain
5. Dealing with current stressors
6. Integration

Given Harvey's educational level, I introduced EMDR simply as a treatment for pain by explaining pain as a problem that starts in the body, but which is maintained in the brain. I added that the longer we experience something, such as pain, the more our brain activity is modified by that and the stronger the "pain memories become," just like learning to ride a bike. I explained that the bilateral stimulation component of EMDR activated the sensory part of the brain, where pain was stored, and that it could disrupt the brain activity which maintains pain. With luck this might lead to reduced physical discomfort and emotional distress, and increased feelings of self-control. I added that the activity in this part of the brain was not changeable by cognitive methods, which was why attempts to tell yourself to ignore the pain or that it's all in your head were ineffectual. Harvey could accept that his brain was involved in his pain and that this did not mean he was crazy, and that targeting the pain this way was something he had not tried.

We rated the pain as the #1 problem since all of Harvey's other problems were stemming from this. Harvey agreed that if we could help him get some control over his pain, everything else should become more manageable. When we targeted his pain (at the second session) Harvey's negative cognition (NC) was "I can't control it" and his positive cognition (PC) was "I can learn to control it" with a validity of cognition (VoC) of 2. I asked Harvey to describe his pain in terms of how it felt, what size it was, shape, color, etc. Harvey described the pain as a burning pain which he saw as a red cylindrical object, with a consistency of Play-Doh, which seemed to open out at the bottom, with a SUDs (subjective units of disturbance scale, or pain rating) of 8/10. I instructed Harvey to "just notice that" along with the auditory bilateral stimulation (BLS) and "let whatever happens happen." As I used continuous BLS, I did not stop to check the SUDs but checked in without ceasing BLS and advised him to "keep noticing" until he did not report any further improvement after two consecutive sets. From the first check-in, about 60 seconds after commencing BLS, Harvey noticed improvement ("The pain is released—it's starting to ease off.") After a total of five minutes, when the changes had stabilized, I instructed Harvey to "take a break" and "just reorient yourself to how you are feeling in your body and your mind now." After another brief pause, I asked Harvey to rate his pain again. He went quiet for a few seconds and seemed to be looking for something. Finally, with a mixture of disbelief and pleasure, he declared, "I'd have to say it's no more than a 2." He started moving his right leg tentatively and realized that the pain had completely gone from his leg. "There's nothing ... it's great!" he exclaimed. He also described feeling a bit light-headed and "spacey"—typical effects of BLS. Harvey's VoC increased to a 5/7 (even though Harvey declared he felt the best he'd ever been, he was not ready yet to believe that the changes he was experiencing were not some kind of trick or illusion on my behalf). I acknowledged that such an improvement might seem miraculous, advised Harvey that these changes would likely continue for some time and that when the pain returned it would be different, both in terms of its intensity and how it felt, and to be on the lookout for these and any other changes. I also gave Harvey a copy of my *Change Your Brain, Change Your Pain* CD and told him that it included bilateral stimulation and guided instructions to help manage pain flare-ups in between sessions. Harvey did not have any red flags about self-use of BLS (e.g., complex dissociation).

At the next session Harvey reported that the pain relief had lasted 12 hours, and that when the pain came back it was indeed different. He also reported that he had been more active, and that he had "overdone it" on a couple of occasions, leading to increased pain, but this was okay because that was what he'd chosen to do. He'd also found the CD helpful, not just for his pain but also for sleeping. He was pleased that it gave him an alternative to medication. Harvey said that he was not the sort of person who believed in such things, but that after our last session he'd realized that anything was possible.

I asked Harvey what he thought of the changes he'd experienced after just two sessions, and what this might mean for the future. Harvey replied that he felt very surprised, but hopeful. He added that he had been feeling more confident, and that he had "a new attitude" although he did not know where it came from. In an attempt to help Harvey own the changes that he was experiencing, I told him that whatever he was experiencing came from him and that anything I did was just facilitating his capabilities. I added that the experiences of injury, pain, and disability had obviously had a very negative effect on his self-esteem and that part of our work would be to help him get that back. We did some more EMDR on the pain, and this time it reduced to a "0". Harvey's VoC increased to a 6/7. We also targeted Harvey's loss of confidence in his health. The NC about this was "I'm vulnerable" and the PC was "I can get better." Again, Harvey's distress reduced and his belief in the PC increased.

In the following sessions Harvey stopped taking antidepressants and his reliance on painkillers also decreased significantly. After he stopped taking the antidepressants his blood pressure reverted to normal, for the first time in over five years. He reported that he was calmer at home. His employer had found him a part-time position in a warehouse which was appropriate to his physical capabilities and still in the kind of environment where he felt comfortable. The EMDR did not restore Harvey entirely to his former self; he still had pain and limitations as to what he could do physically. Harvey still did not know what the future held, but he reported feeling more relaxed that somehow things would work out. He felt more able to focus on his relationships with his wife and children, and felt that the pain was more of a nuisance rather than something that occupied center stage in his mind.

In this chapter we have introduced EMDR as a treatment for chronic pain/MUS on the basis of its efficacy with PTSD, which overlaps significantly with pain, the AIP model, and a growing body of research regarding this application of EMDR. We've reviewed EMDR as a therapy in terms of what defines it as a method and how it can be applied. We've identified seven tasks or goals which reflect the unique demands and treatment goals of this population and how they guide treatment. Armed with this theoretical and practical knowledge, we are now ready to venture into the practicalities of EMDR treatment of chronic pain/MUS.

PART TWO

EMDR PAIN PROTOCOL

5

Phase One: History and Treatment Planning

The first (history) phase of treatment can be summarized as the who? what? where? of therapy. Who is the client, what is their problem and where did it originate? What memories or events are causing the client's problems? Other "what?" questions include what current stressors are impacting on the client? What does the client need to learn in order to overcome this problem? The therapist must understand the background of whatever symptom or problem brings the client into therapy. The length of time that a client has struggled with the problem, and the timing of their decision to seek help are important. Why are they asking for help now? Therapy cannot commence without a workable, mutually agreed upon description of the problem (case conceptualization), so the therapist needs to hear the client describe the problem and transform that into something that both can work with. The history phase also involves the establishment of the therapeutic relationship: a boundaried emotional connection that acts as both a vehicle and a container for change, regardless of what method is being employed.

Purpose of history taking

As with other types of problems, treating pain begins by taking a history of the problem and relevant life events. The purpose of taking a history is to get a sense of the life of the problem, including duration, patterns, treatments, effects on mood and functioning, and current stressors. Because pain is often associated with illness or injury, the history taking must address how the pain started and any causal injury or illness processes. The history taking also involves more than just recording the history of the client's presenting problem. Many chronic pain sufferers have endured adversity prior to the injury that caused their pain, and the therapist should extend their inquiries well beyond the client's sometimes limited narrative of injury and pain. I start this process before the first session by emailing all new clients an intake questionnaire to complete and send back to me before we meet (see Therapist Resources section). At the end of this stage the client and therapist should have a mutually agreed upon definition of the problem and goal of treatment.

Chronic pain/MUS is often part of a cluster of problems including previous trauma, emotional regulation problems, deficits in self-care, etc. History taking should be client-centered, in the sense that although it is ostensibly a therapist-driven process aimed at helping the clinician define the goals of treatment (as per the seven tasks described in the previous chapter), it's also often the first time the patient has ever had to tell their story. As much as possible the clinician should let the client tell their story in their own way and simply gather and organize the information they need as it emerges. Giving the client space to tell their story, revealing as much or as little as they feel ready to, can be incredibly healing for patients whose pain journey (let alone life before) has been traumatic. Of course, it's not just what the patient says and how they say it that's important. It's what they don't say, can't remember, or can't forget.

Duration of the problem

How long has the client experienced physical pain? Generally speaking, the longer a person has had pain, the more helpless and defeated they feel. They may have become accustomed to living with significant levels of physical discomfort and physical impairment—but they are not happy. Any long-term major stress probably means the client has sleeping problems, fatigue, and their ability to work, love, and play may be significantly reduced. The longer the client has struggled with the problem, the more tired and less resourced they are likely to feel. Chronic pain sufferers are generally quite tense, physically and mentally. In some cases, this will be obvious as evidenced by restlessness, irritability, depression, concentration problems, etc.

With higher functioning clients, they do not display their stress so visibly, but the likelihood is that their nervous system is under considerable strain and that they are experiencing increased physiological arousal not dissimilar to that associated with PTSD.

Diagnosis

The medical diagnosis is the primary lens through which most clients understand their pain and some assessment of this needs to be made before considering psychological aspects. What is the client's medical diagnosis? Does the client understand the diagnosis? What does it mean for their general health and functioning? Is there any uncertainty about the diagnosis? If so, what effect is this having on the client's coping and adjustment? Is there a need for additional medical investigations? Assuming all relevant medical investigations have been completed, how consistent is the client's pain with their diagnosis? Is there is a component of the client's pain that is not accounted for by their medical diagnosis? If so, what is their attitude to that? What are the implications of the diagnosis for the future? Is the medical diagnosis accompanied by other health problems, including related mental health problems?

Clients with multiple diagnoses and long histories of health problems, investigations and treatments are more at risk of having experienced medical trauma such as misdiagnosis, surgical mishaps, etc. Rates of PTSD as high as 50% have been reported in recipients of surgery, with factors such as complications, re-admissions, and multiple surgeries increasing the risk.

Treatments and outcomes

Most chronic pain sufferers will also have an extensive history of medical treatment which will form part of their narrative about their view of life, self-efficacy, health, and well-being, etc. What medical investigations and treatments has the client received? How satisfied is the client with the treatment they have received? Even if unsuccessful, does the client feel that everything that could be done has been tried? Does the client feel guilty because of treatment failures? Does the client feel angry at the medical profession for failing to heal their pain? How supported does the client feel by the treatment system? Has the client been dismissed or invalidated? If so, is this triggering of earlier experiences of not being seen or heard associated with developmental abuse or neglect? How much responsibility is the client taking for self-management? Has the client been traumatized by some aspects of their medical treatment?

Trauma history

Given the overlap between trauma and pain, it is important to screen for trauma. The types of trauma most commonly associated with pain include physical and emotional neglect in childhood, physical and/or sexual abuse, combat exposure, and work-related accidents. When there is a clearly defined trauma associated with the pain, such as an accident or assault, the client will generally already be accepting of the link between their pain and trauma, even if they may not fully understand the ramifications. Clients with complex trauma histories (e.g., chronic physical or mental abuse, neglect, etc.) may have repressed or dissociated from their childhood trauma and thus not volunteer it or link it to their current health problems. Such clients often prefer to see their presenting pain as a simple symptom of injury which can be "fixed" by medical treatment. Consequently, probing pain clients about potential trauma where it is not volunteered needs to be done sensitively. Attachment deficits are not traumatic per se, but they are so common in chronic pain sufferers that their absence is the exception. Poor attachments lay the foundations for compartmentalization: separation of mental and physical elements of functioning, maladaptive emotional regulation strategies (e.g., addiction, overwork), and consequent allostatic stress.

As Maureen Kitchur notes, "Unless there is solid evidence to the contrary, clinicians would be wise to assume that virtually all clients carry with them some degree of developmental fixation or stuckness." What sort of emotional milieu did the client grow up in? Was the client's family a place where they were supported to reach the normal developmental milestones of adulthood and healthy functioning? What attitudes is the client likely to have formed toward themselves and their health from their family? Jim Knipe asks clients, "Who did you have to be to survive in your family?" This question is a great way of accessing the defenses that the client had to develop that probably still contribute to their poor self-care, etc. Was the family a place where it was okay to be sick or vulnerable? Was the family a place where it was okay to ask for help? Or was the client's family a place where they learned maladaptive attitudes and behaviors to survive? If the latter, what are those attitudes and how might they be preventing the client from coping more effectively?

Present life circumstances

What are the client's current life circumstances? How stable are they? Does the client have access to adequate economic resources, food, and shelter? What social supports do they have? Many chronic pain sufferers are struggling with unstable life circumstances, which adds stress and makes it hard to focus on health and self-care. Clients are not going to easily be able to practice meditation (for example) when they don't know where their next meal is coming from, or the bailiff is knocking on the door. Where the client is struggling with significant current stressors, these may need to be dealt with prior to attempting desensitization of past pain related trauma. This might mean providing support, psychoeducation, resource development, etc.

Personality

Hippocrates said, "It's far more important to know what person the disease has than what disease the person has." In addition to what happened, we also need to consider who it happened to—our patient's personality. The term comes from the Latin word *persona* and literally means mask. Understanding personality is important because it helps us know who we are working with—strengths, weaknesses, emotional style, traits, etc.—beyond just a damaged human being. Many, if not most, adult survivors of childhood adversity manage to get through life without developing disease, injury, or chronic pain/MUS. Is there something different about people who develop chronic pain/MUS? What heritable traits, dispositions, and aptitudes characterize your patient and how might these have shaped their response to trauma and adversity in unhealthy ways? How might an understanding of your patient's underlying personality help you formulate more individualized treatment strategies?

In the 19th century sufferers of chronic pain/MUS were viewed as hysterics: neurotic (anxious, sensitive, less able to synthesize thoughts and feelings, more suggestible) individuals who coped with their emotional responses to adversity (or in Freud's case, unacceptable sexual impulses) by repressing unpleasant memories, which then got "converted" into physical symptoms (see Chapter 1).

More recently, studies using Cloninger's Temperament and Character Inventory (TCI-R) have found that individuals with higher harm avoidance and lower self-directedness are more at risk of chronic pain. High harm avoidance refers to a tendency to be fearful, pessimistic, sensitive to criticism, and requiring high levels of reassurance. Low self-directedness often manifests as difficulty with defining and setting meaningful goals, low motivation, and problems with adaptive coping.[1] These characteristics fit neatly with those associated with trauma survivors: anxious, self-critical, chronic need for approval (never expressed directly), avoidance of novel stimuli, denial of personal needs, a tendency to adopt goals that are based on others or survival needs, as opposed to more personal, growth-oriented needs. Not surprisingly, these characteristics are also found in other approaches, such as schema therapy, where researchers have found schema based on shame, failure, incompetency, and vulnerability to be linking with chronic pain/MUS.[2]

Despite their thin or absent scientific credentials, popular accounts of mind-body dis-ease and stress align with the above personality attributes of chronic pain sufferers quite closely. Louise Hay, bestselling author of *You Can Heal Your Life*, describes a personality style based around unresolved resentment and guilt as the basis for many illnesses.[3] Jon Kabat-Zinn, author of *Full Catastrophe Living*, describes a personality style centered on doing rather than being.[4] John Sarno, MD, author of the bestselling *Healing Back Pain*, describes chronic pain/MUS sufferers as "... people who don't think much of themselves; they have a constant need for approval; they are conflicted, prone to anxiety, and quick to anger. They have no patience."[5]

There are other phenomena to be considered. In Chapter 2 we saw how Dell identifies hypnotizability as a characteristic of individuals who are more likely to dissociate when faced with overwhelming stress. According to Dell, highly hypnotizable individuals have an innate capacity to distance themselves mentally (dissociate) from unpleasant feelings (whether traumatic or not).[6] Associated with this they have a greater ability to compartmentalize conflicting aspects of personality (one part knows something bad happened, another part doesn't). This idea represents something of a return to the 19th century ideas about hysteria, but it has other implications regarding our understanding of personality. Such individuals are often conflicted: it is intolerable to be that hurt, vulnerable person in that hurt, vulnerable body. This conflict is often resolved by developing a coping self which attempts to present a more okay version of the self to others. According to Frank Putnam, this capacity to adopt different selves to cope with different circumstances is an innate capacity—we put on our "work face" when we leave home in the morning, or our "hanging out with friends face" on card night. Putnam also posits that most personalities host numerous, sometimes discrepant versions of themselves to a greater or lesser degree.[7] The neurotic can also be calm, confident, and effective, under the right conditions. The domestic violence perpetrator is often the person everyone turns to for help at work.

The more traumatized an individual is, the sharper the divide between different aspects of themselves and the less smoothly they will transition between different states. They may also harbor a "secret self" where needs perceived as unacceptable are harbored and attended to. Generally speaking, trauma survivors' (and many chronic pain/MUS sufferers') sense of self is fragmented, prone to self-destructive and sometimes high-risk behavior, and socially isolated. On the whole, they are innately sensitive and prone to anxiety, but feel ashamed of themselves for being this way. Most are hypnotizable to some degree. Consequently, they will lean toward dissociative strategies as a defense mechanism. Some will develop coping strategies which are remarkably creative and even mature for, say, a five-year-old child. But in order to survive, they have had to become someone they are not: someone who appears to have no needs, or someone who is adept at morphing into who they imagine others need them to be. They live outside their bodies—while we all sometimes push our physical limits, for trauma survivors this is a way of life. They may not trust anyone, meaning they can never access the support that can only be felt through a deep emotional connection. They may avoid new experiences for fear of negative consequences, trapping themselves in a closed loop of repeating past patterns. In general, personality is thus best viewed as a balance of fluid, multi-faceted, opposing forces comprising visible and invisible elements, which may be more or less integrated, depending upon the degree of adversity the individual has experienced.

In person such individuals may (or may not) appear greatly concerned about their current symptoms but make light of (or ignore) early adversity. They may prefer to talk about external circumstances rather than feelings. There is often a narrative of having coped with early adversity very well, only for everything to come crashing down when they got sick. If only they had not fallen ill or gotten injured, everything would still be okay. The challenge is to avoid being seduced by the coping self and make space for the secret self, both of which are valid facets of the whole persona.

Coping strategies

The kinds of coping strategies the client employs will of course reflect their personality. What dissociative strategies are they employing, and how effectively? Do they avoid their pain? Do they see it as an opponent to be conquered? How well are they able to balance physical activity levels against the impact of their pain? How well do they pace themselves when it comes to activity? How does the client manage the emotional aspects of their pain? Are they repressing their feelings and then experiencing uncontrollable emotional outbursts, or do they simply feel overwhelmed? How well have they been finding new goals and activities to replace those lost due to the effects of pain? From a therapeutic standpoint the question becomes: What knowledge would the client need to access within themselves which would allow them to adopt more flexible and adaptive coping strategies? For example, is there any evidence of a wise adult part that could help the client make better health choices without totally sacrificing the goals they have set for themselves?

Note: History taking does not have to be completed before commencing treatment. However, it should give you enough information to assess what kind of therapeutic interventions your client needs and in what order. Clients with complex medical/trauma histories and/or poorly managed pain are often exhausted and rarely ready for EMDR immediately. Clients who can't identify trauma that might be relevant to processing EMDR may benefit from hypnotic uncovering of target material (see Chapter 12).

The following case history illustrates how chronic pain can coexist with developmental trauma and the importance of taking those traumas into account during the history taking and case conceptualization.

Bridget developed chronic pain after twisting her back the wrong way in her job as a factory worker. Although her physician could find nothing worse than a small disk bulge, Bridget's injury was causing intense low back pain, tingling sensations down her right leg, and difficulty performing even the most basic of physical tasks. Bridget's pain was not responding to rest, physiotherapy, or medication; in fact, it seemed to be getting worse. As the months wore on, Bridget felt increasingly disbelieved by her doctor and frustrated by the failure of treatment. A spiral of pain, stress, sleeplessness, and fatigue developed, and Bridget felt increasingly despondent and depressed.

Bridget had endured and coped with much adversity in her life prior to her current injury. Bridget was raised by harsh, controlling parents—her mother's idea of love was that her daughter should be grateful for being fed and having a home. Her father was an absent and distant figure who preferred drinking with his friends to interacting with his family. When he was home, there was tension in the air, which would occasionally erupt into violent arguments. Consequently, Bridget learned to withhold her feelings and to try and attract as little attention as possible. Bridget was a sensitive person and it took considerable effort to detach herself from the emotional conflict she sensed around her. She sometimes felt as though she was watching the world from inside a television. At other times she found it hard to tell what she was feeling at all.

In order to escape her chaotic home life, Bridget left school as soon as she was legally allowed and found work in a supermarket. She developed a romantic attachment with a boy she met at work and fell pregnant to him when she was 18. They set up house together and Bridget tried to build the home she had always wanted. But he turned out to be an angry, unstable young man with the same violent tendencies as Bridget's father. After several miserable years with him, Bridget finally summoned up the courage to leave. She had a couple more failed relationships before deciding that she was better off just trying to raise her daughter by herself. Bridget spent the rest of her adult life as a single mother, trying to support herself and her child single-handedly.

Bridget's personality reflected her life struggles; she found it difficult to trust people and prided herself on her self-reliance, although she would do anything to help someone in need. Bridget saw this self-reliance as a strength—as she put it, "If you don't depend on anyone, you can't be hurt." Bridget was also very tough-minded with herself and prided herself on her ability to keep going no matter how tired or stressed she felt. Before being injured she had a high tolerance for pain and had once worked through a shift despite having a fractured wrist. Bridget always put her responsibilities ahead of herself. However, Bridget's superficially strong exterior really covered up a very insecure, self-doubting persona. Bridget had deep unexpressed feelings of shame and worthlessness about herself—why else would her parents have treated her so badly? It was in this context of self-denial, working hard to live up to her responsibilities, regardless of her own personal needs, that Bridget's injury occurred.

Bridget's pain was greater than could be accounted for by her physical injury, and it didn't make sense medically. Bridget had no concept of her pain other than in terms of the injury that triggered it. But when the history is taken into account, Bridget's pain becomes less mysterious. As a result of her stressful past, Bridget had always suffered from anxiety, autonomic nervous system problems (sleeping problems, energy problems), and emotional disconnection. Blood tests would almost certainly have revealed biochemical abnormalities involving cortisol and serotonin (neurotransmitters involved in fighting infection and pain). Bridget's emotional disconnection meant that she tended to ignore her needs and that she had no effective means of regulating her emotions or their impact upon her pain and suffering. Her sleeping problems meant that she had no energy and probably decreased immune functioning.

EMDR or adjunctive strategies?

The whole purpose of history taking is to formulate a good case conceptualization and an effective treatment plan. The typical chronic pain patient is going to present with some combination of childhood adversity, trauma, and illness.

There are six primary sets of events or circumstances that are common to trauma-pain sufferers, ranging from simple trauma to attachment and complex medical issues. The general rule is that the more of these factors a client presents with, the more likely EMDR will need to be preceeded by and integrated with adjunctive strategies (see Figure 5.1). For example, a generally healthy person who has whiplash as a result of a car accident, but no other significant trauma, would probably benefit from standard EMDR. But if they were also affected by earlier trauma, attachment deficits, and other health problems, they would probably need help rebuilding their energy levels, managing negative affect, resourcing, and ego-strenghtening, all of which requires more than standard EMDR reprocessing.

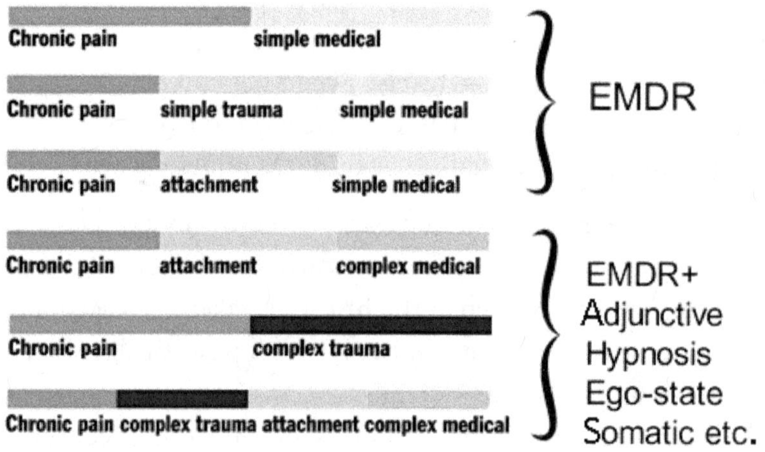

Figure 5.1 EMDR or adjunctive strategies?

Case conceptualization and treatment planning

The outcome of the history taking is a good case conceptualization. How ready is your client for EMDR and which of the seven tasks described in Chapter 4 does your client have to overcome, and what is their most urgent problem? If the client does not appear ready for EMDR, what adjunctive strategies might you use first? (See Chapters 12 and 13.)

In addition to the seven tasks, the case conceptualization should also include an assessment of the client's resources and strengths. What personal qualities and strengths does the client demonstrate? Even the most depressed, guilt-ridden client also has a story of survival and small successes that they have probably minimized. Other resources include how much access the client has to their emotions. What is the client's emotional range and capacity? (The more access the client has to positive emotions, the easier it will be to generate antidote resources in the installation phase.) How well is the client able to detach from their emotions? (Necessary for the desensitization phase.) How able are they to concentrate? (Also important for the desensitization phase.) What about support? Work?

Assuming the client is ready for EMDR, the problem then becomes which problem to target first. Shapiro recommends targeting the earliest memory or trauma on the basis that this often represents the foundation of the client's current presenting problems. The nexus between current symptoms and past trauma is not always so clear with pain sufferers, particularly where the pain is associated with physical injury, even though the client may have suffered some adversity in childhood. In such cases, it can be more effective to start with the present pain, and once that is under control, work backward. Getting the client's present pain under control is akin to creating safety in a PTSD sufferer—without the freedom from threat that improved pain control affords, the chronic pain sufferer may be anxious to participate in the processing phase of therapy. Someone with complex trauma and pain following an accident at work may regard pain as their main problem and not want to work on their childhood trauma until well into therapy. A client with a simple trauma-related pain (e.g., a frozen shoulder following a motorbike accident) may have no qualms about reprocessing their accident trauma immediately. Wherever trauma is contributing to pain, the therapist has to assess the severity of the trauma, and the client's readiness, and start with where the client is at. If the client does not appear ready for EMDR due to exhaustion, inadequately controlled pain, lack of safety, or hyperarousal, then EMDR may need to be preceded by adjunctive strategies such as safe place, feelings container, and other hypnotic and somatically based strategies.

Sara presented complaining of depression, suicidal ideation, flashbacks, pelvic pain, self-harming behavior, and self-loathing, on top of a history of severe childhood sexual abuse at the hands of a male relative. Sara's abuse had involved repeated vaginal intercourse and witnessing a chicken slaughtered by the perpetrator and being warned that would be her fate if she told anyone what happened. Sara's mother did not believe her when she reported the abuse, and Sara still struggled to find the acceptance and love she craved from her mother. Despite these problems, Sara had managed to marry and have a son, build a career as a successful teacher, and rise to the level of principal. Sara's husband turned out to be an angry, abusive man and Sara eventually left him. She had been a success as a teacher, though, and had won awards for her innovative ideas. About 12 months before coming into treatment, she suffered a breakdown and had only recently managed to go back to work as a youth counselor. She found that this work triggered flashbacks of her abuse, which seemed to involve more and more details as time went on. Sara's flashbacks also involved intense physical symptoms, including heart palpitations, pelvic pain, bodily aches, and fatigue. She found these episodes so distressing that sometimes she cut herself just to get some relief. Sara was very ambivalent about seeking help and trusting someone, but she was also intelligent enough to know that she needed help.

Despite the horrific abuse she'd suffered, Sara displayed many resources. She was clearly intelligent, as evidenced by her career. She was very resourceful in the sense that she could generally find who or what she needed to solve problems in her life. She provided a home for a female friend and a drug-addicted son. She had a strong sense of humor. She loved caring for animals—she had collected stray cats. She could detach from her feelings, sometimes consciously, sometimes not—she described how she had succeeded as a teacher by cutting herself off emotionally from her narcissistic, critical mother.

Although it was evident from the first session that this was a case of complex trauma, involving the full gamut of symptoms and issues that these cases typically involve, it nevertheless took months to complete the case conceptualization. Many of the earlier sessions were taken up with stabilization and managing present crises, or teaching Sara emotional management skills, installing resources, building safety, etc. Sara also had to be encouraged to believe that she deserved to feel normal and not suffer. This involved a range of strategies, including working with positive and negative ego states: getting her to reflect on her thoughts, feelings, and attitudes whenever she engaged in self-destructive or unhealthy behavior or sometimes just quietly reminding her that everyone has the right to look after themselves and enjoy feeling comfortable in their own body. It's really beyond the scope of this book to give a detailed account of the steps involved in interventions such as ego state therapy, but the Client Resources section at the back of this manual contains several worksheets designed to assist clients to improve their self-care. The following treatment plan was formulated:

1. Taming the pain
2. Emotional regulation
3. Self-care
4. Uncovering the meaning of the pain

5. Dealing with current stressors
6. Trauma processing
7. Integration

The desensitization work was not commenced until almost a year into Sara's treatment, and it began with targeting her present pain and using short sets to ensure she did not slip into a dissociative state. After each small set, considerable time was spent helping Sara understand and feel comfortable with the effects of the BLS. This included offering her suggestions when she could not answer questions regarding her feelings. In the early stages of the desensitization work, the focus was on helping her to feel comfortable with being in her body and experiencing feelings so that she could eventually learn that there were other ways to manage feelings than dissociating or self-harm. It also goes without saying that the development of a strong therapeutic relationship based on sensitivity, pacing, acceptance, empathy, and boundaries was developed.

Migraine as a somatoform disorder

Michener's paralysis following the plane crash (Chapter 2) illustrates a conversion reaction (now known as a functional neurologic disorder), wherein intense unprocessed affect is somaticized. In Michener's case, his paralysis could easily be linked to the trauma of the plane crash, as can many trauma-related pains (e.g., vaginismus in a sexual abuse survivor, whiplash in a motor vehicle accident survivor). In such cases, assuming there are not too many additional trauma or health problems, the standard EMDR trauma protocol is often all that is required. However, in many other cases, the connection between present pain and past trauma is less direct. How do the vague pains of fibromyalgia, the gastrointestinal problems of IBS, or the headaches of migraine sufferers relate to the childhood adversity that so many sufferers of these conditions have experienced? Are there discrete memories that are suitable for EMDR processing or do these symptoms warrant a more indirect approach?

Migraine headaches are typically defined as a neurological disorder based on a combination of genetic factors and sympathetic nervous system dysfunction.[8] To some degree they can also represent a type of somatoform disorder.[9] Consistent with this, PTSD has been identified as a possible etiological factor in some migraine headaches.[10] Migraine headaches are also often associated with other somatic symptoms (especially fatigue and gastrointestinal problems).[11] Many migraine sufferers are also affected by osmophobia—a sensitivity to noxious odors, which can be a trigger.[12] Migraine severity has also been found to be associated with a history of childhood physical abuse, anxious/avoidant attachment, PTSD, and shutdown dissociation.[13] Based on Schauer & Elbert's (2010) defense cascade model, shutdown dissociation involves transition to dissociative immobility when fight-flight is not an option.[14] Not surprisingly, shutdown dissociation is more common in individuals who have been exposed to chronic physical or sexual abuse.[15]

Headache sufferers typically present with a range of physical and psychological complaints, of which the migraines may be a major or minor concern. Given the connection with dissociative shutdown, assuming all possible physical causes have been ruled out, migraines should be regarded as a form of somatoform dissociation. Steve Marcus's headache protocol describes a method of treating migraines incorporating diaphragmatic breathing, head compression, and BLS.[16] However, he cautions that treating headaches involves much more than a protocol and that targeting the headache directly (with EMDR) can exacerbate the problem.[17] Marcus recommends beginning with a full assessment of the etiology of the headache, including the "where, what, and when" of how it commenced, whether there has been head trauma, exposure to noxious chemicals, etc. As with treating other dissociated affect, safety, affect tolerance, resourcing, and titrated exposure are essential.

Laura, a woman in her late 50s, sought help addressing lifelong anxiety and panic attacks, lack of sense of self, and episodic migraines. Laura grew up with an abusive alcoholic father who made her feel inadequate and like someone who had virtually no right to be here. She tried to earn his love by being who he wanted her to be, even joining the air force to be the son he always told her she should have been. By some stroke of luck, she married a man who was very kind to her, but their only child was born with cerebral palsy, and because of her personality, Laura took sole responsibility for caring for him. Although she had access to government funded carers, making sure that her son's needs were met was nevertheless an exhausting 24/7 responsibility. She described a lonely life (she had no time for friends because of caring for her son), full of fear and anxiety. Over the years Laura saw various psychologists and even a psychiatrist, without success. After her husband died suddenly, in her late 50s she decided to try therapy again, and somehow found me. Rapport was quickly established; Laura was a smart, funny woman and we "clicked."

Laura's treatment (which would ultimately last three years) began with the most pressing issue—the trauma and grief of her husband's recent death—which responded well to EMDR. Following that, we began slowly peeling back the layers of her life, including her childhood abuse and its effects on her sense of self, the demands of caring for her son, and the changes in her life associated with the loss of her husband. Remarkably, although Laura could not stand up for herself, she had no difficulty fighting for her son's rights and would fly into a rage if one of his carers failed to treat him according to her high expectations.

Laura responded well to some parts working to help integrate her wounded child part. She cried a lot for what that little girl had to endure. She started to find an inner voice which could guide her in making better choices about her needs ("I'm not a silly person—I can trust myself."). She learned, via a combination of parts work and somatic inquiry ("If your headache could speak, what would it say?"), that her headaches were really her body saying she needed to give herself permission to be angry for herself. Alongside this she was learning to listen to her heart and develop a stronger sense of self. One day, just before her 60th birthday, she realized that two-thirds of her life were over and that she was exhausted from caring for her son ("I want it all and I want it now."). She made the difficult decision to place him in full-time care so that she could have a life. She felt a mixture of guilt and relief about this, but she knew in her heart that it was the right thing to do. She took up yoga, joined a knitting group (where she made some nice new friends), and booked an overseas holiday (the first in her life). She continued to experience some situational anxiety, but never to the point of panic attacks, and her migraine headaches decreased to the point of no longer being an issue.

An integrated approach

As the above cases illustrate, EMDR alone is rarely sufficient. Treatment of chronic pain/MUS almost always requires an integrated approach including EMDR, hypnosis, ego state work, and somatic strategies.[18] Additionally, many clients will be receiving concurrent medical treatment, physical therapies, and other alternative approaches, which can bring their own kinds of trauma. Medical mismanagement, discrimination, and invalidation are common experiences.[19] Where there is a history of extensive medical and allied health involvement, always evaluate the following: 1) How in control does the client feel of their medical/other treatments? 2) How congruent is that treatment with their needs? 3) How respected does the client feel about their treatment? 4) How well are they attending to physical self-care, such as diet and activity? 5) What are their expectations regarding the healing process?

There are four broad streams to treating trauma-related pain, which mirror the stages of standard treatment of complex PTSD. Namely: therapeutic relationship, resourcing, trauma processing, and integration. The difference when applying this approach to pain/MUS is that the treatment often starts with a medically unexplained symptom, which may be quite disconnected from traumatic antecedents in the patient's consciousness. Consideration needs to be made as to what extent the somatic symptoms might be of traumatic origin and how to help the patient make this connection. In many cases organic pathology will also be present, with sometimes quite significant effects. The psychological effects of illness and pain also need to be addressed. In addition to affect regulation, traditionally a core element in the treatment of CPTSD, more somatically focused pain management strategies may need to be developed. These may be developed through hypnosis, EMDR resourcing, somatic work, and ego state work. Directly or indirectly, the aim is to facilitate increased affect management and decreased reliance on dissociative coping strategies (although these may still have a place).

Hypnosis is an intrinsic element of EMDR practices and processes—it has to be because of the nature and involvement of dissociative responses in survivors of trauma. Dissociation is an inherently hypnotic phenomenon, as evidenced by abrupt shutting off of information, sequestration of content, and defensive dissociative modularity (compartmentalization).[20] Any effective treatment must incorporate and address the hypnotic quality of dissociative processes. Consistent with this, hypnosis is an adjunctive element to many treatment approaches, including psychoanalysis, CBT, and EMDR.[21] Elements of EMDR, such as the therapeutic relationship, floatback, safe place, EMDR check-in, resourcing, and future template, all owe their origins to hypnosis (the EMDR check-in can be viewed as a form of trance ratification). Recipients of EMDR also often enter trance-like states following EMDR—even van der Kolk described his response to EMDR as "hypnopompic." Additionally, more distinctly hypnotic interventions, such as guided imagery or other evocative strategies, can supplement EMDR for patients with treatment resistant pain (see Chapter 12).

Despite the many similarities, EMDR appears to address dissociative phenomena in a way that is fundamentally different to hypnosis.[22] For example, EMDR interventions such as the cognitive interweave can summons latent ego states without trance.[23] Hypnosis explicitly utilizes dissociative phenomena in a way that EMDR doesn't. Somatic aspects represent a kind of bridge between EMDR and hypnosis since the success of both approaches rests upon their ability to generate "involuntary responses." In EMDR these might be relaxation, decreased tension, and distancing effects, while in hypnosis it could be relaxation, arm levitation, or catalepsy. Thus EMDR, hypnosis, and somatically focused therapy, and their constituent elements, are overlapping modalities which are highly dependent upon each other for their efficacy.

These elements are delivered in a phased, integrated way, according to the needs of the patient. The more trauma the client has endured (medical or psychological), the more likely they are to have depleted energy reserves and limited coping skills, and the more likely they are to need all these treatment inputs, beginning with the safety of a secure therapeutic relationship (see Figure 5.2). Although it was developed independently, this model is identical to the Phillips & Frederick (1995) SARI model.[24]

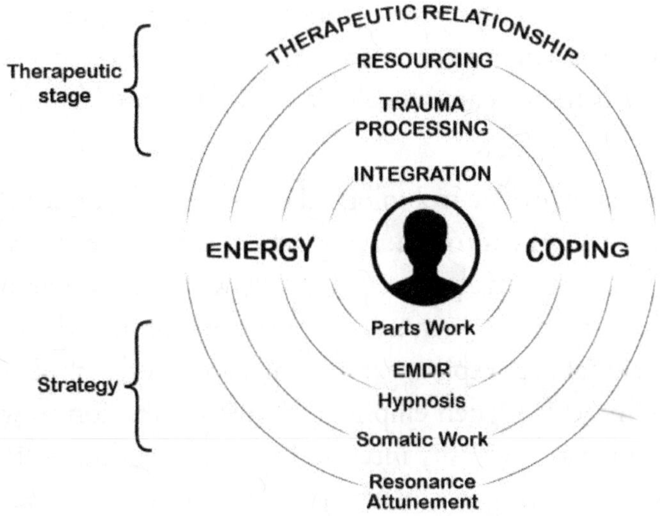

Figure 5.2 Phased integrated approach

The therapeutic relationship

The therapeutic relationship is the crucible within which therapy occurs—its importance can't be overstated. As Harville Hendrix said, "We are born in relationship, we are wounded in relationship, and we can be cured in relationship."[25] Given the contribution that attachment problems make to chronic pain/MUS, it's not surprising that a reparative attachment such as that afforded by the therapeutic relationship might be important.

As discussed in Chapter 2, the attachment system is a central organizing system in the brain wherein infants use their parents for regulating their inner states until their own psychoneurobiologic functions develop. As Siegel has described, these shared states of attunement are internalized and encoded as procedural memory in the child. Securely attached individuals know how to take care of themselves, and how to regulate negative feelings and sensations. Attachment deficits are known to result in disorganized behavioral responses and deficient "body micro-practices" (looking at others, reaching out), as well as impaired regulation of stress and negative affect.[26]

Given the recent discovery of mirror neurons and the capacity for the therapist to moderate the negative effects of attachment deficits, awareness of the impact of attachment problems on mental and emotional functioning is vital in the treatment of physical and emotional pain. A therapeutic relationship incorporating trust, attunement, and acceptance is both the location and the vehicle for healing attachment problems. Siegel has suggested that a good therapeutic relationship may actually help repair neurological deficits caused by childhood attachment problems.

Porges' polyvagal theory provides a neurobiological framework for understanding why attachment is important. When we feel safe, our nervous system enters a ventral vagal state where we can "rest and digest," feel relaxed and able to engage fully with others (and our environment).[27] There are various ways of facilitating such a state. Siegel emphasizes the importance of being mindfully present and being able to explore gaps in understanding with statements like "I don't understand" or "tell me more."[28] Ogden emphasizes paying attention to what's happening in the body, describing therapy as "not only interpreting and attending to the client's narrative and emotions but also participating in and attending to the communication that occurs beneath the words in a body-to-body tete-a-tete."[29] Helen Watkins used to emphasize resonance, a process wherein "the analyst uses his or her entire self (cognitively, affectively, perceptually, and motorically) to develop a replication of the patient.[30]

However you do it, a ventral vagal state is not something that can be willed into existence. In fact, any effort to create a ventral experience likely involves sympathetic activation. Bonnie Badenoch, an American therapist who integrates polyvagal theory with clinical practice, has discovered that the most effective way to respond to distressing affect in clients is to be present more and more without agenda so that mutual coregulation can take place, rather than responding to the urge to shift or "do" something for the client.[31] As Carl Rogers once said, "In my early professional years I was asking the question: How can I treat, or cure, or change this person? Now I would phrase the question in this way: How can I provide a relationship which this person may use for his own personal growth?"[32] This way of thinking about therapy also dovetails with the discovery made by Porges and colleagues that ventral vagal parasympathetic states "lateralize to the right hemisphere."[33] The right hemisphere is important where feelings of embodiment, wholeness, and connection are generated, with oneself and others. Badenoch also recommends just learning two or three techniques/methods well, to the extent that they become embodied, rather than trying to learn a lot of strategies superficially. As these various approaches suggest, resonance, and the safety it creates, comes from a place of profound openness, presence, and acceptance by the therapist.

A beautiful and perhaps unexpected example comes from the story of Freud's last patient, a young Viennese woman whose controlling father took her to see Freud for treatment of depression. Margarethe Lutz recalled experiencing a visceral reaction to the elderly therapist (he would die two weeks later) whom she described as "frail-looking, but full of power." After her father answered on her behalf every time Freud asked her a question, he dispatched him so they could talk freely. Alone with Freud, she experienced an intense and immediate experience of connection; "He looked at me uninterruptedly, and his full participation enveloped me." After hearing her story of subjugation at the hands of her controlling father, including not being allowed to watch kissing scenes at the cinema, Freud lectured her about how growing up involved resisting one's parents and told her to stay seated the next time there was a kissing scene. He repeated this latter instruction three times for good measure. Margarethe took Freud's advice and thus began her journey to freedom and self-hood. As she later summarized it, "Those 45 minutes saved my life."[34] Freud's advice was probably something the house cleaner could have told her; what made it so powerful was clearly Margarethe's feeling seen and understood by Freud; some would say adopted.

Despite its importance, a good therapeutic relationship alone is insufficient. Particularly when treating highly dissociative clients, care must be taken to balance rapport-building with therapeutically active interactions. As Watkins observed, the therapist resonates with "no more than half of his personhood—while maintaining the other half fully rooted in objective reality."[35] Milton Erickson demonstrated this balance between being with and doing. His daughter Betty recalls how, "He never forgot to listen to the patient and hear what he was really saying, which is another skill which he constantly honed. Then he would think about what he, and the patient, had to do to help get the best outcome. People call it speaking the other person's language, but it's more complex than that."[36] I (MG) also try to first meet my patients as people, to get to know them as well as their problems—their strengths, weaknesses, and shared points of interest—before figuring out what I can do to help them.

The more trauma and pain a client has endured, the more likely they are to be exhausted and lacking in effective coping resources and need the safety and support afforded by a strong therapeutic relationship. This creates the ground from which the client can develop more effective coping resources, process trauma, and regain a more integrated sense of self. Some chronic pain/MUS sufferers may be seeking symptom relief without appreciating that this may not be possible to any significant degree without engaging with unprocessed traumatic memories/patterns. The therapist must be able to manage these expectations sensitively but assertively.

Resourcing

Survivors of complex trauma and pain/MUS are generally lacking in energy, effective coping resources, and capacities necessary for normal life functioning. This is not to say that they may not have coped valiantly with the adversity life has inflicted upon them, but that strategies such as dissociation, overactive protector parts, and a "go it alone" lifestyle are short-term coping strategies that ultimately inhibit the development of ego strength and a positive sense of mastery. The trauma remains unprocessed, the psyche remains divided, and the nervous system is exhausted because of an overactive fight-flight response.

Three key criteria for assessing whether a client needs resourcing are exhaustion, lack of affect regulation strategies, and the presence of dissociation. EMDR's ability to catalyze innate information processing capabilities makes it an energy-intensive therapy. Energy is a resource that most sufferers of chronic trauma and pain are lacking. Insomnia, fatigue, and exhaustion result in a decreased capacity to withstand exposure to aversive feelings even in the titrated manner that EMDR permits. The client must also be able to tolerate the affective potent distress that may be triggered during the desensitization phase. Lack of effective affect-regulation strategies risks the client feeling overwhelmed and further traumatized.

The idea that we possess innate resources is one of the defining characteristics of EMDR. Resourcing involves building energy levels and coping skills aimed at strengthening the self and one's ability to cope with adversity. Popular EMDR resourcing strategies include calm/safe place, inner advisor, light stream, CIPOS (Constant Installation of Present Orientation and Safety), and imaginal nurturing, to name a few. Andrew Leeds pioneered the idea of combining short sets of BLS with positive imagery, which he called RDI or Resource Development and Installation.[37] Shirley Jean Schmidt developed the Developmental Needs Meeting Strategy (DNMS) for addressing attachment deficits in sufferers from complex PTSD and dissociative disorders.[38] The comprehensive resource model employs a combination of grounding strategies (e.g., breathing) ego state work and relational factors, within a neurobiological framework, to facilitate safety and integration.[39] Most of these interventions were developed with the needs of trauma sufferers in mind. When treating pain/MUS resources for managing somatic distress, such as antidote imagery, pain container or post-BLS somatically based imagery are also likely to be necessary (see Chapter 9 and the therapist and client resources sections at the rear of this book).

A more common problem is the presence of overwhelming pain which absorbs the attention and inhibits the client's ability to respond to BLS. Here resourcing in the form of hypnotically enhanced imagery and suggestions for pain relief can be necessary prior to attempting EMDR. As discussed in Chapter 2, trance phenomena such as depersonalization, amnesia, and ego states are intrinsic to somatization. Dissociative trance phenomena are often associated with increased responsivity to hypnotic strategies (e.g., guided imagery, positive memories, and direct suggestion), which can be leveraged. See Chapter 12 for more information about how to employ hypnosis for pain relief.

In all but the most seriously unwell, the body is a primary source of resources. As Ogden notes, "Somatic resources are the physical functions, actions and capacities that provide a sense of well-being and competency on a physical level, and in turn positively affect how we feel."[40] The body is also a storehouse of physical and emotional learnings: from learning how to ride a bike to learned socio-emotional responses. One way of harnessing somatic resources is paying attention to bodily sensations in the present and using bodily signals as the evolutionary survival guides they are evolved for. For example, noticing sensations of anxiety in the stomach and listening to their message of needing safety, or a lack of energy in the torso signaling a need for rest. Just the act of paying attention to your body (within tolerable bounds) can be healing because of the connection it entails. Another way is to access memories of activities that stimulate feelings of efficacy and focus on them to help recapture those feelings in the present. In EMDR, resources derived from memories or imagery may install via pairing with BLS or hypnosis. When a client is very unwell, external resources may also need to be accessed to nourish and support the body (e.g., support, exercise, diet, strategies for enhancing restful sleep, etc.).

Resourcing occurs at every stage of treatment. For example, during the history-taking phase, resourcing might be necessary if a client is assessed as lacking in the ego strength or stability to engage in EMDR (e.g., calm place or antidote imagery). During the desensitization stage, resourcing might be employed to help contain overwhelming effects (e.g., CIPOS or the butterfly hug). During the closure stage, resourcing might be employed to guard against future episodes of pain or distress (e.g., future template and/or antidote imagery).

Trauma processing

Resolving trauma-based somatic and affective responses that maintain pain/MUS is where EMDR comes in. Generally speaking, there are two types of EMDR pain candidates: healthy, relatively untraumatized individuals who have developed pain following a single recent trauma, and survivors of long-term trauma and pain who tend to be exhausted and affected by multiple health problems of known and unknown origin. The former can often engage in trauma processing with little or no time devoted to the development of a therapeutic relationship and/or extensive resourcing. I have seen trauma and low-grade whiplash pain cured in one session in someone who was relatively well and stable. I have seen temporomandibular joint disorder (TMJ) associated with complicated grief processed in one session, again in a person who was otherwise healthy and free of serious trauma. Even a seriously injured person can benefit from EMDR with stunning rapidity if they are blessed with good family background, personality, and health. Schneider et al.'s (2008) report of a German motorcyclist, whose phantom limb pain and PTSD resolved following seven sessions of EMDR, is a dramatic example. This man's leg was horrifically amputated at the hip following a collision with a truck. Prior to commencing EMDR therapy, he was heavily reliant on opioids after years of failed standard care. But he came from a loving, emotionally healthy family, he had a loving wife, and he had good underlying health. Following seven sessions of EMDR his PTSD was resolved, he was off most medication, and he was ready to consider new vocational possibilities.[41]

Far more commonly, pain/MUS sufferers present with complex trauma histories, combined with overlapping injuries, illnesses, and traumatic medical interventions. They are overwhelmed, exhausted, and without hope. Trauma processing needs to be preceded by the gradual rebuilding of energy levels, safety and stabilization work, and the self/identity.

Integration

Because so many sufferers of pain/MUS are survivors of neglect or adversity, compartmentalization (unintegrated ego states) is common. We all have ego states—parts or aspects of ourselves that manage different situations. Shirley Jean Schmidt (1998) defines ego states as "specialized neural networks that hold specific packages of information related to behavior, affect, sensations and knowledge of our life experiences," often specific to developmental stages or circumstances. As discussed in Chapter 2, one of the oldest conceptualizations of parts is that it involves a division of the personality between an Emotional Part (EP) and an Apparently Normal Part (ANP). Collectively the parts make up the whole person, although some would say that the true self is a separate entity that is not defined by survival responses. Different parts (another term for ego states) are responsible for coping with different situations. For example, there might be a wounded (often exiled) child who holds feelings of vulnerability and needs connection, and a strong adult (protector) who manages social and vocational tasks. The problem with the parts is that they have different goals, and they don't work together. The adult protector is working hard to keep the person safe but never has time for the wounded child. Every now and then, when the adult part is tired or their guard is down, the wounded child emerges and overwhelming feelings of sadness, helplessness, and worthlessness emerge. The adult does not recognize where these come from but instead redoubles their efforts to work hard, earn love, etc.

Unintegrated parts are never in the same room (or body) at the same time—there is only ever one "on stage" at the same time. The result is that whatever need is being met is at the expense of another. As Phillips (2000) notes, "Conflicts between different parts of the self can cause physical and emotional systems. If the inner state of conflict is strong enough, pathways to healing may be blocked by ego states that are at odds with one another."[42] Until those parts are identified and their needs met, any pain relief will tend to be temporary. The integration that comes from parts work also reduces conflict, stimulating a calmer, more unified mental and physical self.

Wade and Wade (2001) recommended the integration of ego state work with EMDR based on the idea that personality is associative and dissociative (depending on the strength of the relationship between the ego states) and that EMDR needs to incorporate ego state therapy to address the effects of trauma and/or attachment deficits on personality development (degree of separation between ego states).[43] Ego state work involves identifying a person's ego states or parts and facilitating their working together in a way that benefits the whole person. For example, Tracey, a trauma/pain sufferer, was not responding to EMDR. In response to a cognitive interweave in which she was asked if there was a part of her that wasn't ready to change, she identified a hard-working strong part of herself which she labelled her "Southport girl"—reflecting her origins in a working-class area of England. This strong part had been essential to her survival, and she was anxious about what might happen if she let go. We acknowledged that part and got her permission to stand down for a while. We were then able to access a softer, more needy part of herself who wasn't allowed to be seen ("little Tracey") by making a connection between feelings of sadness and loneliness (an affect bridge). Following this, she was encouraged to pay attention to her child's part and let her know that she was aware of her and ready to give her what she needed. At this point Tracey started sobbing uncontrollably—little Tracey's years of lonely waiting for someone to show up were over. During this time, I did nothing other than verbally support the inner connection that was being made by saying things like "that's it ... that's it ... just being with yourself now ... just noticing ... that's it ..." After some minutes of this, when Tracey seemed to have "gotten it" I gently reinforced her feelings of integration, wholeness, and presence hypnotically. I let her know that she was one now and that she could feel that in her body. As a result of this work, Tracey became more self-aware, more whole, more able to hear when her body said "no" and more able to live in a balanced, self-nurturing way. Her strong part wouldn't have to work so hard anymore.

Ego state work can be conducted at any stage of treatment but is generally only possible once the client has some degree of emotional stability and some strategies for controlling their pain/MUS. Having said that, viewed from an ego state lens, EMDR targets could be said to represent ego states and cognitive interweaves a way of accessing more resourced ego states. Lawrence (1999) argues that all resourcing that accesses inner resources constitutes a form of ego state work.[44] The net result is decreased dissociation, inner conflict, and more cohesive functioning. As Shirley Jean Schmidt puts it, "Ego-state therapy helps the inner system pull together as a team to work towards the same goals."[45] In most cases, parts work aimed at integrating conflicted ego states (e.g., a workaholic ANP vs. a vulnerable EP) is essential to fully integrate changes and facilitate a balance between mental and physical survival needs. Parts work may also be necessary during therapy to circumvent stuck processing or at the end of therapy when the changes the client has made need to be enshrined in a more integrated sense of self.

The above phases are not necessarily strictly linear or always necessary: a well-integrated client may be ready to engage in EMDR processing without any resourcing; a more complex client may need resourcing through all phases of treatment. A relatively stable client may benefit from ego state work prior to EMDR. In the messy real world of therapy, there may be a lot of backward and forward between different elements of treatment. The general principle is that the less energy and coping skills the client has, the more EMDR will need to be supplemented by other modalities. Treatment must be relational and client centered.

6

Phase Two: Preparation

The preparation phase involves engaging the client in the treatment process and preparing them to participate in the desensitization and reprocessing of their pain, assuming they are ready for EMDR. While there is some overlap with the history phase, the preparation phase also involves certain distinct tasks, such as safe place (where needed), resourcing and self-control techniques. The client's need for these elements will have been established in the history-taking phase. The aim of the preparation phase is to ensure that the client can participate in treatment safely. This is especially relevant for individuals whose pain is linked to trauma, present stressors (e.g., domestic violence, uncontrolled pain), and/or emotional regulation issues. Additional tasks include providing the client with some explanation of the treatment and obtaining consent.

The preparation phase involves engaging the client in the treatment process. This can be difficult—not because the client doesn't want to be helped but because many chronic pain sufferers feel helpless and hopeless as a result of failed treatment, dashed hopes, and the seemingly interminable reality of their pain. The therapist must **sow seeds of hope**. This can be done by introducing pain ameliorating strategies, such as BLS, pendulation, antidote imagery, etc. (see Therapist Resources section). It can also be helpful to judiciously express some truisms along the lines of *"Your body is designed to heal," "Healing is always possible under the right conditions,"*

"Healing takes time." But this should be done with care not to overwrite the patient's need to express their feeling of hopelessness, frustration, etc.

Chronic pain patients are usually struggling with their feelings, as trauma survivors are generally, but with the added stressor of their pain. Is anxiety a shameful emotion or a normal response to uncontrollable circumstances? What about guilt—how does one parse normal guilt about not being able to "carry one's weight" from pathological guilt for having needs? Is this person allowed to be angry? What part is activated when they are angry? What is the function of anger? Is feeling "depressed" a problem or a symptom of something else? Is there anywhere in the patient's life where they feel safe to explore these and other feelings?

Teaching patients about the meaning of their emotions within the safety of the therapeutic relationship (see below) is vital for helping them learn to live more congruently with their physical and mental selves. Remember, most chronic pain sufferers come from families where emotional expression was stunted. At some point it can be very helpful to initiate a conversation about emotions and what their purpose is (see the "Normal emotional stages and reactions to pain" handout in the Client Resources section). Of course, judiciously supporting your patient to understand and express their feelings, in order to better cope, is a task that will occupy a significant proportion of their treatment.

Safety

Safety is a basic human need which has been and continues to be challenged in trauma and pain survivors, a fact which must be recognized and attended to. Safety issues can arise as a result of unresolved trauma and present life circumstances. Where the pain is associated with past trauma (such as child physical or sexual abuse, combat-related injuries, industrial accidents, etc.), clients may feel unsafe because of the effects of intrusive trauma-related memories. Traumatic memories often incorporate an intrusive somatic element, meaning the client is constantly being thrust back into a situation where they felt physical and emotional pain and were helpless to do anything about it. These individuals may need to learn some self-control skills (see below) to provide a source of protection against the intrusive thoughts and feelings.

Safety issues can also stem from inadequately managed pain wherein the client experiences intense and unpredictable pain flare-ups. Recurring pain flare-ups involve constant activation and deactivation of the fight-or-flight response as the body reacts to the onset of pain, and then gradually relaxes when the pain subsides. This form of "attack from within" can be extremely stressful as it threatens the most basic aspects of physical living—the ability to feel comfortable and secure in one's own body. Lack of safety can also result from decreased physical capacities, including the ability to work and perform physically demanding tasks of living. The ability to move and use the body to manipulate physical objects in the world is as basic as learning to walk. To lose this ability is to be sent backward in time to a helpless, dependent state where one has to depend on others to get basic needs met. Most adults find this anxiety-provoking and shameful. All chronic pain sufferers have a safety issue as a result of the impact of uncontrolled pain on their physical integrity. In this sense, regardless of what has gone before, pain represents a present stress/small "t" trauma.

As we have seen, lack of safety is generally associated with hyper or hypo-arousal, vagal states which are antithetical to health and well-being. Some degree of safety is thus a vital prerequisite for effective participation in psychotherapy and the new learning that is necessary for healing.

One of the most powerful "interventions" for creating safety is the therapeutic relationship, a concept with which every therapist is familiar, yet was never taught in most graduate schools. The therapeutic relationship is not as the term suggests a "thing;" it is a process, a mind to mind, heart to heart encounter between two people. It's a grown-up version of what's supposed to happen between a parent and their child: attunement, presence, acceptance, nurturance. Watkins (1996) identifies resonance as a right hemisphere (though not entirely) aspect of attunement and as key to ensuring that treatment is aligned with the patient's needs and capabilities.

> *"When the therapist, through resonance, takes into herself the patient's problems and co-experiences them in many psychological spheres, the patient reciprocates by co-resonating with the therapist and taking back into himself the objective understandings of the clinician—in the same spheres. This constitutes true experiential insight (not only intellectual understanding), which occurs in much less time than in traditional therapy."*[1]

In recognition of the centrality of emotional communication, neuroscientist Allan Shore describes attunement as "right-brain to right-brain communication."[2] But from a therapeutic standpoint, being empathic is only half of the equation; there needs to be a balance between "being with" and "doing to." When treating survivors of complex trauma, the therapeutic relationship, and the safety it affords, becomes an essential element of treatment. We must, therefore, find a balance between doing therapy and being with our patients.

One of the biggest obstacles to the therapeutic relationship is an overactive left hemisphere in the therapist (but also often the patient), the part of our brain that wants to fix things. Some modern manual-based methods, or at least the way they are taught, are in danger of overemphasizing this aspect of therapy. In addition, chronic pain sufferers with a strong need to be "fixed" will pull therapists' fixer parts (which we all have) forward. Most chronic pain/MUS sufferers are used to being "done to," whether from abusive parents, critical teachers, or authoritarian treating professionals. They may adopt a helpless position in therapy: "*I am hopeless/helpless, nothing has ever worked, and I doubt there is anything you can do for me.*" Failure to manage the demand characteristics of patients who present like this can lead to premature application of interventions, with, at best, no ill-effect, and, at worst, a rupturing of the therapeutic alliance. The therapist is pursuing a therapeutic agenda that the patient is not ready for. Even seemingly benign strategies such as "safe place" can be unhelpful if introduced before the patient is ready. The patient will either try to comply in order to be a good patient, or, if they are brave enough to admit it's not working, conclude that they have failed again.

Ultimately, if you can offer a safe space where your patient can express their reality and become more aware of unconscious aspects, with gentle guidance and support, including safe places and affect management skills when necessary, you will have afforded them a unique healing opportunity.

Safe place

A more explicit intervention is the evocation or creation of a safe place or person. The aim of this is to give the patient a resource for entering a ventral vagal state where they can rest, reconnect, and recharge. This can be facilitated by inviting the patient to remember a place or a set of circumstances that engender feelings of safety and calmness.

"Is there anywhere you can go or anything you can do where you feel safe from the trauma/pain?"

If the client cannot think of anything, the therapist can offer some suggestions.

"Some people feel better when they are doing something they enjoy that takes their mind off the pain; some people like listening to the soothing sounds of nature, such as the ocean, or rain on a roof, and some people feel better when they can talk to someone who understands.

"Do you have anything like that in your life?"

Hopefully this will stimulate the client to think of a place or situation where they feel safe. The therapist then gets the client to talk about that place, what it means to the client, and why they feel safe there. As the client tells the therapist about their safe place, which is often the first time they have ever talked about it to anyone, they are self-validating their own safe place resource. The therapist should also reinforce the client's ability to access their safe place:

"Good ... everyone needs a safe place, somewhere they can go to escape and relax."

After the therapist has established a good description of the client's safe place, the therapist should reinforce the mental and emotional connection the client feels with their safe place by asking them to imagine it: notice how it makes them feel, what positive thoughts it evokes, and feeding back to the client in a very soothing, hypnotic voice their connection with that place.

"So, can you think of your safe place [or person] now ... where it is ... what it's like ... any colors ... sounds ... smells ...

"And how you feel in your body when you think of it ...

"And then think of a word or phrase that describes how being in that place makes you feel."

(Clients generally respond with things like "peaceful," "safe.")

Install or ground the safe place verbally as follows:

"And now I want you to keep thinking of that place ... and how it makes you feel ... and what it makes you think about yourself ... and remember all the times that you've been to that place ... and how you felt when you were in that place ... and how you feel now just thinking about that place ... and know that that is your place ... where you can go whenever you want to or need to ... and even if you can't get there physically, you can know that that place is inside you ... and you can find it ... just by thinking of it ... and how it makes you feel ... and those words ... and you can find it whenever you need it ... and you will know when you need to go there ..."

If you are trained in hypnosis, this kind of verbal installation will come naturally. As discussed in Chapter 2, many chronic pain/MUS sufferers, especially those who display dissociative phenomena, are susceptible to suggestion via trance (see also Chapter 12). You can also install the safe place by instructing the patient to ***"think of that"*** (once they have identified and described the feelings they associate with their safe place) and pair it with BLS. We know from the work of Amano & Toichi (2016) that BLS can enhance access to positive imagery.[3] However, where the patient's connection with the effects of the safe place feels weak, verbal reinforcement may be necessary.

Occasionally clients will report that they have no such place in their life and never have. A calm place is sometimes the best that can be achieved.

Safe place for clients with no safe place

If the client really is unable to identify any safe place, past or present, the therapist can offer to help them create one. The best safe places are those that involve emotions, so you want to create something that has some emotional resonance with the client rather than something purely imaginable. At this stage the therapist should refer to the information obtained in the client's history taking. Did the client mention any people, places, or activities that might hint at a resource or safe place in the history taking? If not, the therapist should ask the client about what sports or interests they have, and how those activities make them feel. Or what people or places they might like to meet or see, and why. Movies and book characters can be another source of material. The more the therapist can learn about the client's interests, hobbies and activities, likes and dislikes, the easier it is to create a safe place. After eliciting some ideas and imagining some possibilities, the therapist says,

"Okay, so now I'd like you to get comfortable ... just let your body go limp in the chair ... and notice your breathing ... the gentle rise and fall of your chest ... and the feeling of the chair supporting your weight ... and with one part of your mind you can listen to the things that I say ... and with another part of your mind you can drift off ... into your own thoughts ... or stay here with me ... whatever feels right for you ... noticing your breathing ... the gentle rise and fall of your chest ... and as you notice your breathing ... you can be reminded of how your body takes care of itself ... so naturally ... because you are part of nature ... and all living things understand the importance of safety ... animals retreat to their lair ... birds fly to their nests ... even flowers close up at night ... and people need to feel safe too ... naturally ... Robin Hood had his forest, Cinderella had her castle ... Robinson Crusoe had his cave ... and you have ... [name person, activity, or place identified earlier] and when you think of [name of special person, activity, or place] ... you can know that is a safe place [or person] for you ... that you can go to ... naturally ... whenever you

want or need to ... and notice how that makes you feel ... what sensations in your body ... go with the knowledge that you are safe and sound ... in your special place ... with nothing to do and nothing to worry about ...

"... And if there are any obstacles between you and [name safe place or person] ... you can remove them ... however seems appropriate ... so that there is nothing in between you and your special place ... and you can see your way clear ... naturally ... to your safe place. And as you move past those obstacles ... and approach your safe place ... you can notice the details of that safe place ... What does it look like? ... Does it have a sound? ... Or a smell? ... What colors do you notice? ... And how does it make you feel ... in your body ... and is there anything extra that it needs? ... Add it in ...

"And imagine yourself enveloped in that safe place ... naturally ... safe and sound ... And whenever you want to or need to, you can think of that safe place ... and go there to be safe ... so take some time now ... all the time that you want ... to enjoy that place ... and then when you're ready, you can return to the present ... knowing that you can return to that place whenever you want to or need to ..."

The client should be in a nice state of trance by now. The therapist should allow the client a few minutes to reorient themselves and then discuss this experience. Assuming it was a positive one, the therapist should advise the client to practice thinking of this place and exploring it more fully in their mind and the feelings that it gives them. My *Calm & Confident* app also contains a powerful semi-hypnotic process to help anchor clients safely in their own body.

Safe place for clients facing present threat

Where lack of safety is due to present circumstances, such as abuse, uncontrolled pain, or other external stressors, the therapist should either help develop safety or give the client resources to cope. A woman living with an abusive spouse might need self-esteem building to build up the courage to leave. A chronic pain sufferer struggling with attacks of acute pain might need assistance developing strategies to minimize the pain (see self-control strategies below). A trauma sufferer facing ongoing victimization may need help developing resources to protect themselves.

Nina suffered from pelvic pain which started after she was bullied at work over a period of several years, followed by the birth of her first child. Although Nina left the workplace where the bullying occurred, she continued to feel very anxious whenever she was confronted with conflictual situations. In her current life she was being bullied by an older sister, who was constantly criticizing her mothering and putting her down with her parents. Nina was a very family-oriented person and her sister's criticism and its effects on her relationships in the family caused her great distress. She described feeling as though the weight of the whole family was on her and "If I fall down, the whole family will fall down." Nina's sister's attacks also triggered her pelvic pain episodes, which would result in her suffering from vaginal pain, fatigue, and body aches, so much so that she might have to spend the day in bed. Nina was also having problems with the principal of her son's school, which also acted as a trigger for her traumatic stress and pain. Nina had seen countless doctors for her pelvic pain, only to be told that there was nothing wrong. Eventually her physician referred her to me. After taking a full history, it was clear that Nina's pain was a manifestation of the bullying trauma she had suffered, and that it was being triggered by present hostile circumstances. A safe place was developed around Nina's home and marital relationship. Added to this, Nina was taught some verbal assertion skills with which to ward off her sister's attacks. Following this, Nina was able to participate in EMDR, focusing on targets to do with her present stressors (conflict with sister and principal) and past trauma (the bullying). I had her practice defending herself against her sister's verbal attacks imaginably (future template). This resulted in Nina being able to stand up to her sister and the principal, and a cessation of aggression toward Nina. Nina also felt more confident and secure, and her pain attacks ceased.

Given the high percentage of chronic pain/MUS sufferers affected by developmental deficits, it can also be helpful to link the patient with a safe person, nurturing figure, etc. This could be a parent, relative, teacher—anybody who makes the client feel safe and loved. It could be someone from the past, dead or alive, or someone from the present or an imaginary figure.

"Can you remember someone from your life who made you feel safe?"

"If you can't think of anyone, is there someone you remember from watching a TV show or the movies?"

If the patient can't remember anyone real or imagined, reassure them and say:

"Okay, let's give your imagination a little help here. Try holding that question in your mind again ['Who is my safe person?'], but don't think about it too much, just trust your unconscious mind to find it for you ... now notice the BLS and see what comes."

Initiate BLS and repeat phrases ***"Just trust your unconscious mind," "Let whatever comes come"*** and wait for a couple of minutes. Every now and then say something like, ***"Don't think about it too much—just let whatever comes come."***

This open-ended, indirect approach often results in something "popping up" from the patient's subconscious that they had forgotten or not considered. Let's say the patient suddenly remembers their old aunt Gemima, who used to look after them after school, including fresh-baked cookies and milk.

"Great, so just remember Aunt Gemima and how she made you feel about yourself, and notice where you feel that in your body, and really allow yourself to feel connected with Aunt Gemima, and what she wanted you to know about yourself. Just noticing where you feel that in your body ... and breathe that in ... fill yourself up with those safe loving feelings ... more and more with every breath you take ... Safe .... Calm ... just finding that within yourself now ... Maybe allowing an image of Aunt Gemima and how she made you feel to form in your mind ... and committing that to memory. So that you can access this memory of Aunt Gemima anytime you want to or need to."

Because of the high levels of trauma and attachment problems, and the inhibiting effects of the latter on the development of a healthy ego, the need for a safe place or person is ubiquitous in chronic pain/MUS sufferers. Children (and adults) need to feel "seen, safe, soothed, and secure." The challenge is choosing the right moment to introduce this intervention. If the patient expresses significant feelings of isolation and anxiety, and their pain/MUS is tolerable, then finding a safe person should be considered a priority. Safety is such a basic human need it should supersede all other therapeutic goals, including sometimes even those that the patient has prioritized (e.g., "I need to get back to work"). There are various ways of doing this, e.g., Dan Brown's Ideal Parent Figure Protocol[4], Manfield's dyadic resourcing, and parenting practices of Dan Siegel.[5]

If the patient is wracked with uncontrollable, inadequately managed pain, then this rather than unmet developmental deficits would be a priority. But both will need to be addressed sooner or later.

Jessie, an exhausted female chronic pain sufferer, was very teary and emotional at her first session. She had recently suffered a major relapse after years of turmoil and finally winning her health back. Now she felt tired, anxious, helpless, and hopeless. Many of her physical symptoms were medically inexplicable (fatigue, headaches, burning, tingling sensations in her extremities) and this heightened her sense of anxiety and loss of control. She felt confused and frightened as to what was wrong with her. Although I already had most of her history thanks to my intake questionnaire, Jessie took the opportunity to express a combination of more information about her struggles with treatment providers and her anxieties about her health. After about 30 minutes of this with no visible reduction in her distress, I pondered how best to spend the remaining 30 minutes of our first session. I could continue listening empathically and hope this might have some effect, risking her leaving the session with little or no benefit, or interrupt her and do something to give her some relief, risking breaking the attunement (which felt non-existent) and also possibly failing due to the level of distress Jessie was in.

I decided to offer an intervention aimed at reducing Jessie's physical and emotional distress reasoning that: a) this would give her some immediate relief from her overwhelming distress, and b) it would provide a foundation for changing her feelings of helplessness. I suggested the following:

"I hear you, Jessie. We've got about 30 minutes left. How would it be if we did something that might help you feel less discomfort and distress?"

Jessie nodded silently through her tears.

"Great, so can I ask you to just focus on whatever discomfort or distress you are feeling now ... and where you notice that most in your body ... and what it feels like ... what size, shape, and color those feelings have ... just getting a felt sense of the distress as clearly as you can ... [repeat as necessary] and then when you've got that I'd like you to move your attention to a part of your body that feels free of distress ... where there's no discomfort ... where everything feels normal .... so normal that you don't notice it ... until I draw your attention to it ... and just notice what that part feels like ... how relaxed the muscles feel there ... how right everything feels ... and what that feels like ... what size, shape, and color those feelings have .... Just getting as strong a felt sense as you can of that area of comfort

[repeat as necessary] and then when you've got that, bring your attention back to the area of discomfort/distress ... and imagine that as you bring your attention back to the area of discomfort, you are bringing with it some of that awareness of comfort and relief ... and pay attention to that area again for a few moments now ... and notice whatever you notice ... whether it feels the same or different ... and whatever you notice is fine ... and then when you are ready, take your attention back to that area of comfort and notice whatever you can about it, like you did before [I repeated this process of directing Jessie's attention backward and forward between her discomfort and her comfort about three times].

I noticed that Jessie's facial expression and posture relaxed slightly as we did this process. After no more than 10 minutes I instructed Jessie to:

"Great. Now take a deep breath, relax, and just notice what's happening now. Does that area of discomfort feel the same or different to when we started?"

Jessie reported that she felt less anxious and that she saw the calmer feelings as being the color green. I commented that green is a natural color (I knew she loved nature) which symbolizes tranquility, hope, and optimism. My intention in explaining the meaning of green was to deepen Jessie's sense that she could connect to healing resources. Jessie seemed curious about this and the expression on her face had changed from defeat to curiosity. Nevertheless, she expressed some anxiety as to how long these effects would last. I reassured her that they can last anywhere from a few hours to forever, and that she could listen to the recording of this exercise that I had made whenever she needed to access these feelings in future. At her next session Jessie excitedly told me that she had listened to the recording under different conditions and surprisingly found it to generate even more powerful feelings of calm than it did in the session. She was more hopeful that things could change.

This exercise utilizes pendulation, a process developed by Peter Levine. See the Therapist Resources section for a complete script.

Self-care

Another aspect of safety is the client's ability to care for themselves. Many victims of pain and neglect exist in a state of self-neglect: failing to eat, sleep, or pace themselves properly. They may have unsatisfactory relationships based on being there for others rather than a healthy mutual exchange of affection and support. They may believe that "getting the job done" or "keeping everybody happy" is more important than their needs. They may regard working without rest as a sign of strength. These attitudes and behaviors obviously reflect maladaptive attitudes and ego states. They also undermine healthy functioning and exacerbate injury and pain.

The therapist can and should take the role of advocate for better self-care. She is in a unique position to do this. But it must be done in cooperation with the parts that drive workaholism, chronic people-pleasing, self-punishment, etc. As discussed in Chapter 2, parts are aspects of the self that have evolved to deal with different aspects of life (not separate selves). In trauma survivors (including emotional neglect/abuse) these can take extreme forms divided along separate physical, emotional, and mental lines. Parts represent a dissociative response to the lack of opportunities for integration associated with growing up in circumstances of danger and/or inadequate attachment.

In ego states terms, a person's parts might simply consist of an EP and an ANP, or using IFS terminology, a manager, protector, firefighter, or exile.[6] IFS labels parts based on the tasks the different ego states are responsible for.[7] Different parts usually involve different states (levels of arousal, behaviors, and aims). For example, a workaholic (protector) part might represent an attempt to cope with feelings of vulnerability or worthlessness (e.g., "As long as I'm busy I don't have to feel" or "As long as I'm busy I'm worthwhile"). Such a part will likely feel threatened by the suggestion to take better care of oneself since this would leave the inadequate shame-based part unprotected. So rather than saying, "You are too hard on yourself" (which would be perfectly fine, just not terribly therapeutic), she could negotiate with the workaholic/self-punisher part by saying something like:

"Would it be okay if we talk with your workaholic part (or whatever name you give it), Sharlene? I know you have been working very hard to keep Sharlene safe, and that you must be tired from all those years of constant toil. If we could find another easier way for Sharlene to feel okay about herself, would you be interested in being able to stand down a bit?"

The aim is to "unburden" the protector part and create space or access for working with the vulnerable parts it's protecting. Commencing this process assumes that the therapist has developed some understanding of the protector part's positive intentions and fears about what would happen if it stopped doing its job. It also comes with helping the protector part understand that the context has changed, that there is now an adult self that can support and heal burdened parts, and that the present is different to the past, the patient is bigger, stronger, etc.

The IFS term for this process is "unblending." As the terms suggests, it's about creating more space between the parts and the self within that patient's parts system.

Assuming the part acquiesces, you then propose something like the following (based on information the therapist has gleaned from the client about their ability to self-care):

"I want you to know that I know more about protecting myself than you might realize. Remember that time I took a holiday and didn't open my emails once? Or that time I accepted a compliment? Or that time I said no to someone because I was tired? I know I don't always get it right, but I am learning to look after myself better, and I promise you I will do this more in future if you can just stand back and give me a chance. This would be better for all of us—how does that sound?"

Assuming the patient agrees, you might follow this with a discussion about how they can do this and what additional help or resources could help:

"Tell me more about that part that was able to say no."

"Where and when do you notice that you are more able to express your needs?"

"What happens in your body when you feel able to express your needs?"

"Who in your life is supportive of you expressing your needs?"

The important point is that rather than pulling for self-care, which would likely antagonize the part that needs to do that, you have facilitated a rapprochement between different parts with opposing needs. The workaholic (protector) part is going to be much more willing to allow self-care if it knows that there is an alternative (and better) way of fulfilling its objectives and it feels consulted about the change process. Note: these practices have their limitations when working with severe dissociation such as DID.

This is a very abbreviated sample of a process which can be found in some form in many parts approaches. The above example is derived from Schwartz's IFS.

Other approaches involve accessing a safe person.

Another ego state approach is Shirley Jean Schmidt's DNMS.[8] Schmidt uses an ego state approach to strengthen a patient's connection to three healthy parts of self—a Nurturing Adult

Self, a Protective Adult Self, and a Spiritual Core Self. These Resources are based on real experiences a patient has had of nurturing and protecting a loved one, and peak spiritual experiences—so that patients understand their Resources are real parts of self, not just imaginary helpers. Importantly, her work includes dealing with barriers to self-love and connection associated with maladaptive introjects ("I'm unlovable, worthless" etc.).[9] Parts work is generally necessary in the preparation stage, where there is evidence of compartmentalization and/or other dissociative phenomena (e.g., amnesia, depersonalization), because of the likelihood that that patient never had the opportunity to develop a sufficiently resourced self to benefit from standard EMDR. Remember the AIP model posits that EMDR facilitates the emergence of adaptive information—but what if the patient never had an opportunity to develop that adaptive information? Attempting EMDR in such clients without first addressing dissociated ego states usually ends up stuck or looping.

Self-control techniques

Clients with uncontrolled physical or emotional pain, who also have emotional regulation problems, may need to learn self-control techniques prior to engaging in treatment. This is particularly important when treating complex trauma where the client is likely to experience strong negative emotions in between sessions which they need to manage. Self-control techniques are also important for helping clients cope with incomplete sessions. In the treatment of emotional pain and trauma, self-control techniques can include breathing exercises, emotional distancing techniques, and distraction.

Breath awareness

Breath control techniques are one of the oldest and simplest methods for alleviating physical and emotional pain. Focusing on the breath gives clients something soothing yet visceral to focus on. The act of breathing also involves a cycle of stress and release (as the person breathes in and out) which can act as a natural pain relief circuit.

1. *Assume a comfortable position.*
2. *Begin by attending to whatever physical sensations you notice in your body.*
3. *Try and "just notice" whatever is happening in your body in a detached way without thinking about it or analyzing it too much.*
4. *JUST NOTICE whatever you're feeling ...*

5. *And notice your breathing, the gradual rise and fall of your chest with each breath that you take. Notice how your chest expands with each in-breath and deflates with each out-breath. You may notice that there is a slight feeling of tension with each in-breath, and a feeling of relief with each out-breath ...*
6. *As you focus on your breathing, you might like to think about how NATURAL breathing is, how CONNECTED breathing makes you feel with your body and the rhythm of life. You might also enjoy the realization that breathing happens AUTOMATICALLY, without your having to make any special effort.*
7. *And now imagine that with each in-breath, you're breathing in life and relaxation, and with each out-breath, you're breathing out stress and pain, NATURALLY.*
8. *And as you continue to focus on your breathing, you may also notice the rate of your breathing slowing down, as your mind becomes more detached from your everyday consciousness.*
9. *If any other thoughts or feelings intrude into your awareness of yourself, just notice them and let them go by.*
10. *Notice if anything changes about how you are feeling, including your awareness of what you are feeling. If nothing seems different, that's fine too.*
11. *Just keep breathing and keep noticing. Whatever you feel or notice, just observe it and let it go.*
12. *Continue doing this for 15 to 20 minutes.*
13. *At the end of that time, give yourself a few moments to gradually reorient yourself.*
14. *If you have been able to maintain your attention on your breath reasonably consistently, you should notice mild feelings of detachment and lightness; some people notice other sensations, such as tingling or numbness. Whether you do or not, regular practice of this technique will help you learn how to experience your pain differently, in ways you might never have imagined.*

Bilateral stimulation

Another self-control technique is to take the bilateral stimulation/dual attention element of EMDR and use it as a pain management technique. This is an obvious and safe application of bilateral stimulation given its proven ability to reduce physical tension. (Exceptions are DID, psychotic, and epileptic clients.) Bilateral stimulation/dual attention for pain relief simply involves teaching the client to focus on their pain while simultaneously concentrating on a bilateral stimulation (audio tones or tapping) and "letting whatever happens happen."

Before doing this it can also be helpful to explain the role of bilateral stimulation. A simple explanation which integrates theories about EMDR with brain science is to adapt McCulloch's orienting response theory (note: this is about explaining the role of bilateral stimulation, not AIP). I explain that the brain is a kind of input-output device which reacts differently to different experiences (or inputs). I explain that one of the main ways the brain responds is emotionally (output), and give examples such as pain causes unhappiness, music triggers happiness, sitting by a waterfall triggers relaxation (as per Figure 6.1).

Clients can easily understand how the emotional response to these stimuli is automatic and fairly predictable. I then explain that the problem with relaxing stimuli such as music is that they only make you feel good while you are doing them. I explain that this is because once the brain gets used to something, it habituates to it. Basically, once you have heard Beethoven's 9th Symphony a couple of times, you're actually half hearing half remembering the next time you listen to it. Because you're not fully attending, it's easy for your attention to drift back to unpleasant present stimuli such as physical pain. (This explanation concurs with most people's experience.)

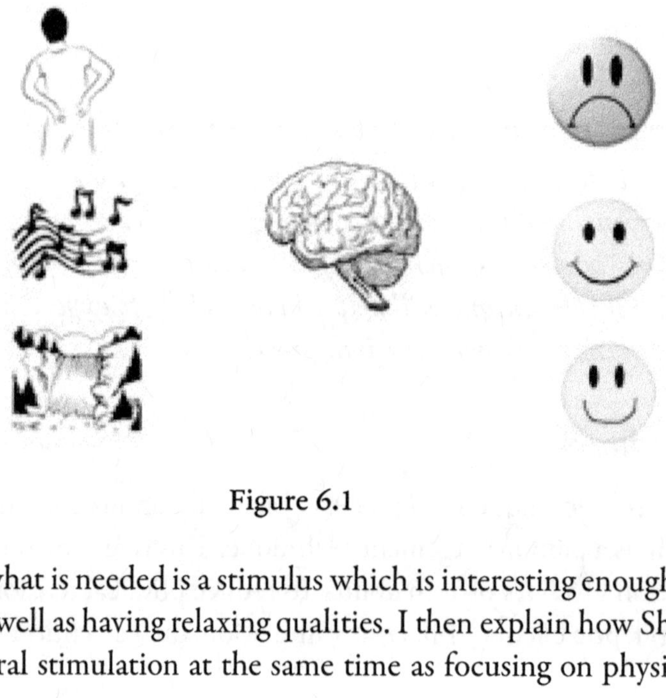

Figure 6.1

I then explain that what is needed is a stimulus which is interesting enough to hold your attention indefinitely, as well as having relaxing qualities. I then explain how Shapiro discovered that focusing on bilateral stimulation at the same time as focusing on physical or emotional pain seems to do this. People cannot maintain their attention on their pain while simultaneously focusing on bilateral audio tones. This sets up a chain reaction of emotional responses from the brain's first response, curiosity ("What is that?" "Where is it?"), to relaxation once the brain realizes it is not a threat (as per Figure 6.2). Voila, you have modified an output and a painful memory. For a full version of the wording associated with this explanation, see the "BLS rationale for pain" in the Therapist Resources section. I tend to use this explanation when using auditory BLS for non-traumatic pain. While not inconsistent with the AIP model, I think it provides a better explanation than the AIP.

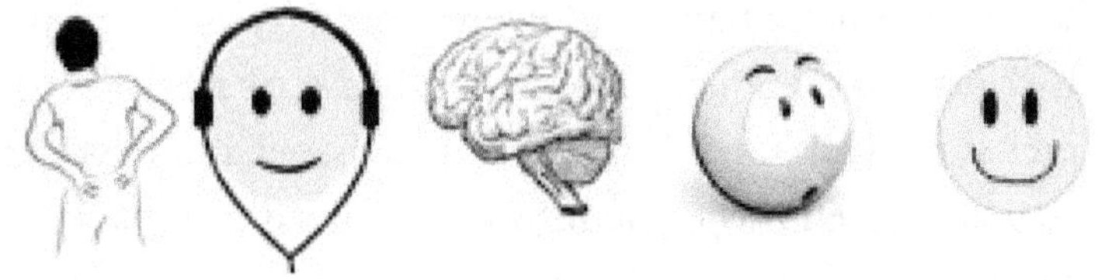

Figure 6.2

Then show the client how to use bilateral stimulation to reduce physical pain.

1. *"Think of a physical or emotional pain you'd like relief from."*
2. *"Notice how and where you feel the pain in your body."*
3. *"What image goes with those feelings?"* (If prompting needed, say, *"What do they remind you of?"*)
4. *"Now, holding the image of your pain in your mind and how it feels, concentrate on the bilateral stimulation and let whatever happens happen. Just listen to the audio tones and notice what happens in your body."*
5. The therapist does this for 30–60 seconds and then instructs the client to *"take a break,"* and asks, *"What do you notice now?"*
6. Most clients will report feeling more relaxed, or that the pain seems smaller or further away. If the client is struggling to notice any changes, it can be helpful to suggest other physical and mental possibilities to help clients recognize changes following BLS (see the "Effects of BLS menu" in the Therapist Resources section).
7. Instruct the client to *"notice that"* and continue with the bilateral stimulation.
8. Repeat until the client reports feeling completely free of pain or no further changes are occurring. Return to normal EMDR protocol.

9. If the client reports "nothing" at step 5, prompt them by asking, *"When you say 'nothing,' what do you mean?"* (No change or no pain?) If the client reports no change, check that this is really the case and that they have not merely failed to notice feelings of relaxation (however slight), decreased tension, decreased pain, feeling as though the pain is further away, etc. Remember that it is almost impossible NOT to experience some sensory shift following correctly applied BLS.
10. Once the client has achieved some pain reduction with BLS, they can be offered self-use of BLS as an ongoing pain management strategy.

For clients with non-traumatic pain, and even simple trauma and pain, this is a safe and highly effective self-control technique. Note that self-use of BLS for pain relief is NOT re-processing. The target is not a traumatic memory and associated thoughts and feelings, but a visceral present experience. Even if the client has unresolved trauma, you can avoid this being triggered by keeping the client's focus on their present experience and their SENSORY changes following BLS.

The use of BLS to alleviate non-traumatic pain involves the creation of a "target within a target." This pain target does not have to include all of the information included in a normal target. A feeling/sensation, image, and SUDs is sufficient. Once the client has learned how to control their pain using BLS, the therapist can return to the issue of reviewing the negative cognition and installing the positive cognition. Figure 6.3 shows the difference between processing a pain target and processing a normal trauma target. NB: This "target within a target" does not have to include all the information such as NC, PC, etc., just whatever the client is reporting is happening in the moment to moment processing.

You are working extensively, possibly for weeks, with the client's mental representation and/or experience of their pain, and how that changes following successive rounds of BLS, looping back repeatedly to the felt or imagined sense of the pain, as opposed to a trauma. Once a stable state of improvement is attained, you can progress to reviewing the positive cognition, installation of positive cognition, and closure.

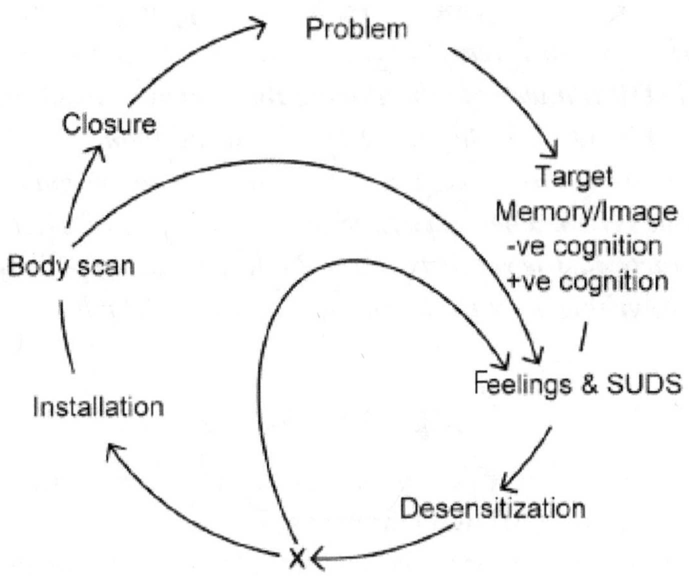

Figure 6.3 Target within a target

See Chapter 12 and the EMDR+ and the EMDR– strategies at the back of this manual for more pain control strategies.

Pain and the AIP model

Prior to commencing reprocessing, it can be helpful to explain chronic pain in terms of the adaptive information processing model. This model posits that human beings possess an innate information processing capacity wherein experience normally gets transformed into new learning. Trauma involves feelings of overwhelming terror which persist long after the trauma has ended. Sooner or later the person needs to realize that it's over and they survived. Like trauma, pain is a response to an event—it means there has been an injury, and normal functioning may be disrupted. There's also a kind of physical threat in the pain itself. Like trauma, chronic pain can be thought of as a failure of adaptive information processing—the body has not healed as it should. Like in trauma, chronic pain also involves memory and neurological changes which maintain feelings of discomfort long after the event which initially triggered the pain. The following is an example of how to present these concepts:

"Pain can occur for many reasons. We generally understand pain as a signal that something is wrong physically. However, sometimes pain can continue longer than expected,

despite medical treatment. Pain can persist because of fatigue, stress, and biochemical and neurological changes. As a result of these changes, the pain becomes 'locked' in the nervous system. EMDR is a way of stimulating the nervous system to facilitate healing, like in the picture (Figure 6.1). Because EMDR utilizes non-verbal methods (BLS) to stimulate change, it has a more direct effect on your nervous system and it stimulates the parts of your nervous system where pain and stress are mainly stored (e.g., the emotional brain, the sensory cortex). The result is you feel relaxed and hopefully less pain, without really having to do anything more than concentrate and ... let whatever happens happen."

Expectations

The final task of the preparation stage is to address the client's expectations. This can involve anything from explaining how EMDR differs to cognitive or "talk therapy" approaches, to their hopes (or fears) about the treatment process. Chronic pain clients often have low treatment expectations because of previous treatment failures. Because of the way EMDR works, that is not necessarily a problem—i.e., the change is not dependent upon the client believing in the treatment. However, it can be a problem in the body scan stage when the client needs to be able to notice any changes in how they feel. Clients with low expectations may fail to notice small but important changes which the therapist needs to start a healing trend. We will talk more about how to neutralize this and help clients maintain an objective, curious stance in the chapter on desensitization. But knowing how to redirect the attention of clients with low expectations toward difference or changes (tracking changes) is vital. Remember that you are using a method which SHOULD produce relaxation and decreased arousal in anyone who is not highly dissociated or alexithymic. For now the best thing is to reassure the client that things can change and just to have an open mind. The therapist can say something like,

"EMDR works differently to other treatments and it can work where other treatments have failed. Even if this treatment cannot completely eliminate your pain, EMDR often stimulates feelings of relaxation, which always reduces pain. The most important thing is to have an open mind and let whatever happens happen."

After the first or second session I also give my clients a copy of my "Pain management recipe" (see Client Resources section). This is basically a summary of all the necessary treatment elements, why I think they are important, and the fact that even with all the right elements, healing takes time. Whenever the treatment feels stalled or stuck, it usually means there is a deficit of one of these elements.

7

Phase Three: Assessment

The assessment phase of EMDR therapy involves the selection and construction of "targets" for reprocessing. A target is a uniquely EMDR concept which refers to the memory or memories identified as most responsible for the patient's current symptoms. In addition to past memories, targets can also involve present stressors or triggers (e.g., inadequately managed pain), or future events (e.g., imagining coping better). The target is constructed out of relevant images, sensations, emotions (including SUDs rating), and cognitions associated with the memory. Normally it also involves the elicitation of a positive cognition and a VoC. Assuming the patient has been assessed as ready for EMDR, accurate identification of targets for reprocessing facilitates optimum treatment outcomes. It's like the surgeon who has to distinguish between primary and secondary cancers when deciding which tumor to cut out. Identifying and removing the primary cancer is going to be much more beneficial for the patient's long-term healing. Unfortunately, it's rarely so simple when treating chronic pain/MUS. In this chapter we will review some of the issues associated with identifying and constructing EMDR targets prior to reprocessing.

EMDR targets come with benefits and risks. Used appropriately, EMDR targets provide a kind of BASK (Behavior—Affect—Sensation—Knowledge) summary of the presenting problem which enables the patient to identify unrealized aspects (people do not tend to think of themselves in terms of meta-cognitions such as negative self-beliefs or schemas) and participate in the titrated exposure at the heart of EMDR reprocessing. Used unwisely (e.g., prematurely, too rigidly, or with bad target selection), EMDR targeting can take the treatment off the rails. Some of the pitfalls and variations to address them will also be covered in this chapter.

Memory

When treating pain associated with simple PTSD, the target is likely to involve a single memory of a recent life-threatening event wherein the patient experienced overwhelming feelings of terror and helplessness and possibly injury. Constructing the target simply requires guiding the client through the image, distilling the core belief schema including NC and PC, assessing the VoC on a seven-point scale, detecting the associated emotion, measuring the SUDs and the emotion, and finally locating the body sensations. The standard trauma protocol is often sufficient in such cases.

Simone sought help after the vehicle which she was driving was struck by a truck. The impact caused Simone's vehicle to spin out of control before coming to rest on the side of a busy freeway. Although Simone was not seriously injured, she developed low to moderate whiplash pain, anxiety and flashbacks. Coincidentally, three of her close friends had been killed in a collision with a truck a year earlier. Simone's image was of the truck filling her windscreen. Her negative cognition was "I'm going to die." Her positive cognition was "I survived" (VoC: 2/7). Her emotion was terror, which she felt in her chest. Since shortly after the collision, she had developed pain in her neck and upper back, of no identifiable origin, which her physician had diagnosed as whiplash. Should her target incorporate this pain? I asked her what was more distressing, the pain or the emotion? She chose the emotion, so her target for reprocessing was no different to what one would use with the normal trauma protocol. If she had said the pain, I would have substituted that for the emotion and the SUDs rating would have been based on the intensity of the pain rather than her emotional distress.

Protocol variation:
Substituting sensations for emotions (TICES).

When targeting present pain, the pain sensations may be used instead of the emotion in the target set-up. In terms of the "E" in TICES (Target—Image—Cognition—Emotion—Sensations), the pain is the negative affect including how and where it is felt in the body. While there is inevitably negative emotion associated with the pain, this is not generally the focus when targeting present pain. It would be if targeting how the pain makes the patient feel about themselves, which is a different problem involving a more standard application of the TICES. It is the author's experience that asking the client to identify their pain sensations after asking them how the pain makes them feel is unnecessary and can be confusing. This variation aims to facilitate a more client-centered, affect-laden target which is sufficient for reprocessing.

In cases where the trauma preceded the pain by a long time, or childhood neglect, it may not be so easy to link predisposing traumatic circumstances to the pain. An adult who was neglected as a child who develops chronic low back pain due to overuse might not have a memory that relates to their pain even though their pain is ultimately connected to their neglect (they never learned how to get their needs met, which contributed to their getting hurt). In such cases, the childhood material may not be incorporated into the target until its relevance becomes more obvious to the client, which may be later in therapy.

The first consideration is obviously to assess whether the target is going to involve a traumatic memory or not. The information garnered in the history phase will guide this decision.

- Was there a traumatic event associated with the onset of pain, such as an accident or assault?
- Were there traumatic events following the pain (e.g., medical mishaps)?
- Is the pain itself a kind of trauma?

Pain which is associated with a traumatic memory can be targeted with very little variation of the standard EMDR trauma protocol, i.e., a memory, a feeling, and a negative cognition. The only variation is that the feeling may involve physical and emotional pain. For example, a woman who was crushed by some equipment at work saw the memory of the falling equipment as her image, and "I'm going to die" as her negative cognition, but for the feeling she labeled pain (which she had felt ever since the accident).

Protocol variation:
Targeting pain.

EMDR targets can range from past trauma to present pain, to the effects of pain. Although pain/MUS sufferers frequently have other trauma in their background, which may or may not be directly related to their current pain, the impact of present pain is often of primary concern. For the patient, uncontrolled pain is a safety issue, a kind of threat from within, which makes them feel unsafe in their own body. It must be neutralized or brought under adequate control to permit focusing on other issues. Facilitating pain reduction by targeting present pain helps with client stabilization (sense of mastery) and preparation for trauma work. Targeting present pain involves changes to the TICES which are further discussed below.

When targeting present pain, the image may be constructed on the basis of sensory descriptors ("If your pain had a size/shape/color, what would it be?") and associated imagery ("Is there an image that goes with that?") where there is no direct trauma. Additionally, clients who have never addressed their trauma (and may not be ready to) may even find it safer to focus on physical pain/MUS rather than painful dissociated memories. Where pain is part of an unresolved traumatic memory (e.g., whiplash pain), or where there is unrelated trauma, and it is unclear where to begin with EMDR, ask the patient which problem they want to focus on first, the trauma or the pain.

Other targeting considerations

Non-traumatic pain, such as chronic low back pain, arthritis pain, etc., does not generally involve a trigger memory in the way that trauma-related pain does. For therapists working with the general population, this will be the majority of cases. Since non-traumatic pain often does not involve a trigger memory or event, it does not lend itself to targeting in the usual (i.e., traumatic protocol) way. In fact, the present pain IS the trauma—it's an intrusive, disabling, distressing, and uncontrollable threat to normal functioning and identity.

Associated with that there may be EMDR targets linked to the effects of the pain: lost functioning, response-ability, and role capacity (e.g., "I'm useless," "I'm a burden"). The image would be based on the client seeing themselves as unable to perform activities that related to their sense of self.

There are, however, other ways of constructing a target for reprocessing—for example, a target image can be constructed based on the client's perception of their pain. Asking the client what size or shape the pain is, whether it's hard or soft, and so forth, can evoke a visual image of the pain which can be used in place of a memory for the desensitization target. Many clients have never really verbalized their pain and simply getting them to describe it can be a powerful intervention.

Quite often other small "t" traumas emerge following EMDR treatment of apparently physical pain. Adele developed chronic pain in her wrist after many years working as a data-entry clerk on computers. As a result of her injury, Adele had to quit her job, which made her feel anxious and like a failure. She developed symptoms of depression, including sleeping problems, fatigue, irritability, and lack of motivation. Adele wanted help to feel less depressed, cope better with her pain, and hopefully get her life back to normal. In therapy Adele was reluctant to reveal too much about her life; she glossed over her childhood other than to reveal she was a middle child of three from an intact family where affection was not shown much. "Just help me get back to work—that's all I need," she demanded. In such circumstances, even though I might suspect there are deeper issues, I have found it best to commence treatment with what the patient wants and is ready for. I provided Adele with some EMDR (BLS really) targeting her pain (size, shape, color), coupled with some resourcing imagery, pendulation, and general advice about pacing. Adele found this very helpful and her depression and pain improved to the extent that she could return to work (in a new job) on gradually increasing hours. Adele felt very happy to be working again and her confidence and mood improved week by week. Unfortunately, after she increased her hours one week, her pain flared up and she had to reduce her hours. This triggered a return of those old feelings of failure. By this time Adele felt more trusting and she casually mentioned how disappointed her mother was about her inability to work normally. This led to a more in-depth discussion about Adele's childhood which revealed that Adele's mother had always put her down and discouraged any expression of pain or vulnerability. Adele's mother's attitude to life was summed up by the mantra "you've gotta be tough." Adele had also left school early and not risen to the same levels of professional achievement as her two siblings. Her mother was always subtly reminding her of her two successful siblings. Adele craved her mother's approval and sought to win it by working in a professional capacity. She did not care how much typing she did, or how tired she felt, so long as she could maintain her employment and hopefully win the approval of her mother.

This added history led to some EMDR work around how Adele's mother made her feel. The target was an image of Adele's mother saying "you've gotta be tough" when she told her that she'd had to reduce her hours. Adele said this made her feel like she couldn't do anything right. The negative cognition was "I'm not good enough." The positive cognition was "I'm alright" with a VoC of 2. The negative feeling was a tight sensation in Adele's abdomen—in addition to the pain in her hand. After a couple of sets of BLS Adele exclaimed, "I can't do everything," and said that she realized this was what her mother made her feel she should do. When asked to review the positive cognition she was able to endorse it as 5/7. When asked what stopped that from being a 7/7, Adele said that her injured hand really did limit what she could do, but that she realized that this wasn't her fault.

Another technique, in addition to obtaining a description of the pain based on its size, shape, and color, is to help the client make an association between the pain and a sensory memory. For example, "What does the pain feel like?" "What does the way it feels remind you of?" Questions like these generally evoke an imagined, free-associative image, e.g., "a red balloon," "a hot poker," "a knife," etc. Once you have got a meaningful image of the pain, you have something to work with. Balloons can be punctured; hot pokers can be plunged into buckets of iced water; knives can be made blunt. A small percentage of highly left-brained people will have difficulty with this exercise—to them pain is pain and it's pointless to try and pretend it's anything else. For such folk it may be best just to target the pain directly as it is felt. Also see the EMDR strategies in the Therapist Resources section.

Many chronic pain/MUS sufferers are "walking DSMs", having survived physical or sexual abuse, emotional neglect, adult trauma, accidents and injuries, and multiple health problems. It's not uncommon for them to be affected by a mix of diagnosable medical problems and diseases of stress. They are more likely to be suffering from CPTSD than PTSD. Targeting options are many, ranging from past trauma/adversity (e.g., childhood memories), present triggers (e.g., pain, health fears) to future template/resourcing (e.g., healing imagery, coping strategies).

Melissa presented with pain associated with chronic ulceration in her mouth and esophagus, plus joint pain, skin rashes, stomach pain, neuropathic leg pain, and fatigue. Melissa was also a survivor of emotional deprivation in childhood, emotional abuse from her father and an older brother, family breakdown, childhood asthma and eczema, various other infections, and being raped as a teenager. Among other things she was diagnosed with orofacial granulomatosis/oral Crohn's disease. She presented as anxious and depressed, and also confessed to struggles with bulimia and self-harm. She was experiencing a lot of anxiety about the effects of her health problems on her future well-being and clinical levels of dissociative symptoms. She met the criteria for a diagnosis of CPTSD. CPTSD demands an integrated approach where EMDR is supplemented with extensive resourcing, ego state work, and hypnosis. Extensive safety and stabilization may be necessary to commencing EMDR processing of traumatic material. I made a rough list of possible targets and asked Melissa where she wanted to start.

Melissa indicated that her past and present health problems were what was troubling her the most on the day of our first appointment (I already had most of her history from the intake questionnaire I give all new patients, which she had thoroughly completed). After reviewing her story and reasons for seeking help, we both agreed that while there were many problems she needed help with, what she needed most was some help managing her symptoms and feeling more hopeful about her future. So the first intervention I did with Melissa was a resourcing exercise where I simply instructed her to focus on her present symptoms and think of something that could alleviate them. I then commenced BLS. Following this, Melissa reported that she felt calmer and could experience a sense of quietness within herself that felt new. Her PC, which we backloaded, was "I can relax." Subsequent targets would follow the flow of her treatment which was quite dynamic. For example, at the following session we targeted the memories of her brother's emotional abuse—a source of much of her insecurity and distress. Many sessions later we targeted the rape. Target selection was determined by what Melissa was ready for from week to week. Most targets were never completely reprocessed in one go—her presentation was too complex for that—and we would return to them repeatedly over the course of several years of therapy.

To summarize:

1. **Pain Associated with a Traumatic Event:** If the client's pain is associated with traumatic stress, the assessment phase involves identifying the trigger memory associated with the client's physical pain. For example, a phantom limb pain sufferer might have as their target an image of the accident in which they lost their leg, a negative cognition, and either an emotion or physical pain as the affect. An injured war veteran might see their pain in terms of the events surrounding their injury and the feelings they had about themselves at the time. Where pain is associated with a traumatic event, it (the memory) can be incorporated into the "target" as part of the affect, instead of emotion.

   Where the pain is associated with CPTSD, there are likely to be multiple target possibilities associated with past trauma/adversity, present pain/safety issues, and present and future coping needs. In these circumstances the development of targets requires considerable flexibility involving different positive and negative cognition themes, sensory vs. emotional focus, omitting elements such as the PC, etc. (see following pages). As we saw in Melissa's case, EMDR processing is often fragmented (it's impossible to completely process some targets sequentially) and integrated with resourcing and other therapeutic interventions.

2. **Pain Not Associated with a Traumatic Event:** If the pain is not associated with a traumatic event, there may be no single trigger memory. In this case, the therapist can construct a "target" based on the client's perception of their pain. A pain-based target can be created by simply asking the client to describe their pain in terms of a size, shape, color, and so forth (see below). The negative cognition relates to how the client feels in relation to the pain—in this case the pain is the traumatic memory. It is not always necessary or desirable to obtain a negative and positive cognition prior to commencing processing this way. For one thing, if the pain is associated with a medical condition, clients may not necessarily have a negative cognition. Later, when the client reports feeling better, a positive cognition can be evoked and installed (e.g., "So, when you think of the pain now, what do you realize about yourself?"). As indicated by Adele's story, non-traumatic pain can still be linked to emotional problems, and these can be processed in the normal way when they emerge.

Negative cognition

The negative cognition relates to how the trauma or pain makes the client feel about themselves. In the case of trauma-related pain, the negative cognition is likely to follow traditional lines—"I'm helpless," "I'm going to die," etc. In the case of non-traumatic pain, the negative cognition is more likely to relate to the pain or the injury that caused the pain, e.g., "There's something wrong with me," "I'm helpless/out of control," etc. This will involve clients' attitudes or beliefs about themselves around their pain. There are differences in the conceptualization of the negative cognition. In trauma-related memories, the negative cognition is considered to be irrational since the trauma is over and the person has survived. However, chronic pain sufferers often are faced with uncontrollable pain and they often do have something physically wrong with them. In this case, the negative cognition is valid, but it still needs to be diluted so that the dominant thought is of okayness rather than not-okayness. Pain and injury should not be the dominant aspect of a person's self-concept. Clients can learn to control their pain. Clients can learn that even though they have an injury or disability, they are still whole persons.

> **Protocol variation:**
> **Negative and positive cognition.**
>
> Shapiro has categorized EMDR negative cognitions into different themes. Lack of safety/vulnerability, control/power, responsibility/feeling defective (Shapiro, 2012, p. 84). Trauma survivors tend to endorse NCs with themes of lack of safety/vulnerability, and control/power, while pain sufferers typically endorse NCs with themes of responsibility and feeling defective (Grant, 2021, p. 107). While any client-centered NC is adequate, and there are always issues of safety and control, it is the author's experience that the negative cognition only needs to be proximate to how the pain makes the client feel about themselves and/or their ability to control it.

Shapiro has divided negative cognitions into 3 themes: lack of safety/vulnerability (e.g., "I'm trapped," "I'm going to die"); lack of control/power ("I'm weak/helpless," "I'm trapped"); and responsibility/being defective (e.g., "There's something wrong with me"). These themes determine the type of negative cognition clients are likely to have depending on whether their pain is trauma-related, or more medical. Basically, if the pain is trauma-related, the negative cognition is more likely to have a theme of safety/vulnerability. If the pain is more medically related, the negative cognition is more likely to reflect lack of control/power and/or feeling defective. Awareness of these themes and their relationship to trauma vs. pain is important when eliciting the negative and the positive cognition, particularly if the client is having difficulty finding the words to best describe how the pain makes them feel about themselves.

Below is a list of the kinds of negative/positive cognitions which often come up in the treatment of pain.

Lack of safety/vulnerability

- I'm not safe
- I'm trapped
- I can't escape
- I'm alone

Lack of control/power

- I am not in control
- I am powerless/helpless
- I am a failure
- I can't cope
- I can't control the pain/my feelings

Responsibility/being defective

- I'm bad/not good enough
- I'm weak
- I'm hopeless
- I'm useless
- I'm a burden
- I'm defective
- It's all my fault
- I deserve to suffer

As in EMDR treatment of post-traumatic stress, the structure of the questions used to create the target is important—it invites the client to consider their pain from a detached awareness standpoint. For example, one of the first questions of the treatment phase is "When you think of [trauma/pain], what does it make you feel?" Notice how this question sets up a mental separation between the problem and the client's emotions. It's very different to asking, "How do you feel?" which essentially collapses the pain into the client's felt sense of self. This wording sets up a separation between the client and the problem and elicits a less emotionally loaded description of the problem. There is, however, no need to seek a description of the pain until you get to the treatment phase.

When working with medical pain, do not spend too much time getting a perfect NC and PC if the client finds this difficult. It takes the client "off the track" in terms of their emotional preparedness for EMDR processing and it is often somewhat easier to obtain after the client has started noticing positive changes following BLS. This is one of the differences between pain and trauma: trauma memories are easily activated by talking about what happened, but because pain memories are more visceral, talking too much can actually take the client away from feeling what is happening. For example, Peter, an alexithymic man, found it hard to describe how his pain made him feel about himself and after years of being in pain, he could not imagine ever being able to have any sort of control over it. But after a few minutes of BLS he was surprised to notice feelings of relief unlike anything he had ever experienced before. Now when asked how he felt about his ability to control his pain, he cautiously admitted that he might be able to learn how to control his pain (VoC of 2/7). Sometimes I dispense with the negative cognition in the assessment phase, preferring to commence dual focus bilateral stimulation as soon as possible, in the interests of engaging clients whose motivation may be low. I only do this with non-traumatic pain and with clients who present as relatively free of other major trauma or structural dissociation. Once the client has begun to notice some change happening, a positive cognition can be evoked by asking the client to appraise their perceived ability to control their pain. The surprised client may not at first be able to attribute what has happened to anything they have done—they should be reassured that any improvement they are feeling comes from them and their nervous system responding to the bilateral stimulation. Once the client realizes this, even if they don't understand it, they are much more ready to believe that they can control their pain (or at least learn how).

Positive cognition

The positive cognition is a statement about how clients would like to feel about themselves in relation to their pain (e.g., "I can cope," "I'm alright," etc.). The positive cognition should have some grain of truth to it (e.g., "Sometimes I can control my pain"). It is not, in my experience, easy to get chronic pain sufferers to develop positive cognitions but they are a useful goal to have if they can be developed. The positive cognition is evoked by saying something like,

"When you bring up that picture or incident [or think of the pain], what would you like to believe about yourself, now?"

Validity of Cognition

The client should rate how strongly they believe in the positive cognition on a scale of 1 to 7. Ideally the client should have at least some belief in what they are saying.

"When you think of the pain, how true do those words____ [clinician repeats the positive cognition] feel to you now on a scale of 1 to 7, where 1 feels completely false and 7 feels totally true?"

If the client says they can't believe that they will ever be able to control their pain, challenge this. Most chronic pain sufferers are occasionally able to escape their pain, either through distraction or even sleep. Ask the client,

"What about when you're asleep? What about when you have a hot shower?" etc.

Most clients will admit that they don't feel their pain when they're asleep and/or that there are times during their waking life when the pain is different. If the client is having difficulty with the PC, it is okay to proceed without it. You can backload it following successful reprocessing (e.g., "In the light of the changes you have experienced, what statement could you make about your belief in your ability to control your pain now? What would you say?").

> **Protocol variation:**
> **"Backloading" the positive cognition.**
>
> Chronic pain sufferers who have struggled with pain for many years may find it difficult to endorse a PC with any degree of believability. It is more efficient and effective to dispense with the PC in the set-up stage and "backload" it after successful reprocessing. Once the client has achieved some degree of relief and control, they generally find it much easier to endorse PCs such as "I can cope," and "I can control the pain."

Partial positive cognition

Progress can be slow when working with pain, especially medical pain or pain associated with complex trauma. Clients may not feel it is realistic to say "I can control my pain" with any degree of confidence. In this case, it can be more appropriate to use a partial positive cognition such as "I can learn to control my pain" and strengthen or upgrade this later on when the client has had more positive experiences with EMDR.

Subjective units of disturbance scale

It is helpful to quantify the pain so that a baseline measure can be established by using the Subjective Units of Disturbance scale. For instance,

"How bad is the pain on a scale of 0 to 10, where 0 is no pain and 10 is the most pain you can imagine?"

If clients have fluctuating pain levels, it can also be useful to inquire whether their current pain levels are typical, above average, or below average. The therapist can work with whatever pain the client reports in the moment—it isn't necessary to get the client to feel the worst pain.

Target "memory"

If targeting present pain, an image of the pain based on its sensory/affective qualities may be a more appropriate image than a memory. There are three lines of questioning you can use to help clients get an image of their pain:

1. Getting the client to describe their pain in purely sensory terms, e.g., ***"If the pain had a shape, what shape would it be?"*** (repeat for size, density, color, temperature, etc.) See the "Pain words" list in the Therapist Resources section for a list of possibilities.
2. Getting the client to describe their pain in terms of an association with something they have previously experienced: ***"What does the pain feel like? What does the pain remind you of?"***
3. Getting the client to describe their pain in imaginal terms: ***"Can you draw a picture of the pain?"***

You may use one or all of these questions to help the client get a mental representation of the pain and thereby start to connect with it in the detached way that is necessary for EMDR reprocessing (as much as anything, this is the whole point of getting an image, NC, PC, etc.). Remember, the purpose of the image is simply to help bring the patient "on track" sufficiently for the pain to be reprocessed. It doesn't have to be perfect. Also allow for the fact that some people may find this difficult, even impossible. If the patient responds by saying something like ***"It's pain—how can I draw it?"***, don't pressure them, but consider that there is a level of alexithymia and dissociative avoidance that probably permeates most of this person's responses to negative affect. In this case, helping reduce dissociative barriers to the body will be a major component of the therapy, interspersed with brief EMDR interventions.

Future template

Patients with persistent pain will usually need resources for managing ongoing pain. Resources can comprise pain ameliorating imagery, emotional regulation strategies, beliefs about general healing, ego-strengthening activities, or memories and hope. These are typically incorporated into a future template which can be installed via EMDR processing (or hypnotically—see Chapter 10).

The future template refers to skills or resources that the client may need to cope with future episodes of trauma or anxiety. The future template involves getting the client to think of future episodes of trauma or pain, think of what they have learned about coping, and imagine themselves using that skill or resource to cope with the problem. The best future templates are derived from the client's remembered positive experiences of feeling better either through EMDR or some other strategies they have learned. For example, Colin, the Vietnam veteran we met in Chapter 4, learned to control future pain episodes using bilateral stimulation. His skill in focusing his attention and allowing his nervous system to respond to the bilateral stimulation, together with the positive cognition "I can control my pain," represented his future template. Nina, the bullying victim we met in Chapter 6, learned assertion skills as part of her future template. Chronic pain sufferers often find pain antidote imagery useful as part of their future template. This might involve creating a mental image of relaxation or feelings of relief, and installing this with bilateral stimulation. The best antidote imagery is derived from the client's felt experiences of relief following BLS (see the section on how to build resources somatically in Chapter 9). It could also involve installing more adaptive attitudes and beliefs about the client's ability to cope. We will look at this more in the installation phase.

8

Phase Four: Desensitization

The desensitization phase is where "the rubber meets the road" in EMDR. Here the patient is invited to focus on the selected pain-related target coupled with BLS in a detached, non-judgmental way. Changes in the sensory-affective experience of the problem are noted during check-ins until they plateau (not always at a SUDs of zero). These changes are crystallized in the positive cognition—a new, more adaptive belief the patient adopts about themselves. As with other phases, certain variations are necessary to reflect the unique demands of chronic pain/MUS, including strategies for addressing more muted physiological responses to BLS, the need to consider different BLS modalities, the need to extend the length of EMDR "sets," and continuous BLS. In this chapter we will review these adaptations.

Desensitization

The desensitization phase represents the heart of EMDR treatment. Here all the assessment and preparation is brought to a head in a pivotal series of focused attention/bilateral stimulation sessions wherein the client concentrates on their pain while simultaneously concentrating on the bilateral stimulation. The client should be made aware that there is nothing they have to think of or do once the bilateral stimulation starts, that they should just notice what they're feeling and let whatever happens happen.

"We can't predict how your nervous system will respond to the EMDR stimulation, so try and adopt an open mind and just notice the sensations of your pain as best you can. Initially, the intensity of the pain may not seem to change, or it may even increase; this is just the pain response shifting in response to the stimulation. In the unlikely event that the pain increases to an intolerable level, just raise your hand like this [show stop signal]. Remember, your nervous system knows what to do, so there's no need to try and make it happen, just notice and just let whatever happens happen.

"What we will be doing often is a simple check on what you are experiencing. I need to know from you exactly what is going on, with as clear feedback as possible. Sometimes things will change and sometimes they won't. There are no 'supposed tos.' Just notice and just let whatever happens happen."

The next step is to instruct the client to think of their pain (memory or image), the negative cognition, and where they feel it in their body, focus on the bilateral stimulation, and let whatever happens happen.

"So, can you think of your pain now, the way you have described it ... and your negative thoughts ... and where you feel the pain in your body ... and just notice ..."

Bilateral stimulation

If using auditory stimulation (recommended), instruct clients that they may listen with their eyes open or closed. It's not uncommon for clients to report that their eyes moved in response to the auditory stimulus. The therapist should check that the client is really focusing on what is happening in their body in a non-judgmental way rather than what they think is happening or what they expect to happen or what they remember. In other words, the therapist has to be able to recognize whether or not the client is in a mindful state. There are easily observable clues: respiration slows down (after an initial increase), speech slows down, and the content of speech becomes more reflective of here and now bodily states than past memories. Observe the client during the bilateral stimulation—look for changes in facial expression and body posture. The attuned therapist may also be able to sense when the client is feeling different by his or her own reactions. The best way to do this is to try and stay with the client during the bilateral stimulation. When you feel like you need a break, the client probably does too. Cease BLS after something seems to be happening or enough time has elapsed that something ought to be happening (usually between 30 and 60 seconds). When you ask the client "What do you notice now?" you should not only be looking for words that indicate the client is feeling different, but words that indicate the client is in a "here and now" state with their body (e.g., statements like, "My body feels more relaxed" or "I notice that my breathing has slowed down"). It can be helpful to volunteer suggestions if the client is finding it hard to describe their reactions to the BLS. Highly left-brain clients, who are usually disconnected from their bodies, may need longer to "get into" a non-verbal experience such as BLS. Continuous BLS is recommended for clients who have difficulty noticing or experiencing sensory changes in response to BLS (see below).

Instruct the client to "take a breath" and ask them to notice what they feel in their body.

At this point, many clients will report their pain feels duller, softer, further away, or just less distressing. If the client has trouble identifying changes, you can offer possibilities, e.g., "Some people report the pain seems less, some that it just seems further away, or smaller ... what do you notice?" You can also offer possibilities from the "Effects of BLS menu" in the Therapist Resources section at the end of this manual. This sense of relief or distance from the pain is maintained by repeated instructions to "just notice" during additional sets of BLS.

Continue until a relatively low, stable level of distress has been achieved.

If using auditory BLS, it can also make for smoother processing to not stop the BLS during the initial few check-ins, and maybe go for several minutes until the client's changes seem to plateau. This helps keep avoidant/alexithymic clients "on track" and allows them more time to tune into changes stimulated by BLS. This variation of the standard protocol is based on the fact that although pain fluctuates, it tends to be experienced as more unchanging over time than traumatic stress. Longer BLS thus gives the client more opportunity to experience change and each check-in ("What do you notice now?") helps them notice that change.

Installation (positive cognition)

Once a stable level of relief has been achieved, even if only mild, ask the client to review the negative "I-statement" they made at the beginning of treatment (if a negative cognition was obtained). As a result of feeling less distressed/more relaxed, clients generally find that this has changed and the positive cognition can be tested and installed. Depending on what aspect of the pain you are working with, the PC may relate to safety/vulnerability, control/power, or responsibility/feeling defective.

"Do the words [positive cognition] still fit or is there another positive statement that would feel more appropriate?"

If you did not obtain a PC in the preparation stage, simply ask the question:

"Based on the changes you have experienced today, what would you say about yourself now?"

Don't be afraid to suggest possibilities (e.g., "I can cope," "I can control my pain," "I am okay").

Instruct the client to think of the positive cognition while focusing on how they feel now, and a brief (no more than 30 seconds) set of BLS.

Review the VoC until a relatively stable 6 or 7 is achieved. In the treatment of trauma a VoC of 7/7 is recommended. Because of the variable and ongoing nature of chronic pain, and the potential impact of injury factors, this is just not always possible. Sometimes even a 5/7 is the best that can be hoped for. This is still a lot better than nothing and not necessarily an indication of unprocessed trauma. Like desensitization, installation continues until there are no longer changes and the VoC is stable. Blockages such as stalled processing, shifting pain targets, dissociation, and the limiting effects of physical pathology are common and necessitate creative use of cognitive interweave and other skills. See Chapter 11 for details about how to cope with these.

A closer look at bilateral stimulation

Although visual bilateral stimulation is the norm when using EMDR, audio and tactile BLS may be employed where visual BLS is contraindicated for whatever reason. Where pain is the primary target, audio BLS may also be advantageous. Auditory stimuli have long been used for healing purposes and have been found to be helpful in the alleviation of pain and insomnia.[1] The effects of auditory stimuli have been found to be more rapid and longer lasting than visual stimuli.[2] Phenomenologically, audio BLS has a more visceral impact than visual BLS.[3] In terms of evolutionary function, the human ear is one of the oldest structures and an organ of survival because of its role in detecting non-visual stimuli.[4] Audio BLS has been shown to be effective in the treatment of PTSD related chronic pain/MUS. My 2014 study of 11 chronic pain sufferers, nine of whom met the criteria for PTSD, found audio BLS to be effective.[5]

Another variation when targeting present pain is to extend the length of EMDR sets and do check-ins without ceasing BLS (continuous BLS). While briefer sets give PTSD patients time to rest and recover between sets, they may take them "off the track" in the treatment of pain. Continuous BLS gives patients with entrenched physiological responses more time to engage with and respond to BLS, making it easier to experience effects. Most sufferers of chronic pain/MUS are also alexithymic or dissociated to some degree and continuous BLS gives them more opportunity to notice often subtle changes in their body.

> **Protocol variation:**
> **Continuous audio BLS.**
>
> Continuous audio BLS may be an effective alternative to eye movements when targeting present pain. The speed of the BLS should be sufficient to attract and hold attention but not too rapid as to be overstimulating. EMDR check-ins can be performed without ceasing BLS. Because of the entrenched, chronic nature of symptoms in complex pain, changes may be subtle and slow in coming. Continuous BLS allows for the gradual accumulation of minor sensory changes and gives dissociated or alexithymic clients more time to attune to BLS and experience its effects. Check-ins should be conducted every 30–60 seconds or when non-verbal changes are noticed or if you feel unsure about what is happening.

It's also very important to pay close attention to what's happening in the body during EMDR. Apart from anything else, the success of EMDR therapy depends on the client's ability to notice changes in the sensory-emotional elements of their problem following BLS. Another reason to pay close attention to physiological responses to BLS in the treatment of chronic pain/MUS is because changes may be smaller and take longer to occur, due to exhaustion and decreased ability to respond to novel stimuli. Because of alexithymia and dissociation, just asking patients ***"What do you notice now?"*** following EMDR sets is rarely sufficient. Failure to detect such changes represents a lost opportunity in the sense that it can appear as though nothing is changing when in fact it is. Much closer tracking and active facilitating of changes is required. So, the standard EMDR check-in of ***"What do you notice now?"*** needs to be supplemented with additional questions, observations, and suggestions. For example:

"Tell me more about that."

"Do you notice anything else?"

Observe: ***"I notice that your breathing seems to have slowed down."***

"You look more relaxed."

Suggest possibilities: ***"Does the pain feel softer? Smaller? Further away?"***

"Do you feel lighter?"

Once the patient has reported substantial changes, and you want to help the patient integrate them, the positive effects of BLS can also be installed by pairing them with BLS or hypnotically or both. The author typically uses the following hypnotic phrasing to reinforce the effects of BLS: ***"So you're sitting in the chair, feeling relaxed, feeling more comfortable, feeling more connected with yourself, more whole, more together, mind and body as one ... all together now ... that's it ... because you are learning how to feel more integrated ... that you can be safe ... that you can heal. And I want you to take a moment and really notice what this feels like ... a new way of being in your body that can become part of your experience of yourself more and more every day, in many ways ... something you will enjoy noticing ... just taking a few quiet moments to notice that for yourself now ... that's right."*** This verbal refreshing of post-BLS changes gives the patient an added opportunity to consolidate their new learnings and is an under-emphasized area in the way this method is currently taught.

Protocol variation:
Tracking and facilitating effects of BLS.

Because of dissociation and alexithymia, it should not be assumed that clients are sufficiently self-aware to notice any and all changes. Close attention should be paid to both the client's self-report and non-verbal signs during EMDR check-ins. Observe changes in facial expression, decreased respiration, posture, etc., in addition to the client's feedback. Questions that direct awareness to the body ("What do you notice now?") and hold it there ("Just notice that.") are useful.

In patients with more complex presentations, phase four may need to be titrated by combining EMDR processing with other interventions. Exhausted individuals may need a break from processing in favor of a more cognitive engagement. CPTSD sufferers are rarely capable of sustained intensive trauma processing and desensitization needs to be accompanied by other inputs such as the flash technique, brainspotting, deep brain reorienting, ego state work, hypnosis, or psychoeducation.

For patients with persistent pain due to serious injury or illness, self-use of BLS outside of therapy can also be helpful. This simply involves provision of auditory recordings of BLS for the patient to use for purposes of relaxation, self-soothing, etc. My apps are a convenient and inexpensive resource in this regard (see the Resources section at the rear of this book). Apps which incorporate a blend of BLS, music, and guided imagery have been found to be helpful in the management of chronic pain/MUS.[6] Despite concerns about the unregulated use of BLS, which this is not, there is no research to show that it is dangerous. On the contrary, over 20,000 downloads of my apps have generated a handful of reports of adverse responses, of a temporary nature, managed by cessation of usage of the app.

Protocol variation:
Self-use of BLS.

In patients with persistent pain, self-use of audio BLS "at home" may offer a safe and effective means of self-soothing. BLS is known to stimulate physiological changes associated with relaxation, decreased worry, distancing effects, and even sleepiness. For appropriate clients with ongoing pain, self-use of BLS gives them a safe, effective tool for alleviating pain, stress, and insomnia which often persists in between treatment sessions. Self-use should be introduced as a self-soothing strategy (not DIY EMDR) after the client has experienced positive effects of BLS (e.g., relaxation, etc.) in session.

BLS can also enhance the client's response to other treatment inputs—for example, Jerry found that listening to auditory bilateral stimulation when applying heat pads seemed to enhance their impact on his pain. Louise found that listening to bilateral stimulation helped take her mind off her pain and fall asleep more easily. Many clients report feeling drowsy after listening to auditory BLS and many of my clients find listening to auditory BLS helps them fall asleep. In addition to its relaxation effects, auditory BLS seems to interrupt anxious rumination associated with sleeping problems.

Every client can benefit from BLS so long as they can focus mindfully on the stimulation and are able to discern its impact upon their nervous system—sometimes with a little guidance from the therapist. Clients who apparently don't find the BLS helpful have often simply not attended to it with the right mindset (e.g., clients who devote their mental energies to assiduously trying to figure out what is causing the sounds rather than just listening with an open mind).

I mainly use auditory stimulation with pain. My 2014 study involving 11 chronic pain sufferers (including traumatic and non-traumatic pain) found that auditory BLS was as effective as visual BLS in alleviating the subjective element of pain in seven of the subjects with gains maintained at six months in four of the seven for whom follow-up data was available.[7] Auditory BLS is both more "visceral" in its impact and, of course, more easily adapted to self-use. Self-use involves giving the client the option of using BLS to assuage stress and pain in between sessions. Once the client has experienced the beneficial effects of BLS in session, so long as they do not have complex PTSD, they are ready and primed to make use of it independently.

A recent study involving 60 chronic pain/PTSD sufferers using apps incorporating BLS found nil adverse effects.[8] This is contrary to what the AIP model predicts—that one memory can spontaneously trigger other memories to surface under conditions of dual attention/BLS. There are several possibilities as to why this doesn't seem to happen very often with self-use of BLS: 1) Just focusing on one element of one issue (anxiety, pain, inability to sleep) does not involve sufficient engagement with the memory to trigger the kind of free association that normally occurs during EMDR desensitization; 2) While the situation/symptoms that the individual is seeking relief from (as above) might ultimately be trauma related (e.g., childhood emotional neglect), the memories/feelings are sequestered by dissociative processes which inhibit access; 3) The situation/symptoms that the individual is seeking relief from involve stressful but non-traumatic present circumstances (e.g., physical pain, conflict). So, while it seems prudent to assume a stance of caution on the basis that some traumatized individuals could experience unwanted intrusions as a result of self-use of BLS, the evidence thus far is that self-use of BLS is benign. Working models of EMDR also support this—the primary effects of BLS are deactivation of the orienting response, relaxation, working memory effects, etc.

In summary, when treating chronic pain/MUS, the desensitization phase of EMDR requires considerable flexibility and input from the therapist compared with "standard" EMDR. These include strategies for addressing more muted physiological responses to BLS, the need to consider different BLS modalities, the need to extend the length of EMDR "sets," continuous audio BLS, actively tracking and facilitating changes following BLS, titrating desensitization with other therapeutic strategies, and the option of self-use of BLS (by patients).

9

Phases Five to Eight: Installation to Closure

In phases five to eight the patient is assisted to adopt the positive cognition, based on sensory/affective changes experienced in the desensitization phase and any resources necessary for future coping, as tested by the VoC and relevance to the original target. The work is checked to ensure there is no residual trauma and additional processing/resourcing provided. During the active phase of EMDR therapy, incomplete sessions are not uncommon and strategies have to be implemented to accommodate symptoms in between sessions. While patients may report that they feel free of emotional distress, some may continue to experience residual physical discomfort due to the physiological effects of serious injury and/or chronic illness. Resourcing and future template are often necessary to help them cope following active treatment.

What is a resource?

A resource is any skill or ability that can be used in coping with pain. A person might have a good imagination, which enables them to dream things up to change their pain. Or they might remember something they saw or experienced which made them feel better, and use that memory to change how they feel. Resources come from a combination of innate characteristics and past experience. Below is a list of general resources that can be harnessed to help a client overcome their pain.

- Imagination
- Affect range
- Experience of overcoming adversity
- Energy

Creating and nourishing resources to help clients face the challenges of life is one of the most important tasks of EMDR, or any psychotherapy. But it bears remembering that resources are not something external that you "bolt on" to the client (like a spare set of fuel tanks); they are, in fact, an outgrowth of personal development, integrated with trauma processing and the reassociation and reorganization of the client's inner life that takes place in therapy. Over 50 years ago Milton Erickson declared that long-term change was impossible without these processes. For this reason I much prefer to create resources based on the client's previous experience and memories, because they involve internal reassociation and they are more likely to "fit" the client's current needs and readiness.

Imagination

Imagination is one of the oldest and most popular resources. Techniques such as guided imagery, visualization, and hypnosis all draw on imagination. Imagination is the ability to see things other than as they are. Imaginative people are able to enter into fantasy easily, and leave unpleasant realities behind. Imagination is a right-brain creative activity. An imaginative person finds it easy to create a mental image of their pain, and then manipulate that image so that their mental perception of their pain is altered. Harry imagined his pain as a big red balloon, and then deflating the balloon by releasing a pressure valve. As the air escaped from that big red balloon, Harry could imagine his pain shrinking too. Julia, a more left-brained person, found this idea ridiculous. She much preferred keeping busy as a way of coping with her pain. The trouble with this approach was that it did nothing to alleviate Julia's pain and it actually made it worse in the long run by preventing her from ever relaxing. In EMDR Julia learned she could feel different as a result of attending to the bilateral stimulation. Basically the therapist helped increase her affect range. Other imaginative strategies include visualizing a control room in the mind where one can "dial down" the pain, imagining an anesthetic mist which can neutralize the pain, imagining something cold (e.g., ice) for "hot" pain, and something hot (e.g., a warm bath) for coldness or stiffness. One of the most comprehensive summaries of pain imagery can be found in Hammond, 1990, p. 45–84.

Affect range

Affect range is the ability to experience different feelings. The more feelings a person is capable of feeling, the more emotional resources they and the therapist have to draw on. As the great philosopher Baruch Spinoza famously said, "The more capable the body is of being affected in many ways ... the more capable of thinking is the mind." In an era dominated by Descartes, Spinoza was ahead of his time in realizing that what happens in the body has a greater effect on how we see ourselves and the world than what we think. This idea underpins the central mechanisms of EMDR wherein sensory-emotional responses to bilateral stimulation form a basis for new, more adaptive attitudes and feelings. It's also consistent with the concept of embodied cognition, a hot topic in neuroscience in recent decades. After learning how to focus on the bilateral stimulation and the changes it stimulated in her body, Julia began to be more aware of her emotions and more able to take action to manage (rather than simply avoid) negative feelings. Different moods involve different physiological states. If a person can feel joy or laugh, they can escape their pain—or at least the emotional component of their pain. Affect range is a product of temperament and family history. A person is more likely to have a good affect range if they were brought up in an emotionally accepting environment.

People who were raised in emotionally repressive circumstances may have a limited affect range. Andrew Leeds has noted that some people may actually be phobic about positive feelings—especially shared positive affect.[1] Leeds notes that such people may appear superficially to be coping well, but there is really no emotional foundation to their behavior. People like this, who are generally survivors of chronic neglect and/or abuse involving insecure or unstable attachments, need extensive emotional tutoring to learn to recognize and integrate positive emotional experiences (see Chapter 6 of *Change Your Brain, Change Your Pain*—"How to reconnect with your feelings"). You could begin by asking them what experiences give them joy or pleasure, especially experiences which involve sharing with others. The latter may take some time to uncover, but where the parents have failed, there is usually a relative, a teacher, or some other mentor figure. You need someone who made your client feel safe and who was consistently available for a significant period of time. Jessie never felt wanted by her parents, but she found a mother figure in a widowed neighbor who, in return for a bit of companionship every afternoon after school, gave her all the attention a young girl could want. Jessie laughed as she remembered how Mrs. Jones would peel off a 10-dollar bill from a wad she kept in her freezer and send her to the shop to buy a loaf of bread and something for herself with the change, but it was never about the money. If the client cannot think of anyone real, see if they can remember someone from TV who represented a parent figure they would have liked. Then ask them to remember or imagine being with this person, and how they feel when they think of this person. To help anchor the feelings, take your time with this. Also ask the client to notice where they feel the positive feelings in their body. Get the client to describe them in terms of size, shape, color, etc. Ask the client if there is a word that summarizes how this memory makes them feel (it will usually be something like "safe" or "secure"). The more you can help your client to re-experience this positive shared affective experience, the more you are helping them to relearn that they can have good feelings and that those feelings can be shared and trusted. This opens the client up to receiving more emotional support, having experiences which stimulate different feelings to those associated with the pain, learning that they can have other feelings than pain and depression. Some traumatized clients have literally forgotten how to have fun. Lucy was depressed after losing her high-powered job due to a back injury. She was angry at herself because all she wanted to do was lie on the beach and read Jackie Collins novels when she should be taking stock and reading some of her motivational texts to help prepare herself for a new future. Knowing that she had not had any sort of real holiday in several years, I gently said, "Maybe you need to enjoy Jackie Collins for a while and then when you're feeling more stable you can go back to the motivational texts."

Experience of overcoming adversity

Adversity can be destructive, but it can also be instructive. Overcoming adversity can lead to the development of hardiness, and the realization that one is strong and capable of surviving. Louis's elbow was smashed when he tried to protect a man from being assaulted. As a result of this injury Louis couldn't work for several months, and his girlfriend left him, taking their son with her. Louis was reduced to living in the back of his car. It was the hardest nine months of Louis's life, but eventually his elbow healed and he found work as a gardener. Unfortunately, about six months after he'd started his new job, Louis damaged his back while lifting a trailer. The doctors told him that he could never work as a gardener again. Louis was devastated—he'd loved the gardening position. As bad as he felt, Louis remembered the earlier time when his partner had left him, which seemed much worse, and he thought, "I can survive this." After another difficult six months, where he learned to live with pain all over again, Louis eventually found work as a train driver. Louis's ability to overcome adversity was based on an ability to look beyond the present circumstances, adapt, and set new goals and determination (see also: "How to build resilience," Chapter 11 of *Change Your Brain, Change Your Pain*).

Energy

Many sufferers of trauma and pain are anhedonic—they have lost the ability to derive pleasure from lived experience and are depressed, tired, and unmotivated. Pierre Janet used the term "aboulia" to describe this loss of mental energy, although in trauma and pain sufferers it probably also involves some degree of alexithymia. In Freudian terms one could say there is a loss of libido (the energy associated with survival and procreation). Regardless of how you define it, the result is the same: fatigue, withdrawal, hopelessness, decreased sense of future. Such persons feel totally unresourced. While there may be good reason for feeling tired and depressed (pain, lack of sleep, lost ability to function), surviving depends upon finding or stimulating the energy to develop resources to combat the effects of trauma and pain.

The simplest source of energy is interest. Any thought process or activity which generates feelings of safety and/or interest and excitement automatically accesses energy as well as taking the person's mind away from their predicament. The best resources are those which trigger positive affect. This is the basis of traditional resource interventions such as guided imagery and pleasant events scheduling. However, in order to benefit from such activities, the client must be able to see outside the confines of their negative, often pain-focused mindset, and they must be able to experience the positive affect that, say, walking on the beach normally triggers.

Accessing energy necessitates drawing the client's attention away from their problem-focused view of life and toward things which they find pleasurable or satisfying. You can facilitate this by engaging the client in a conversation about activities and interests they find enjoyable (regardless of whether or not they are currently doing them). A traumatized foreign aid worker with low back pain and fatigue was sleeping up to 16 hours per day and had withdrawn from all social and recreational pursuits. Hanna had even let her gym membership lapse. The only "recreational pursuit" she could identify was watching forensic police shows on TV. But a thorough review of her activities in the last month produced a recollection that Hanna had swum in the ocean twice lately (after recently relocating to a seaside town). Hanna's eyes lit up when she recalled how she used to enjoy swimming as a child and how much she enjoyed rediscovering those feelings. "What effect did swimming have on your energy levels?" I asked. "And what effect do you think it might have if you did it again?" Being reminded that she could be energized by enjoyable activities helped Hanna discover a resource she did not realize she had. Milton Erickson's work with "the African Violet Lady" is a classic example of this process. (See Mary's story in Chapter 12, or search for "the African Violet Lady" on the internet.)

Affect-based resources

Affect-based resources are memories, learnings, and emotional states that incorporate an active coping stance. An affect-based resource could be a memory of having overcome past adversity, or a memory of a safe place which generates feelings of peace and safety when accessed. Or it could be an image derived from feelings of relaxation induced by bilateral stimulation. In EMDR an affect-based resource is a mental state that incorporates feelings of confidence or calmness in the face of adversity. For example, after Leanne focused on the bilateral stimulation in EMDR, her back pain disappeared. When the therapist asked her what she felt now, she stated, *"Nothing."* When the therapist asked her to say more about this, she said it felt like a white light had come into her body—a very pleasant feeling she had had before during a near-death experience. The therapist then asked her what word or positive thought went with that image and that feeling. *"I can be healed,"* Leanne replied. *"Just think of that and just notice now,"* said the therapist, before commencing BLS. After about 30 seconds of bilateral stimulation, the therapist asked Leanne what she noticed now. *"Peace,"* she said. *"I know I can find peace whenever I need it." "Good,"* said the therapist, *"just think of that,"* and again Leanne focused on the white light and the thought that she could have peace whenever she need it. Following this Leanne reported feeling even more strongly connected to that feeling of peace and the positive cognition. The therapist instructed her to practice this at home, in conjunction with the bilateral stimulation.

How to build resources somatically

As Leanne's story illustrates, a powerful way of building resources for clients with ongoing pain is to create associations with positive bodily states. When a client reports decreased pain following bilateral stimulation, they are experiencing both an absence of discomfort and usually also increased feelings of relaxation and well-being. These feelings can be used as a basis for developing strong, affect-based resources. This is done by asking,

> ***"What does that feeling remind you of?"***

Or,

"So, what do you notice now … What's there now where the pain was before …? What has come in its place …?"

Usually (hopefully) the client will report sensations like:

"softer," "smaller," and "more relaxed." See "Comfort words" in the Therapist Resources section.

The therapist then instructs the client to

"just notice that"

and restimulates.

Following this, assuming the feeling is maintained, the therapist then instructs the client to

"think of something that feeling reminds you of … What does it feel like? What's it like?"

This usually stimulates a free association to dreamlike imagery such as a sponge, a cushion, a small red dot, etc. There is often a non-logical quality to this imagery, but it is loaded with positive affect. Then instruct the client to

"think of that"

and restimulate.

Then ask,

"What do you notice now?"

If the client reports the healing imagery is stronger or at least maintained, then instruct them to

"stay with that …"

and restimulate.

If the image changes, don't worry, just instruct the client to

"just think of that"

and restimulate.

If the image fades or is too weak, instruct the client to

"make it stronger, or think of something stronger ..."

and restimulate.

It may take several sets with changing imagery before the right imagery is settled upon. In some cases, it has taken me two or three sessions to arrive at a stable effective imagery. The therapist can tell when the client has discovered a reliable, stable healing imagery when the image stays the same after several sets, and when the client reports no further strengthening of the imagery.

Once a stable healing image is achieved, instruct the client to

"think of a word or phrase that goes with that ..."

Or,

"think of a word or phrase that summarizes that feeling"

and restimulate.

Clients may say something like "peaceful," "relief," or "I'm going to be okay," "I can cope," etc. Sometimes the word or phrase will take the form of a positive cognition and this should be installed in the normal way at this point.

Clients usually report that the healing imagery and feelings feel stronger, like a part of them. Margaret suffered from chronic pain in her hip. During the desensitization phase she reported that it felt like something was rubbing away the pain and reported getting an image of a little polished carved man she had at home. She imagined her pain being rubbed away like the carving being rubbed by all the hands that held it. The positive cognition that she got with this was "I can feel better."

The therapist should be flexible and alert for spontaneous emergence of resources during and out of the client's own processing. For example, a woman suffering from a frozen jaw and neck pain associated with an unresolved grief (NC: "I can't live without him") got an image of her dead grandson living inside her heart and verbalized this as, "Now I can remember him with love." These words and that image were installed as a positive cognition.

Another way to develop resources is by making use of adaptive emotional responses and associations which occur during therapy. For example, after Paul noticed that his pain felt less intense following bilateral stimulation, he was asked to describe what he felt where the pain was before. ("What's there now where the pain was before?") After a moment's introspection, Paul described a feeling of softness, like a ball of cotton wool. The therapist then instructed Paul to think of the cotton wool and a word that he associated with cotton wool. "Soft," said Paul. "Just think of that," said the therapist. After a few sets of this, Paul reported being able to create feelings of comfort just by thinking of cotton wool and the word "soft," while listening to bilateral stimulation. This resource was installed with BLS.

The secret to somatically based resource creation is to direct the client's awareness away from noticing the absence of something (pain) toward the feeling that has come in its place (e.g., softness, relief). The human mind is such a good problem-detection device, it sometimes fails to notice when a chronic condition starts to change. Once the client's awareness has consciously picked up on the post BLS feelings, it is an easy matter to generate a positive cognition and resource/future template. When Paul's therapist asked him how he felt about his ability to control his pain (post BLS changes) he replied, "I can control my pain." Paul's future template was his ability to generate feelings of relief by thinking of cotton wool while listening to bilateral audio tones.

Healing resource (wild card) installation

Another step that can be taken, for clients who develop good pain control with EMDR, is to ask them to imagine the injury that is causing the pain and develop imagery for "healing" the injury. Anything can pop up—it's like a wild card. The client does not need to be in pain to do this processing.

1) Create a target by asking the client to picture the injury that is causing the pain.

   "What does it feel like is wrong with your body that is causing the pain?"

Encourage the client to feel free to use their imagination uncritically. If the client has difficulty describing it verbally, you can also ask them to draw a picture of "the injury that is causing the pain."

2) Then ask the patient to

"imagine something that could heal the injury"

or

"think about what it would take to heal the injury that is causing the pain."

You're looking for material from the unconscious, something like "a wet sponge," "a cloud," or "a healing light." A response such as "an operation" is no good; you need something that comes from the unconscious.

3) "Install" the healing imagery as follows:

Instruct the client to

"think of that [repeat healing imagery]"

while attending to bilateral stimulation. After a few sets, to strengthen it, you can also ask the client to think of a word that goes with the healing imagery, and do a few more sets. Where appropriate, client can use this at home, by thinking of the word and the image, and doing self-stimulation (tapping or tones).

Helping clients who feel they have no resources

Some people report a complete lack of positive experiences, memories, or resources. This false but self-defeating attitude must be challenged, but without arousing the ire of the client. The therapist has to respect the client's view of themselves, while nevertheless make the attempt to change it. For example, to the depressed client with a horrific background of abuse, trauma, and neglect you can simply ask, "So, how have you survived?" Any response to that question (other than "I dunno") is going to involve the admission of some kind of resource. Even if the client says, "I dunno," the therapist should resist the temptation to volunteer suggestions and adopt a neutral but curious stance. For example, "I don't know either, I don't know how anybody could have survived what you have ..." followed by a pause. This restating of the question followed by silence creates pressure on the client to respond. Clients may volunteer achievements and then dismiss them as luck or the result of actions by others. The therapist can make a bridge between the achievement and the client by asking, "So, what might that [achievement] say about you?" It is the therapist's job to help the client redefine themselves.

Future template

The future template is an expansion of the installation phase. It's typically used after the client has completed processing of past and present triggers, but still needs to feel confident about their ability to cope with, say, future health issues and/or pain. The future template is harnessing a fundamental quality of the human brain—its ability to predict. One of the latest theories of consciousness is based on the brain's ability to function as a prediction machine. Just as memories of past experience can influence present perceptions and behaviors, the future can also influence the present through simulation and prediction.[2] In the future template the changes and new learnings accrued in the desensitization phase are tested and consolidated.

The future template would typically incorporate resources for managing future pain that might have been created in the preparation or desensitization stages (antidote imagery, self-use of BLS, memories of coping, etc.). The future template is also a resourcing process. The future template harnesses the brain's inability (at times) to distinguish between what is real and what is imagined, in an adaptive way. The patient is asked what future situation they would like help preparing for, and then to imagine themselves coping with that situation as vividly as possible (including a PC), and then to run a movie of that with BLS. Their response is reviewed and any disturbance is processed in the usual way.

The future template is also a way of checking the work that has been done. If the client struggles with adopting a future template, it may be a sign that they are still lacking something in terms of skills, self-confidence, or ego strength. If the patient reports feeling unable to see themselves coping in the future, simply ask: ***"What's stopping you from seeing that?"*** If the patient feels unsure about their ability to apply what they have learned, 1) validate their anxiety, and explore more if necessary, 2) develop missing skills if identified, 3) run a movie of them applying what they have learned to future episodes of the problem.

An enhancement to the future template when using it to resource patients to cope with chronic pain/MUS is to incorporate an age regression or floatback from the future to the present. Once the patient has successfully imagined themselves coping in the future: ***"Great, and now I'd like you to look back from then to now and review what you have learned, and share that with your present self, so that your present self can know what your future self already knows."***

The future template also involves the maintenance of hope, something which many chronic pain/MUS sufferers have lost. In a landmark text on the subject, Jerome Frank noted that most psychotherapy patients suffer from a sense of hopelessness and helplessness, and that the restoration of hope is the curative factor in psychotherapy.[3] In a recent review article, Colla et al. defined hope as "a human strength that enables individuals to draw on resources in their environment to support pathways toward healthy development and achievement." [4] Hope is a double-barreled phenomenon, representing both a resource and a quality that attracts other resources. As Plato said, "We are twice armed if we fight with hope." Hope springs from feeling able to set goals and believing that life has meaning. For most people, meaning arises from relational factors (i.e., increased access to internal resources as a result of external relationships). Dissociation expert Richard Chevetz, MD, describes how he held hope for a depressed patient:

> *"One woman, after many years of treatment and many crises of suicidal proportion, put it this way as she lingered at the doorway to my office at the end of a session several years ago: 'Stop telling me you hope I'll keep myself safe. What is that? I hate it when you say that, stop telling me you hope. I don't want it. Just keep it away from me.' I replied, 'I hear you, Scylla, and it's also true, I really do hope you'll keep yourself safe. You are really the only one who can do that.' 'Yeah, well I'm sick of you hoping this and hoping that. So just stop it. I don't want any of your hope.' 'I suppose you're not quite ready to acknowledge your own hope.' 'You're out of your mind.' 'Since you don't seem to be ready to have your own hope, could you mind much if I hold on to your hope for you? I will keep it safe until you are ready to own it. And just in case there is some hope hidden inside you in a place where it's not in danger of being dismissed or destroyed, I'll still hope you might find a way to know about it and not to be so frightened of it.' 'I still think you are out of your mind.' And, she left, and came back the next week for her appointment just as I had hoped."*[5]

Hope is intrinsic to EMDR through the AIP model, which posits that people have or can find the resources they need. This is not a new idea—Milton Erickson believed that new experiences are the key to change and that it is the therapist's job to act as a catalyst for these.[6] Erickson developed many ways of doing this, including stories and indirect suggestions. When a patient is feeling too hopeless (which most of my patients do at some stage), I tell them a story about another patient who felt hopeless but kept on with therapy and eventually got better. The implicit suggestion is that if it happened to them, it can happen to you.

The fostering of hope can be a slow and uneven process, which is why, for example, close tracking and identification of changes during the desensitization phase, to fan those flickering flames of change, is so important. At other times, as Chevetz's story illustrates, when change seems beyond reach, the therapist has to hold their feeling about the patient's hopelessness and maintain trust that it will happen eventually. Erickson also emphasized the importance of the therapeutic relationship as a catalyst for change, from the perspective of a collaborative process rather than a controlling one (***"What can I do and what can you do?"***). Sometimes, when treating patients with chronic, multiple problems, it's simply a matter of hanging on to the fact that the patient shows up for their session every week, doing the work, and holding that hope.

Phase six: body scan

The body scan is a recurring feature of EMDR, as the therapist continually checks with the client regarding their felt pain levels. For alexithymic or dissociated clients, the body scan can be difficult and considerable stabilization and awareness skills building may be required before the client can perform this. Some clients report feeling pain when in fact they are remembering their pain because that is what they are used to, but in fact there is little or no pain currently felt in the body. A relaxed face and posture are the giveaway signs. I usually say something like:

"There is a difference between felt pain and remembered pain. Felt pain is in the body; remembered pain is in the mind. Which pain are you really feeling now?"

Clients often say, "Oh, it's in my head."

To which I reply, ***"Well, that's not pain, that's a memory."***

And I redirect their attention back to the body,

"... So, what are you actually feeling in your body right now?"

Alexithymic clients find this backward and forward direction of attention between the mind and the body very useful in learning to distinguish between thoughts, memories, and feelings. Again, if the client is unable to find words to describe what they are feeling in their body, feel free to help them by offering suggestions.

The final body scan for a particular session or course of treatment involves getting the client to attend to how they feel and check that there is no residual pain. When the client reports no pain or it is apparent that the client cannot improve any further, the therapist should say something like:

"Close your eyes and keep in mind the original memory/image and the positive cognition. Then bring your attention to the different parts of your body, starting with your head and working downward. Any place you find any tension, tightness, or unusual sensation, tell me."

Assuming the client gives a clear response, or an acceptable level of discomfort, the processing part of therapy is concluded. As noted, chronic pain clients may not always be able to achieve a zero SUDs and the therapist may need to have imbued the client with resources such as a future template.

Phase seven: closure

The closure phase involves reviewing the session, and/or the client's journey in therapy, and preparing them for the future. At the end of each session the therapist should prepare the client for possible pain flare-ups or intrusive memories (if the pain is part of a traumatic reaction).

"Things may come up or they may not. If they do, make a note of them, and they can be a target for next time. If you get any new memories, dreams, or situations that disturb you, just make a note of them. It isn't necessary to give a lot of detail. Just put down enough to remind you so we can target it next time. The same thing goes for any positive dreams or situations. Even if nothing comes up, make sure to use the CD as often as you feel necessary and give me a call if you need to."

If the pain is not part of a traumatic reaction, say the following:

"We have no way of knowing how long the changes you have experienced today will last. But whatever happens, hopefully you have learned something new about coping with pain. Even if your pain comes back, it may not be the same because of how the EMDR affects the way your brain remembers the pain. So, just have an open mind and let whatever happens happen. Maybe keep a log of any problems and we can work on them next time."

Phase eight: re-evaluation

During treatment, each session should begin by reviewing the client's experience of their pain and related stress or trauma over the period since the last session. Changes in sleeping patterns, physiological arousal, and activity levels need to be screened for, identified, and fed back to clients to avoid a false perception that nothing has changed.

"So, what have you noticed about your pain [or other problem] since our last session?"

If the client does not volunteer material or is unable to identify any changes, the therapist should inquire about sleep, mood, activity levels, relationships, etc., looking for any unusual changes in normal coping and functioning.

The therapist needs to check with clients for any changes in how they have been feeling in terms of the material that was processed at the previous session and use this as a basis for constructing new targets for EMDR reprocessing. It is not uncommon for the image of the pain to change between sessions, as the clients experience changes, particularly if progress is being made.

It can also be helpful to give clients who may be vulnerable or struggling with self-care issues a quick telephone call in between sessions to check how they are going with homework assignments. Paul found it hard to make time to listen to his relaxation audio exercises, but when he received a call from his therapist asking how he was going, it motivated him to put aside what he was doing and invest in his self-care more.

Managing persistent pain

Clients with ongoing pain may also need additional skills and resources for managing pain. Three of the most well-known traditional techniques for overcoming pain are meditation, relaxation, and self-hypnosis. These three strategies can be adopted according to the client's references and personality. Hypnosis is an indispensable adjunct to EMDR treatment of chronic pain, rather like ego state work and somatic experiencing are to EMDR treatment of complex trauma. Hypnosis offers a vehicle for gently building ego and affect management resources that is less energy intensive than EMDR. See Chapter 12 for more information about how to integrate hypnosis into EMDR treatment of chronic pain.

Other skills and activities that the therapist should be aware of include exercise and sleep. Sleep is a huge problem for most chronic pain sufferers and lack of sleep is a major exacerbating factor for pain. Sleeping problems usually originate in response to lack of safety, which can be maintained by persistent pain. Diet may also be important for patients with chronic illnesses (e.g., celiac disease, IBS, diverticulitis) and conditions which involve inflammation (e.g., rheumatoid arthritis, Sjögren's syndrome). See Chapter 11 for information on adjunctive therapeutic elements regarding these issues.

10

EMDR Pain Protocol

EMDR pain protocol script

Since its inception, EMDR therapy has been framed via protocols—structured procedures and processes designed to guide the therapeutic process in the most safe and efficient way. There is generally an emphasis on past memories thought to be driving present distress. There is a detailed order of proceedings (TICES) even down to the specific wording associated with different tasks. However, it's recognized that adaptations may be necessary to meet the needs of different populations.[1] The protocol outlined here includes detailed instructions necessary for processing trauma vs. non-trauma-related pain, including variations associated with targeting present pain, continuous audio BLS, close tracking and facilitating of changes, etc. The more unsure you feel about what to do, the more closely you will want to follow it, but it should be regarded as a guide rather than the only way to do things. People are different—you are invited to modify this protocol according to your style, experience, and of course the therapeutic needs of your patients.

Bruce Eimer (1993) created the first EMDR pain protocol, which guided my entry into this application of EMDR.[2] There are now a variety of pain protocols for phantom limb pain,[3] mixed pain,[4] and headaches.[5] There have also been reports of EMDR being applied to somatic symptom disorder, rheumatoid arthritis, fibromyalgia, CRPS, post-operative pain, and tinnitus. All (or most) EMDR protocols for pain share three common elements: 1) Past/present/future targeting options centering on pain or trauma, 2) Integration with other psychosomatic interventions, and 3) Recognition that EMDR therapy is part of a broader treatment plan involving other disciplines. The following protocol is the product of many years of clinical experience and research.[6]

Pain and the adaptive information processing model

Begin by explaining chronic pain in terms of the adaptive information processing model. For example:

"Pain can occur for many reasons. We generally understand pain as a signal that something is wrong physically. However, sometimes pain can continue longer than expected, despite medical treatment. Pain can persist because of fatigue, stress, and biochemical and neurological changes. As a result of these changes, the pain becomes "locked" in the nervous system. EMDR is a way of stimulating the nervous system to facilitate healing. Even though we might not be able to completely eliminate your pain, EMDR often stimulates feelings of relaxation, which always reduces pain.

"We can't predict how your nervous system will respond to the EMDR stimulation, so try and adopt an open mind and just notice the sensations of your pain as best you can. Initially, the intensity of the pain may not seem to change, or it may even increase; this is just the pain response shifting in response to the stimulation. In the unlikely event that the pain increases to an intolerable level, just raise your hand like this [show stop signal]. Remember, your nervous system knows what to do, so there's no need to try and make it happen, just notice and just let whatever happens happen.

"What we will be doing often is a simple check on what you are experiencing. I need to know from you exactly what is going on, with as clear feedback as possible. Sometimes things will change and sometimes they won't. There are no 'supposed tos.' Just notice and just let whatever happens happen."

EMDR target

Develop the target based on whether pain is trauma-related or not.

a) **Traumatic Pain**

"When you think of the incident that led to your pain, what picture do you get?"

____

____

____

____

b) **Non-Traumatic Pain**

"Can you describe the pain in terms of how it feels physically?" (Suggest size, color, etc., if client needs help describing their pain.)

____

____

"Is there an image that goes with that?" or ***"When you describe your pain that way, what does it feel like? What does it remind you of?"***

____

____

Optional: Where clients are really unable to find words or images to describe their pain, ask them to draw a picture of their pain. Do not be put off by clients' objections that they are not artists; even a dark angry line can be a helpful tool in focusing the client and concretizing the pain.

The point of getting the client to describe their pain is to help them connect with it in preparation for the desensitization state. Once this has happened, there is no need to ask the client to describe it any further—in fact, there is a risk the client will go into an intellectual mode or other form of avoidance.

Negative cognition

"What does the pain (or memory) make you believe about yourself?"

____

____

Positive cognition

"When you bring up that picture or incident, or when you think of your pain, what would you like to believe about yourself now?" Do not dwell on obtaining a PC if it is not readily forthcoming—it and the VoC can also be evoked following successful desensitization/reprocessing.

____

____

____

VoC

Elicit a Validity of Cognition.

"When you think of the pain, how true do those words____ [clinician repeats the positive cognition] feel to you now on a scale of 1–7, where 1 feels completely false and 7 feels totally true?"

1	2	3	4	5	6	7
(completely false)						**(completely true)**

Emotions

Elicit the emotions.

"When you think of the pain and those words_____ [clinician states the negative cognition], what emotion do you get now?" Note, if pain is the main presenting problem, you may substitute that for the emotion (TICE/S).

____

____

SUDs

Elicit the SUDs.

"On a scale of 0 to 10, where 0 is no pain (or distress) or neutral and 10 is the worst you can imagine, how bad does your pain feel right now?"

0	1	2	3	4	5	6	7	8	9	10
(no disturbance)										**(highest disturbance)**

Sensation/location

Elicit the sensation/location. If you have already done this (e.g., when you asked the client to describe their pain earlier), you may go straight to desensitization.

"Where do you feel it [the pain] in your body?"

____

____

Desensitization

"Now I'd like you to focus on the pain (or memory) the way you've just described it, and those words [NC], listen to the bilateral tones, and just let whatever happens happen." Commence BLS (preferably continuous audio and do not cease BLS when checking in with the client until after changes plateau or the client needs a rest).

Say, ***"What do you notice now?"***

____

____

If client reports a positive difference, say,

"That's fine, just go with that."

Continue BLS and review until a relatively stable level of improvement is achieved.

If the client ever responds (particularly after the first set of BLS) that the pain is the same or nothing has changed, check that they are really basing this on a here and now felt sense of the pain rather than a memory of how they usually experience the pain.

Say, ***"Yes, okay, but I need to know exactly what you are experiencing, like when you described it before we started."***

____

____

If the client continues to report nothing is changing: 1) Ask, ***"Would you like to keep going a little longer or try something different?"***; 2) Check that their pain levels are not too high; 3) Vary the BLS modality; 4) Ask, ***"What does it feel like is stopping the pain from changing?"*** (See also Chapter 11, "Dealing with Blockages.") Play the "wild card": ***"Think of something that could take the pain away or make it feel better—don't think about it too much, just hold that thought in your head, listen to (or watch) the BLS, and let whatever comes come."*** This "wild card" target often pulls up unexpected resources which can then be elaborated on and installed in the usual way.

As long as the pain is changing, keep saying, ***"Notice that,"*** after each set of BLS.

When the pain is gone or the changes have plateaued, review SUDs and VoC.

Say, ***"On a scale of 0 to 10, where 0 is no disturbance or neutral and 10 is the highest disturbance you can imagine, how bad does it feel now?"***

0	1	2	3	4	5	6	7	8	9	10
(no pain)										**(highest pain)**

"Does it feel like you can achieve any further improvement?"

____

____

If the pain (or distress) is still a SUDs of more than 0, ask,

"What prevents the number from being a 0?"

"Go with that." Discuss whatever response is given and ask the client whether or not they would like to continue working.

Pause and ask the client what they notice now. If they report feeling better ask,

"Do you want to continue?"

If the client answers "yes" restimulate until the pain has resolved fully or the changes plateau and return to VoC. If the answer is "no," go to installation phase (either creating antidote imagery if client has residual pain or normal installation if pain is satisfactorily resolved).

Installation (antidote imagery)

Antidote imagery (a memory or image which soothes pain) is indicated where the pain cannot be completely resolved by EMDR. If the pain has resolved completely, there is no need for antidote imagery and you should go straight to the normal installation phase. If not, there are two ways to evoke antidote imagery: 1) Imagery based on sensory changes following BLS; 2) Imaginable healing resource. Unless the client is highly suggestible, the most effective antidote imagery is derived from mental associations based on how the client feels rather than suggestions from the therapist.

1. Imagery based on sensory changes

"What's there now where the pain was before? Can you describe those feelings of comfort (e.g., soft, loose, natural, etc.)?"

"What do those feelings remind you of? What do they feel like (e.g., a pool of water, a wet towel, etc.)?"

The idea is to link the feeling of relief to a memory association. Clients will say things like "wet blanket," "a Pac-Man," "an absorbent sponge." Once clients have identified a healing image, ask them to think of a word that goes with that image and install it by pairing it with BLS.

"Now think of a word that goes with that image and go with that."

Restimulate.

"How true does [repeat PC] sound?" (Or "backload" a PC if not obtained earlier.)

____

"Do those words still fit, or is there another positive statement that feels better?"

____

If the client accepts the original positive cognition, the clinician should ask for a VoC rating to see if it has improved:

"As you think of the pain (or memory), how do the words feel, from 1 (completely false) to 7 (completely true)?"

1	2	3	4	5	6	7
(completely false)					(completely true)	

"Think of the pain (or memory), and hold it together with the words__________________ ______________________ [repeat the PC]."

Do a long set of BLS to see if there is more processing to be done.

Finish up by instructing the client to practice BLS and activating and thinking of their healing imagery as often as they can when they are in pain.

2. Imaginal healing imagery

"Think of something that could take the pain away or make it better. Don't worry about whether it seems realistic or not, just let your imagination run wild."

____

____

Commence BLS while the client is still searching for an answer to the question. Cease BLS after 30–45 seconds and ask, ***"What did you get?"*** or ***"What came up?"***

____

____

"How does that make you feel?"

____

Assuming it's something positive, instruct the client to ***"think of that"*** and restimulate with BLS.

If the client can't think of anything, advise them this is just an imaginal exercise and it doesn't have to be realistic. But do not accept answers like "an injection" or "an operation"—these are not sufficiently client-based.

Once the client has focused on the healing image + BLS a couple of times with it either holding or strengthening, ask,

"Is there a word that goes with how you feel when you think of that image?"

____

Resume BLS until the client reports a stable link between the image and the trigger word and instruct the client to practice thinking of their healing imagery as often as they can when they are in pain and to try and find or add a new detail each time they do it so it becomes richer and stronger.

Note: quite a bit of review and reinforcement of pain management skills may be necessary before the client is ready to endorse the positive cognition.

Installation phase

VoC

If you skipped the PC/VoC in the set-up, say, ***"So, if I ask you to think of the changes that have happened here, what belief do you have about your ability to manage the pain now?"***

If you did obtain a VoC in the set-up phase, say, ***"When you think of the pain now, how true do those words____ [clinician repeats the positive cognition] feel to you now on a scale of 1–7, where 1 feels completely false and 7 feels totally true?"***

1 2 3 4 5 6 7

Sometimes the original PC/VoC is no longer a good fit. Ask, ***"Is there another positive statement or cognition that fits better now? If so, what would it be?"***

____

Instruct the client to ***"just think of your pain now and that thought and just notice ..."***

Perform eight slow bilateral eye movements. Check again.

"So how does that feel now?"

____

Body scan

"So, if I ask you to think of your original pain (or distress) now, how does it feel in your body? What do you notice now?"

____

Repeat back positive changes, e.g., ***"softer, smaller, cooler ... that's good."***

You should have already done this, but if any significant discomfort is still reported, restimulate with BLS or create antidote resources if you haven't already.

"Okay, do you have any idea about what's stopping the pain from changing?"

____

____

When the client reports no pain or it is apparent that the client cannot improve any further, say,

"Close your eyes and keep in mind the original memory/image and the positive cognition. Then bring your attention to the different parts of your body, starting with your head and working downward. Any place you find any tension, tightness, or unusual sensation, tell me."

____

____

Closure

"Now that you are feeling better, you are probably wondering how long the effects will last. Experience suggests that these changes can last anywhere from a few hours to being permanent. Even if the pain comes back, it is often weaker because of the way EMDR affects memory. The most important thing is to just have an open mind and pay attention to what you are feeling in the present. Many people find that EMDR helps them feel more in touch with their feelings and this can lead to increased self-care and reduced stress and pain flare-ups.

"You can also use the antidote imagery we created or bilateral stimulation by yourself to control your pain. I am going to give you a recording of this sound. Whenever you need relief from pain (or stress, or even insomnia), just play this app/audio download and concentrate on the negative feelings you want relief from, just like you did here today. The more you practice, the more you will succeed."

Clients with ongoing pain will need resources to help control that pain. See the Client Resources section at the end of the manual for various ideas about how clients with unresolved pain can cope.

Re-evaluation

Reviewing the client's experience of their pain since the last session, ask,

"So, what have you noticed about your pain since our last session?"

____

If the client says nothing, ask more direct questions.

"Have you noticed any changes in your sleeping pattern?"

____

"Have you noticed any changes in your activity levels since last time?"

____

"Have you done anything different or unusual?"

____

____

____

"Have you noticed any changes in your mood since last time?"

____

Inquire about specific areas of the client's life that they have identified as problematical or affected by their stress, trauma, or pain, such as sleep, relationships, activity levels, etc.

"Tell me about _______ [state problem areas] since the last session. What have you noticed?"

____

____

____

It is not uncommon for clients to fail to notice changes because of depression, alexithymia, or negative thinking. Asking detailed, change-oriented questions helps the client recognize those important changes, exceptions, and new trends. The therapist needs to check with clients for any changes in how they have been feeling in terms of the material that was processed at the previous session and use this as a basis for constructing new targets for EMDR reprocessing. It is not uncommon for the image of the pain to change between sessions, as the client's experience changes, particularly if progress is being made.

EMDR treatment of chronic pain is often less "successful" in terms of the kinds of dramatic treatment gains that can be expected from EMDR treatment of simple PTSD. This is not surprising: chronic pain is maintained by injury processes which are not as amenable to change as mental or emotional phenomena. Where the client is left with residual pain to any significant degree, EMDR may need to be supplemented by adjunctive pain management strategies such as sleep management strategies, exercise, resilience building, etc.

This protocol is based on the original EMDR trauma protocol, as developed by Francine Shapiro, PhD.[7]

Desensitization case example

Here is an example of what processing pain with EMDR can look like. June suffered from chronic low back pain after falling down some stairs. Although June was facing significant other stressors (attachment issues associated with being raised in a cult, financial stress, single motherhood), it was apparent that she was a very resourced, emotionally stable person. By the second session it was possible to isolate her current pain among a number of unresolved stressors and target it with BLS (based on June electing her present pain as the thing she wanted to work on first). The session went something like this:

Therapist: "So, can you describe your pain as you feel it right now, including how intense it feels on a scale of 1 to 10."

June: "The pain feels like a dark, solid ball at the lower end of my spine. It's about 6/10 which is a bit above average."

Therapist: "Okay, so can you focus on your pain the way you've just described it, and the bilateral stimulation, and just let whatever happens happen."

BLS (30–40 seconds)

Therapist: "Okay, take a break and when you're ready tell me, what do you notice now?"

June: "Hmmm [sounding surprised and confused], it feels smaller."

Therapist: [without giving her too much time to think about it] "Great, just go with that ..."

BLS (30 seconds)

Therapist: "... And what do you notice now, June?"

June: [sounding even more incredulous] "It's shrunk to like a small pea."

Therapist: [after pausing to let June notice the changes in her pain and setting her up for a positive cognition/resource installation] "Wow, isn't that amazing—see what you are capable of?"

June: "Yes."

Therapist: "And how would you rate the level of the pain right now?"

June: "About a 2."

Therapist: [running low on time] "Good, and do you think you can have less or does that feel okay for you at the moment?"

June: "I can easily live with a 2 for now."

Therapist: [trying to make changes conscious] "Okay, so can you describe how it feels now where the pain was before?"

June: [takes a moment to think] "It feels empty, blank."

Therapist: "Good, and what image goes with those feelings?"

June: "It just feels like an empty space."

Therapist: "Okay, just think of that and just notice."

BLS/DAS (20–30 seconds)

Therapist: "... And what do you notice now?"

June: "I got an image of my favorite holiday place, a snowfield in the mountains."

Therapist: "And how does the memory of that place make you feel?"

June: "Peaceful, free—all that white empty space just makes me feel soooo relaxed."

Therapist: "Good, and is there a word that goes with those feelings?"

June: "Okay. I feel okay."

Therapist: "Just think of that."

BLS/DAS (30 seconds)

Therapist: "And what do you notice now?"

June: "My whole body feels relaxed, and the pain is hardly noticeable."

Therapist: "Excellent. The changes you have experienced may last anything from a few hours to a few days. You should practice thinking of that image and the words that go with it every day. It may help if you do that while listening to the audio bilateral stimulation recording I provided you."

You can also view a video of EMDR treatment of whiplash pain at:

https://overcomingpain.com/workshops/emdr-treatment-of-pain-workshops-2022-23/

The remainder of this chapter comprises a review of the nine key protocol variations associated with EMDR treatment of chronic pain/MUS.

Pain protocol variations

As we have seen, while there is much overlap between trauma and pain, there are also significant differences (e.g., organic pathology, nociplastic pain, medical trauma) which require variations to the basic trauma protocol. Fidelity to EMDR is satisfied when variations are made with a sound rationale and/or research backing. Many of the following variations have been tested under research conditions, albeit limited. Below is a list of the 9 key variations associated with EMDR treatment of chronic pain/MUS.

1. **Pain history**

   As with PTSD, EMDR history taking with chronic pain requires screening for trauma. While trauma is a well-known risk factor for chronic pain (Fishbain et al., 2017; Kind & Otis, 2019), it should not be assumed that trauma is the only factor relevant to present pain or that physical pathology has been completely ruled out as a cause of pain/MUS. Many clients with pain/MUS have experienced some combination of trauma, neglect, health problems, and extensive medical investigations and interventions. The latter can be an additional unique source of trauma, depending on the nature of their condition and other pre-existing vulnerabilities. For example, recipients of surgery are up to five times more likely to develop PTSD than people in general.[8]

   History taking should thus include a medical history, including childhood illness and hospitalizations, medical trauma, and current health concerns. The latter can have implications for their readiness for EMDR. If, for example, the client truly believes that their pain signals an undiagnosed physical illness, EMDR would fail because the pain is "ecological". If the pain involves a significant neuropathic (e.g., post-herpetic neuralgia, post-surgical neuropathy) component, then EMDR processing of emotional aspects alone may be insufficient.

2. **Health status**

EMDR is based on the AIP model, which assumes "an inherent system in all of us that is physiologically geared to process information to a state of mental health" (Shapiro, 2002). But because of the presence of injury or illness, often chronic, it cannot be assumed that sufferers of pain/MUS have ready access to innate healing capacities or that they are sufficiently well enough to participate in what can be an energy-intensive therapy. It is therefore important to assess the client's general health status in terms of whether they have the capacity to engage with traumatic memories in the way that EMDR therapy requires. This is an additional dimension of phase two.

3. **Resourcing**

While resourcing is an element of most applications of EMDR, the increased somatic dimension of pain/MUS, together with the likelihood that clients with chronic health issues may continue to suffer from persistent pain, requires the creation of resources with a more somatic focus. These typically include pain-ameliorating imagery, accessing positive memories of comfort and well-being, and distraction and avoidance.

A useful strategy is to utilize feelings of comfort and relief following BLS (with present pain as the target) as a basis for creating antidote imagery. This simply involves asking the client with persistent pain "What does it feel like now where the discomfort was before?" and "What does that remind you of?" and then pairing their response with a PC and BLS to install. Alternatively, clients can simply be asked to think of something that could take the pain away or make them feel better, and again pair the response with BLS and/or install it hypnotically. Patients who present as exhausted may require resourcing in the form of energy-enhancing and/or affect-management strategies such as relaxation, safe-calm place, imagery, and accessing positive adaptive memory networks to stabilize them sufficiently for EMDR reprocessing.

Additional pain-focused resources include future template and hypnotic inductions aimed at stimulating healing and increased coping and functioning. Clients with persistent pain may need to practice these strategies regularly as part of their self-care (see Chapter 12).

4. **EMDR targeting**

   EMDR targets can range from past trauma to present pain, to the effects of pain. Although pain/MUS sufferers frequently have other trauma in their background, which may or may not be directly related to their current pain, the impact of present pain is often of primary concern. For the patient, uncontrolled pain is a safety issue, a kind of threat from within, which makes them feel unsafe in their own body. It must be neutralized or brought under adequate control to permit focusing on other issues. Facilitating pain reduction by targeting present pain helps with client stabilization (sense of mastery) and preparation for trauma work. Targeting present pain involves changes to the TICES which are further discussed below.

   When targeting present pain, the image may be constructed on the basis of sensory descriptors ("If your pain had a size/shape/color, what would it be?") and associated imagery ("Is there an image that goes with that?") where there is no direct trauma. Additionally, clients who have never addressed their trauma (and may not be ready to) may even find it safer to focus on physical pain/MUS rather than painful dissociated memories. Where pain is part of an unresolved traumatic memory (e.g., whiplash pain), or where there is unrelated trauma, and it is unclear where to begin with EMDR, ask the patient which problem they want to focus on first, the trauma or the pain.

5. **Substituting sensations for emotions (TICES)**

   When targeting present pain, the pain sensations may be used instead of the emotion in the target set-up. In terms of the "E" in TICES, the pain is the negative affect including how and where it is felt in the body. While there is inevitably negative emotion associated with the pain, this is not generally the focus when targeting present pain. It would be if targeting how the pain makes the patient feel about themselves, which is a different problem involving a more standard application of the TICES. It is the author's experience that asking the client to identify their pain sensations after asking them how the pain makes them feel is unnecessary and can be confusing. This variation aims to facilitate a more client-centered affect-laden target which is sufficient for reprocessing.

6. **Negative and positive cognition**

Shapiro has categorized EMDR negative cognitions into different themes: lack of safety/vulnerability, control/power, responsibility/feeling defective (Shapiro, 2012, p. 84). Trauma survivors tend to endorse NCs with themes of lack of safety/vulnerability and control/power, while pain sufferers typically endorse NCs with themes of responsibility and feeling defective (Grant, 2021, p. 107). While any client-centered NC is adequate, and there are always issues of safety and control, it is the author's experience that the negative cognition only needs to be proximate to how the pain makes the client feel about themselves and/or their ability to control it.

Chronic pain sufferers who have struggled with pain for many years may find it difficult to endorse a PC with any degree of believability. It is more efficient and effective to dispense with the PC in the set-up stage and "backload" it after successful reprocessing. Following successful processing, once the client has achieved some degree of relief and control, they generally find it much easier to endorse PCs such as "I can cope," and "I can control the pain."

7. **Continuous audio BLS**

Normally BLS is ceased during check-ins. While these pauses can give traumatized clients a necessary break during trauma processing, they may serve to take chronic pain clients "off the track" in terms of engagement with BLS. Because of the entrenched, chronic nature of symptoms in complex pain, changes may be subtle and slow in coming. Continuous BLS allows for the gradual accumulation of minor sensory changes and gives dissociated or alexithymic clients more time to attune to BLS and experience its effects.

Check-ins should be conducted every 30–60 seconds, or when non-verbal changes are noticed, or if you feel unsure about what is happening. BLS should be ceased when there are noticeable changes, or the client appears tired. This can be after anywhere from 5–10 minutes or more. If you are not sure, just ask the client, "Have you had enough or would you like a little more?" Following BLS, review and reinforce changes (see below).

Auditory BLS may be an effective alternative to eye movements when targeting present pain. The human ear is one of the oldest structures and an organ of survival because of its role in detecting non-visual stimuli.[9] EMDR expert Sandra Paulsen feels that sounds or tapping are more subcortical, subliminal, and affective.[10] The speed of the BLS should be sufficient to attract and hold attention but not too rapid as to be overstimulating. An additional advantage of auditory BLS is that it can readily be used as a self-soothing aid in between sessions for patients with persistent pain (see below). There is research evidence for this variation.[11]

8. **Tracking and facilitating effects of BLS**

The success of EMDR therapy depends upon the client's ability to notice changes in the sensory-emotional elements of their problem following BLS. Because of dissociation and alexithymia, it should not be assumed that clients are sufficiently self-aware to notice any and all changes. Close attention should be paid to both the client's self-report and non-verbal signs during EMDR check-ins. Observe changes in facial expression, decreased respiration, posture, etc., in addition to the client's feedback. Questions that direct awareness to the body ("What do you notice now?") and hold it there ("Just notice that.") are useful. Failure to detect such changes represents a lost opportunity in the sense that it can appear as though nothing is changing when in fact it is.

Positive effects of BLS can also be installed by pairing them with BLS or hypnotically or both. The author typically uses the following hypnotic phrasing to reinforce the effects of BLS:

"So you're sitting in the chair, feeling relaxed, feeling more comfortable, feeling more connected with yourself, more whole, more together, mind and body as one ... all together now ... that's it ... because you are learning how to feel more integrated ... that you can be safe ... that you can heal. And I want you to take a moment and really notice what this feels like ... a new way of being in your body that can become part of your experience of yourself more and more every day, in many ways ... something you will enjoy noticing ... just taking a few quiet moments to notice that for yourself now ... that's right." This verbal refreshing of post-BLS changes gives the patient an added opportunity to consolidate their new learnings.

9. **Self-use of BLS**

In patients with persistent pain, self-use of audio BLS "at home" may offer a safe and effective means of self-soothing. BLS is known to stimulate physiological changes associated with relaxation, decreased worry, distancing effects, and even sleepiness.[12] For appropriate clients with ongoing pain, self-use of BLS gives them a safe, effective tool for alleviating pain, stress, and insomnia which often persists in between treatment sessions. Self-use should be introduced as a self-soothing strategy (not DIY EMDR) after the client has experienced positive effects of BLS (e.g., relaxation, etc.) in session.

The author has created several apps incorporating audio (and visual) BLS (see Therapist Resources section).

11

Dealing with Blockages

What do you do when EMDR processing of chronic pain/MUS stalls or goes "off track"? As with any therapy, incorrect focus, unexpected responses, skills deficits, and dissociative responses can thwart adaptive processing. In this chapter we will review some of the most common blockages to EMDR desensitization of chronic pain/MUS and how to respond to them. Psychotherapy is always a combination of directed focus and random occurrences and the term "blockages" is just a metaphor for those (not uncommon) times when things take an unexpected turn. It will be seen that EMDR treatment of chronic pain/MUS is rarely a straightforward affair and that the need to introduce cognitive interweaves or switch therapeutic approaches is standard.

The 10 most common "blockages" to EMDR processing are:

1. Bad target
2. Alexithymia
3. Pain moves around
4. Pain increases
5. Unconscious fears

6. Dissociation
7. Safety/containment issues
8. Affect tolerance and regulation
9. Ego states issues
10. Physical pathology

Broadly speaking, there are two possible responses to stalled processing: 1) an interweave (assuming you assess the patient as fit to continue), 2) substituting EMDR processing with some other therapeutic modality, until the patient is ready for processing. With some exceptions (e.g., bad target, physical pathology), the solution to many blockages is some sort of interweave. An interweave is anything the therapist says or does to get stalled processing back on track.[1] In contrast to the core EMDR principle of "staying out of the way," interweaves involve the therapist taking an active role in stimulating responses that might not naturally occur for the patient. The first, and perhaps most common, interweaves were cognitive, Socratic questions intended to "pull up" different knowledge or perspectives. But there are now many forms of interweave, including inquiry/questioning, relational dynamics, affect regulation strategies, hypnotic suggestions, ego state work, psychoeducation, and skills training.[2]

"Bad" target

One of the most common reasons for stalled processing in the desensitization phase is that you are working with the wrong target. Simply put, the patient is not ready to process the target you have selected and created. This is a "bad" target in the sense that it is not fit for purpose. Incorrect target selection usually results in looping, shallow changes which are not sustained, and occasionally unexpected abreactions. Bad targets can happen for a variety of reasons, including patient demands ("I just want to work on this pain"), undetected dissociative phenomena, fatigue, unresolved conflict between ego states, and too many choices when working with complex presentations. Adhering too slavishly to time-oriented or worst to least worst memory categorization can also lead to selecting targets that look good on paper, but are misaligned with the patient's current needs. When working with chronic pain/MUS there is often a tension between past and present trauma: childhood sexual abuse might be the worst memory, but the patient's present pain might be a more valid target (since it represents a safety and control issue).

Renee, a high-functioning PhD psychologist, sought EMDR for various life trauma, including chronic health problems and pain. Even though she had recently lost one of her parents and was facing some other major family stressors, she wanted to clear away a lingering collection of traumatic events from her past. Due to her well-developed ability to present herself as emotionally contained, Renee's therapist assessed her as stable and ready for EMDR. She created a comprehensive hierarchy of EMDR targets and commenced desensitization. During EMDR, Renee reported modest improvements, but they were not sustained. Both Renee and her therapist had been fooled by Renee's high-functioning part, which enabled her to present as more ready to process her past trauma than she really was. Discussion of Renee's lack of progress led to parts work between her protector and an exiled part that held Renee's day-to-day needs. After some months of this, Renee became more integrated (mentally and physically) and able to participate in EMDR.

Alexithymia/inability to detect sensory changes

Sometimes clients report that they feel nothing or that nothing has changed following BLS. This can give the impression that the BLS is not having any effect—but only assuming that the client is reporting accurately on what they are feeling, which is not always the case. So try and avoid accepting responses like "nothing" or "it's the same." Given the high levels of alexithymia in chronic pain sufferers, it should not be surprising that many patients lack the ability to discern small changes in sensory/affective distress. A person who has spent years avoiding their feelings cannot be expected to be able to report accurately on the kinds of sensory alterations that drive change in EMDR. The EMDR check-in should thus be treated as a kind of body awareness training where the therapist takes an active role in helping the patient notice changes through direction of attention, observation, and even suggesting possibilities.

Say,

"Yes, okay, but I need to know exactly what you are experiencing, like when you described it before we started the eye movement."

The therapist can even ask,

"Are you sure the pain is NO different—exactly the same?" It's amazing how often clients grudgingly then admit that actually yes, it has changed a little bit. Another question that can elicit more information is to ask the client,

"What was going on in your mind while you were listening to the bilateral stimulation?"

Clients may report that they were not really attending to the BLS at all, or that they were trying to work out "what" the sound was rather than listening to it non-critically. I have a long list of possible sources for the bilateral sounds from such clients, including a metronome, a ping-pong ball, a xylophone, dripping water, etc. Unfortunately, so long as the client is trying to categorize the bilateral tones, they are not likely to be attending to or responding to them in the desired way. In such cases, the therapist needs to repeat the directions regarding listening to the BLS.

When the pain really doesn't appear to be changing, try the wild card target:

"Think of something that could take the pain away or make it better. Don't worry about whether it seems realistic or not, just let your imagination run wild."

And restimulate (without waiting for the client to say what it is they thought of).

This often seems to stimulate change. Following this, the therapist evaluates what the client is experiencing in the usual way and develops a resource.

"So, what came into your mind and what did you notice that time?"

"Good, stay with that."

Another possibility is that there is additional traumatic material that has not been brought to consciousness which is preventing the processing from unfolding. A traumatized hostage victim with trauma-related pain got "stuck" at a certain point in their trauma processing. The therapist then went back to the history to see if he had missed anything. The client then recounted witnessing a friend being tortured by their captors and how helpless and scared this had made them feel. When this was processed, the client was able to return to their original trauma and complete the processing. The floatback procedure can also be helpful when clients get stuck. This simply involves asking clients to focus on the feeling of stuckness or pain and asking when/if they can remember feeling this before (other than in relation to the present target).

If the client still reports the pain is unchanged, this may mean a reprocessing technique is not suitable (their immune system may be too depleted), but first rule out the possibility that they may have failed to attend to the bilateral stimulation properly, or they may not have noticed changes.

Pain moves around

If the patient reports their pain is moving, this may be an indication that frozen affect is being released, or that the problem is just moving to another part of the body (sometimes as part of a dissociative response). With the former, which you should assume unless you have evidence to the contrary, simply instruct the patient to: ***"Just notice that and let whatever needs to happen happen."***

Generally, the pain will cease moving once it finds the part of the body where it belongs. Process it in the usual way (i.e., continuous audio BLS with regular check-ins).

If the pain stops moving or changing during BLS, it can also help to offer some hypnotic interweaves such as: ***"Just let your body find what it needs to heal, and let whatever comes come."***

"Notice any blockages to your healing and trust your unconscious mind to help you find what you need to let go of them."

"Think of something that could make you feel better or take the pain away."

Pain increases

If the client reports that their pain increases following bilateral stimulation (rare), the therapist should cease the bilateral stimulation immediately and check with the client about what's happening. Obviously, increased pain is undesirable for the client and also distressing. A minor increase in pain is not necessarily a contraindication, and further BLS often leads to pain changing in a more positive direction. However, this should be closely monitored and if the increase in pain is distressing, BLS may need to be discontinued altogether.

Sustained, significant increased pain following BLS is very unusual and probably means that there is something wrong with the client's autonomic nervous system (since the majority of clients report decreased distress following BLS, and the theory suggests this is what should normally occur). When this happens, I interpret it as a sign that the client's pain condition is one that is aggravated by stimulation of any kind (e.g., some types of neuropathic pain) and I tend to fall back to more traditional pain management strategies (counselling, relaxation training) and try the BLS again later. One case I dealt with involved a woman with a diagnosis of capsulitis as a result of overuse. This woman reported aversive tingling and pain in her hand following BLS. She also had quite a lot of other stress in her life. I shifted from BLS to a more client-centered approach and used hypnosis and relaxation for pain management. It was also apparent that I had introduced the BLS too soon—the client really needed to talk a lot more about what was happening in her life. A few months later I reintroduced the BLS and the client responded more typically. I would also speculate that increased pain means that the pain is acute and based on real pathology and therefore not amenable to BLS. Secondly, that there is a neurological component or dysregulated autonomic nervous system.

Increased pain can also be a dissociative response from a protector part which feels threatened by the possibility of losing the pain ("being in pain keeps me safe"). In this event, the focus should shift to parts work and finding out what function the part that carries the pain serves, and how its needs could be met in other ways.

"If there is a part of you that needs this pain, I'd like to invite that part to come forward now."

"How old are you?"

"Tell me and [patient's name] more about yourself."

"What do you need?"

"Would you be interested in learning how to help [patient's name] feel safe without hurting?"

The last question should be followed by a combination of skill-building and accessing more resourced adult parts, and bringing them to help out with the situations that the pain protector part has been shielding the self from.

Unconscious fears

Unconscious fears refers to fears the client may have about what might happen if they lose their pain (e.g., that they have a serious illness which has not been diagnosed, or that they might have to suffer some other unknown form of punishment). These should have been picked up in your history and assessment, but it is always worth asking the client if they (or any part of them) is afraid of losing the pain or needs it for some purpose. For example, complex trauma sufferers tend to be afraid of any somatic change and/or may need their physical pain as a substitute for even worse emotional pain. It's also not uncommon for somatizing grief sufferers to view their pain as a way of remembering and caring—"If I don't hurt, it means I don't care." Where a subconscious (or dissociated) fear is discovered, it should of course be validated and then addressed via psychodynamic work, EMDR processing, parts work, and/or psychoeducation. It's generally useful to explore why the patient had to relegate this fear to their unconscious and bring in whatever resources were/are missing in order for them to feel they can cope.

Dissociation

As already mentioned, chronic pain sufferers typically experience some degree of dissociative phenomena such as absorption, amnesia, and depersonalization. Clients with more complex histories may also present with more severe dissociative phenomena, including more severe manifestations of dissociative symptoms found in non-PTSD related chronic pain (e.g., amnesia of childhood) and additional dissociative symptoms such as flashbacks, hypervigilance, and in the most severe cases, identity fragmentation, fugues, analgesia, and paralysis, etc. There are whole books devoted to this topic so all that can be done here is to suggest a few guidelines.

- You should have assessed what level of dissociation your client is experiencing. Although the DES is not a diagnostic instrument and results need to be considered alongside other data, I have observed the following trends:
  - Mild; non-PTSD related pain (score of 10–20 on DES)
  - Moderate; PTSD related pain (20–35 on DES)
  - Severe (score of 35 plus on DES)
- Loewenstein (1991) has listed some behavioral signs and symptoms of dissociation, including eye fluttering, changes in voice tone, mismatch between content and affect, abrupt changes in topic, spacing out, rocking, rhythmic leg or foot tapping, and amnesia.[3]

- You can generally safely target clients with mild levels of dissociative symptoms (e.g., preoccupation with pain and health-related issues, everyday amnesia, mild depersonalization) where the distress levels are within the window of tolerance. But you cannot generally target pain directly where it is associated with moderate to severe levels of dissociation.

- In cases of moderate to severe dissociation you must first facilitate safety and stabilization through emotional regulation skills, affect containment, parts work, etc. This can take a long time.

- Following initial safety and stabilization you will almost certainly need to work with "parts," at the very least the EP and the ANP, in the sense that the client's physical and emotional and intellectual responses are likely to be quite unintegrated. For example, an ANP might express frustration at not getting better while an EP is still struggling with feelings of vulnerability = feelings which are essentially being dismissed by the ANP. Parts work would require identifying these elements of the client's personality, and helping bring the vulnerable EP into awareness and coaching the ANP to be more accepting.

- Dealings with the medical system are usually significant. They may have been the only time the abused child got treated kindly, but they are often retraumatizing for adults with medically unexplained pain.

- Defensive ideas (usually unconscious), such as the body is impervious, are not uncommon and have to be challenged, especially where the client is employing harmful stress reduction techniques such as self-harm, eating disorders, substance abuse, etc.

- Dissociative chronic pain sufferers need help to feel comfortable about living in a body which is both central to their sense of self and yet also the scene of such overwhelming pain. In therapy you need to look for situations where the client feels safe to experience life viscerally and gently and slowly help them do this. For example, tracking bodily sensations and internal experiences in present time while the client recalls an enjoyable activity or experience or in response to safety or grounding exercises.

- Since the function of dissociation is to contain pain, the therapist must offer alternative strategies for containing emotional and physical pain (e.g., a box, a safe where the client can put their pain). Another strategy is to titrate affect by gently directing attention backward and forward between discomfort and comfort (see the pendulation exercise "Containing the pain with pendulation" in the Therapist Resources section).

- Where dissociation takes the form of self-harm, it's likely that you are dealing with a complex dissociative presentation requiring a comprehensive treatment approach incorporating prolonged safety and stabilization, parts work, affect regulation training, EMDR, and possibly hypnosis. Underlying trauma, dissociative responses, and conflict between ego states generally need to be addressed before any significant symptom relief can be obtained.

Safety/containment

People with complex dissociation (with or without chronic pain) have a high need for safety, both physically and psychologically. Safety generally means the absence of internal or external threat, or having some means to protect one's self from threat via a safe place, grounding techniques, self-regulation through breathing, etc. Because the dissociative client is avoidant of their feelings, the therapist can create safety by making the therapy office a "safe place" for feelings. Apart from offering a non-judgmental space, the therapist can facilitate this by tuning in to non-verbal signs and gently reflecting them back to the client. For example, saying to the client, "You sound tired." Constantly avoiding feelings is hard work and tiring. When a client sees that you see what they are feeling, it gives that part of them permission to come out into the open. So always notice the client's non-verbals as much if not more than what they are saying. How much energy are they putting into just surviving? What effect must that be having on their energy levels and feelings? Medically unexplained pain is also a safety issue (i.e., a threatening, scary experience) which they will avoid via dissociation. Dissociation is, of course, a coping strategy which both protects the individual from unpleasant affect but also effectively "fences off" the pain from potentially beneficial inputs.

After a year Sharon's therapy was stuck at the point of recounting how helpless and disabled her pain made her feel. Fragmentary details of a physically and emotionally abusive childhood had emerged, along with her determined struggle to escape through a career in nursing, which came to a crashing halt when she injured her back while lifting a patient. Sharon seemed overwhelmed by both the severity of her ongoing pain and its devastating effects on her physical functioning. Although clearly Sharon was normally in control of her emotions, now she fought to hold back tears of grief and fear. She had put on a lot of weight and, although always heavy, was now grossly overweight. It had been difficult to do EMDR because of her high pain levels and generally uncontained levels of distress which were maintained by ongoing battles with an insurance company which was always looking for ways to avoid its obligation of paying for her treatment. Sharon was single with no children. She lived in her own home which she always managed to keep looking very clean and neat. Her only support was a neighbor who would drive her to medical appointments.

One day, as she took a pause from recounting her distress about the effects of her pain on her life, wanting to probe deeper, I gently said, *"You must be so disappointed with your body, Sharon."* This statement triggered a wellspring of traumatic memories and feelings. *"I don't think I've ever had a sense of harmony with my body,"* Sharon confessed, *"I've always lived in my mind and my body followed."* Sharon recalled how she was mocked for being overweight as a little girl and how for punishment her mother once made her sweep out the front yard naked at age eight. Anyone passing by the narrow street in their rural village could see. Sharon concluded, *"Something died in me that day."* Sharon also recalled how her mother would tie her to a table and beat her up, and how her father would beat her with a leather belt.

This information was so at odds with Sharon's normal presentation, even allowing for the distress triggered by her pain, that I realized then that there were two Sharons, or at least two very distinct sides to Sharon, the wounded vulnerable Sharon who was kept hidden from the world (EP), and the strong, rational Sharon who protested against the injustices perpetrated against her (ANP). This was the part that finally told her parents that they were not her family when she was 30—followed by two days of crying. It was clear that Sharon kept these two parts separate from each other—and that this was working against her overcoming her pain. She could not rest if there was housework to be done, even though it aggravated her pain and drained her precious reserves of energy. After she completed everything to a satisfactory standard, she might collapse into bed for up to two days, exhausted. No matter how hard she fought, adult Sharon could not escape the feelings of weakness and helplessness that the pain and disability triggered in her younger ego state. The work of connecting these two ego states began with my comment about Sharon's attitude toward her body, which effectively sent her EP a message that it was safe to come out—that this person (me) could accept her. From that moment, with my help, Sharon became more and more conscious of her previously disowned physical and emotional needs. Instead of just the adult, the child ego state was also included in the conversation, sometimes through talking directly to her in front of the adult (Paulsen's "Looking through the eyes"), sometimes by talking to the adult about a child's perspective (Knipe's "Loving eyes"). Although Sharon continued to suffer from significant levels of pain, she learned to live with it rather than trying to deny it, and she felt less dominated and overwhelmed by it. She developed a new sense of self that was based on acknowledging the effects of the pain and being more self-caring and compassionate.

Affect tolerance and regulation

Affect tolerance and regulation is a major element of working with complex dissociation. One of the primary ways of assuring affect regulation is to ensure you work within the client's window of tolerance. This can be facilitated through mindfulness and micro-tracking of sensory processes to help the client learn to witness affect and sensation rather than being overwhelmed by it (e.g., *"I notice you look away when you talk about how the pain has changed your life."*). Another useful strategy for containing affect is to try and maintain a dual awareness with the client: "One foot in the present and one foot in the past." For example, when talking about stressful events or memories, always bring the client back to the present by, say, checking in with how they are feeling in the here and now, giving breaks, etc. Of course, your non-judgmental acceptance, understanding, and validation will also help with containing negative feelings—but take time to make sure the client "gets it." Just telling a dissociated client *"It's okay to have feelings"* is useless unless it is backed up with a recognition of the scariness of this and ways of making it safe. Bilateral stimulation can also be used to stimulate relaxation by targeting unassociated present affect (not consciously connected to any memory) with short sets and close monitoring. See also the "Understanding feelings" and "Basic relaxation/meditation" handouts in the Client Resources section.

Ego states issues

The third stage of working with dissociation is developing cooperation and stimulating integration between "parts." With more complex dissociation, the EP and the ANP may be split up into many parts, including vulnerable children, bullies, critics, protectors, firefighters, etc. The EP usually represents the unexpressed hurt and vulnerability the client is carrying. At the very least there will be Type 1 and/or Type 2 dissociation. At its most simple, the task is to help the client to securely connect the part that carries the pain with the caretaker part or the part that can self-soothe, as opposed to flipping backward and forward between these different states. But the process can be complicated by conflicting needs of different parts, e.g., the protector part may not want to face the pain because of the vulnerability this entails. Here are four basic steps for working with parts.

1. Introduce the concept of personality having different parts. You can make this as simple or complex as you feel is necessary, as long as it includes the notion that we all sometimes react differently in different situations, as though there are different parts of our self that cope with different demands of life, and that although helpful to a point, this division can cause inner conflict and division. And that this division arises out of our child self having to cope with insufficient love or security. Explain that this child part is present whenever our adult self feels overwhelmed, vulnerable, or inferior in its current life. The problem is that there is no relationship between the child and adult parts—they exist in an either-or dyad. Getting the parts to work together entails building a bridge so that the vulnerable part of the personality (e.g., hurt, vulnerable child) can obtain what it needs from the strong part (e.g., resourceful adult). "At the moment every time there is a problem, the strong part abandons the vulnerable part and nothing ever gets fixed."
2. Identify and name the parts, e.g., "Is there a part of you that feels confident?" "What would be a good name for that part?" "What would be a good name for the part of you that feels overwhelmed by the pain?" See Paulsen (in Forgash, p. 147) for an excellent discussion of how to "egotize" parts.
3. Obtain agreement from the parts to work together and facilitate a dialog between the parts, e.g., "Is there any part of you which might object to our working on the trauma now?" It's quite likely that a protector part will object to a process which places the rest of the system in a position of such vulnerability. They may need more safety and containment, or a mechanism to communicate with the therapist to shut down the process if things get too "hot." After each session you need to "tuck in" the parts, e.g., "I'd like to thank all the parts that have helped today. Does any part need to say anything before we tuck them in?" (Paulsen, in Forgash, p. 158). Of course, at the next session your review will have to involve checking how all the parts feel about the outcomes of the last session. What does "scared" need to feel better? Can "strong" hear this? What does "scared" need to see from "strong" to feel safe? What does "strong" need to be able to hear "scared?" Meeting places may need to be created (see also Forgash, p. 41).

One part may use pain to avoid therapy (e.g., by producing a headache). This has to be addressed (e.g., "What does that part need to allow therapy to proceed?")

4. Facilitate a process of moving backward and forward freely between the parts, based on sharing of respective needs and resources. Activate the resourced part. "What would (friend, wise adult) recommend?" Where the pain does not respond directly to being connected with positive ego states, additional work such as strengthening safe places and updating frozen ego states to the present (e.g., "You are safe now") can help stimulate new learning and reduced reliance on dissociation (see Phillips, 2000, p. 83–101, for an example).

Physical pathology

With pain you are dealing with a psychobiological problem where the contribution of biological (and/or neurological) factors is significant. With EMDR you are also aiming high in the sense that you are hoping to provide pain relief—with the exception of hypnosis, this is not a major goal of mainstream pain management treatments such as CBT. Generally speaking, the limits of what can be achieved therapeutically are set by factors such as therapist experience, client characteristics, and biology. In one of his most challenging cases involving the treatment of pain with hypnosis, Milton Erickson, perhaps the greatest hypnotherapist who ever lived, took four hours to put a cancer pain sufferer in trance, where he could experience pain relief. But even he was selective about who he worked with. Unfortunately, pain which is mainly maintained by physical pathology, and where there is little contribution from psychological factors, may be resistant to processing or amelioration via psychological methods.

Jim had a crush injury and nerve damage after his foot was run over by a car. Prior to the accident Jim was a well-adjusted successful professional with no history of trauma or neglect. His emotional distress was directly proportionate to his injury, pain, and its effects on his life. In terms of personality he was a rational, unemotional person who tended to view things in black and white. Jim simply wanted pain relief so that he could function more normally.

But he was resistant to hypnosis or imagery-based approaches, mindfulness did little, and he did not notice any changes following EMDR. Jim's case suggests some aspects of CNS functioning may not be modifiable. In addition to a trauma history, personality factors are almost certainly relevant to this, but their exact role is a poorly researched area. My research with how left vs. right hemisphere dominant people respond to EMDR (above) sheds some light on this important topic, especially given the current appreciation of the role of brain functioning in human experience, but we are far from understanding this aspect of the problem.

In general, I have found neuropathic pain minimally responsive to BLS. Neuropathic pain is associated with conditions such as post-herpetic neuralgia (nerve pain following shingles), brachial plexus injury (trauma to this set of nerves responsible for movement in the upper body), amputation, complex regional pain syndrome (CRPS), and spinal cord injury. Jack suffered from neuropathic pain after his spinal nerves were torn in a motorcycle accident over 20 years prior. He lived in constant pain of fluctuating intensity. He had tried everything, from hypnosis to Holosync. Gabapentin helped him sleep a little better. Jack's pain did not improve following EMDR.

If your client's pain does not respond to EMDR, what else can be done? Harnessing the hemispheric lateralization of pain processing, some clients with unilateral neuropathic pain can benefit from contralateral stimulation—applying measured pressure to the opposite location of the body. It is speculated that this disrupts the brain activity which maintains neuropathic pain. The effects are unpredictable and not always immediate. In addition to pain relief clients may report feeling "strange" sensations in the painful limb such as tingling, etc. It's important to reassure them this is normal and even a positive sign as it indicates the pain activity in their brain is being disrupted. Based on my experience and a few case reports, pain relief tends to be limited to a few hours (and conversely any exacerbation), but it is something which gives the client a bit of control and relief, and preferable to medication with all its inherent problems. Because of unpredictable outcomes, you should caution clients before attempting this strategy. You need to check with the client that you have got the exact opposite location and that the amount of pressure "feels right." Maintain the pressure for 10–30 minutes. Check in with the client regularly. See the "Contralateral stimulation" script in the "EMDR– strategies" at the rear of this manual. Obviously this is not suitable for clients who are aversive to being touched, unless there is a relative they trust whom you can teach the process to. I have had several cases (plus reports from attendees at my workshops) where clients have benefited from their partner learning and applying this strategy. It seems possible that with regular application (by a relative or friend) this strategy might trigger some long-term neuroplastic changes.

Hypnosis can also be effective with neuropathic pain such as CRPS. Not surprisingly, progress tends to be incremental and somewhat dependent upon containment of other stressors/ trauma.

Patients should be prepared for this. Regular listening to recorded sessions, such as the "Neuropathic pain script" in Chapter 12, is the most effective approach.

Another approach, which can be integrated with EMDR or used as an alternative with patients who don't respond to EMDR for whatever reason, is Corrigan's Deep Brain Reorienting (DBR). According to Corrigan, DBR targets deep brain stem structures such as the superior colliculus (SC), locus coelerus (LC), and the periaqueductal gray (PAG), which are associated with the orienting response (an ordered neurophysiological response to trauma). The target is the pre-affective shock, that initial neurological response to the trauma (whatever it was) that precedes affective distress and tends to remain frozen in the nervous system.[4] This involves focusing on sensations in the head such as tension behind the eyes, or in the neck, rather than lower bodily reactions, and mindfully tracking those sensations and associated material until they clear. The combination of mindfulness and neurological focus seems to create a distancing effect which facilitates a deeper awareness and ability to connect with unprocessed traumatic responses including neurological, somatic, and affective activity. In chronic pain sufferers this can lead to a release of defensive body memories which may be maintaining pain.

Summary

In this chapter we have reviewed some ways in which processing can become stalled or blocked and how to address this when it happens. Some blockages indicate that the patient is not ready for EMDR and require substituting EMDR for other modalities, while others are amenable to resolution via various types of interweaves. Muted responses to BLS, changes that don't "stick," looping, and difficulty integrating changes are par for the course in this application of EMDR, and fidelity/"getting it right" has to be balanced with flexibility and client focus. Where the client is deemed to be not ready for EMDR, other approaches such as client-centered psychotherapy, the flash technique, brainspotting, hypnosis, ego state work, and sometimes even reviewing sleep and diet may be necessary. As we are about to see, most of these approaches are readily integrated with EMDR.

12

Hypnosis

Many chronic pain clients will continue to experience some level of pain following EMDR therapy. This is quite normal—it is unrealistic to think that someone whose body has endured years of disease, injury, pain, and perhaps multiple surgeries has the capacity to become completely free of pain. Even the renowned Milton Erickson, possibly the greatest pain management therapist of the 20th century, was measured about how much relief is possible when working with this problem. Hypnosis can both enhance EMDR and afford an invaluable adjunctive strategy for managing persistent pain and its effects. Hypnosis draws upon established therapeutic practices, including the use of imagery, the idea that we have two minds, a conscious mind and a subconscious mind, and the idea that the ability to experience trance is innate, common, and beneficial. Hypnosis also involves utilizing dissociative phenomena and trance states inherent to trauma and chronic pain/MUS to create resources. In this chapter we'll briefly review the use of hypnosis as a treatment for pain, the hidden hypnotic elements of EMDR, and how to use hypnosis as an adjunctive therapy to EMDR.

A (very) brief history of hypnosis

Hypnotic states have long been used to stimulate healing and pain relief. In ancient Greece the priests of Asclepius induced unwell people into "temple sleep" via an elaborate ritual which culminated in the sick person being dressed in healing robes and sleeping in a special chamber where the walls were inscribed with the testimonials of people who had previously been healed. The word "hypnosis" actually comes from the word *hypnos*—the Greek word for sleep. There are many other examples of ritual, music, dance, and sacred places being used to induce altered states, throughout history. The phenomenal popularity of alternative medicine shows that even our modern minds remain open to non-rational healing methods.

In the modern era hypnosis dates back to the work of Anton Mesmer (1734–1815) whose view of hypnosis as a way of harnessing a cosmic force (animal magnetism) laid the foundations for the popular view of the hypnotist as a kind of Svengali figure who controls the trance experience through direct suggestion, e.g., "Imagine that there is a dial in your mind that enables you to turn the intensity of your pain up or down." In contrast, Milton Erickson took a more client-centered, naturalistic approach, e.g., "It's so comfortable to watch a plant grow and not see its growth, not feel it but just know that all is getting better ... growing comfortably in all directions." Whatever approach is adopted, hypnosis has substantial physiological effects which can be harnessed for pain control. Two of the most important physiological effects of hypnosis are catalepsy (slowed psychomotor activity) and sensory changes (anaesthesia and analgesia). Remember, increased physiological arousal and physical discomfort are two of the key dimensions of the experience of chronic pain.

What is hypnosis?

Hypnosis is by definition a special mental state characterized by suggestibility, dissociation, and absorption. Some argue whether hypnosis is a "state," or a "trait," but it's generally agreed that it is a state in which a person is more receptive to suggestions than they would be in normal everyday consciousness. Milton Erickson defined hypnosis as:

> *"a communication of ideas and understandings to an individual in such a fashion that he will be most receptive to the presented ideas and thereby be motivated to explore his body potentials for the control of his psychological and physiological responses and behavior."*

(Haley, 1973)[1]

As this definition indicates, hypnosis is not just something the therapist does to the client but rather an interaction between client and therapist. The therapist facilitates a state of receptivity (e.g., relaxation, safety, hope, curiosity), not dissimilar to the preparation phase of EMDR, which enables the recipient of hypnosis to accept suggestions more readily. Hypnosis can also involve taking advantage of spontaneous trance states and/or trance states induced by EMDR. The former involves phenomena such as capacity for distancing, absorption, free association, depersonalization, and compartmentalization. The latter involves a state of relaxed openness and free association typically observed in EMDR clients following dual focus/BLS—what van der Kolk, talking about his experience of EMDR, described as a "hypnopompic" state.

Hypnosis in the treatment of pain involves stimulation of particular mental and physiological phenomena via amnesia, dissociation, time distortion, hallucination, age regression, catalepsy, psychodynamic psychotherapy, and sensory changes, to name a few. Not unlike the AIP model, hypnosis begins by making the client aware that they have more resources than they think. This may be done by the timely use of truisms such as ***"everyone is born with a capacity to heal"*** or ***"everyone has had the experience of being surprised to discover they had an ability they never knew they had"***, or ***"you have a conscious mind and a subconscious mind, and while your conscious mind is very smart, the part of your mind that is infinitely more capable and wise is the part that controls all your bodily systems, without you ever even having to think about it, your subconscious."***

While Erickson felt that everyone was capable of entering into trance, it's generally accepted that some people are more hypnotizable than others. Spiegel has categorized three personality types representing high, medium, and low hypnotizable personality types: Dionysian, Odyssean, and Apollonian, named after Greek gods with matching characteristics.[2] Dionysian (pleasure-seeking) personalities are imaginative, trusting, able to concentrate, have a present rather than past or future focus, and are willing to go with feelings and suspend critical judgment. At the other end of the scale Apollonian (task-oriented) personalities are more cognitively oriented, organized, critical, and logical. They have a high need for control and find it harder to trust and let go. This categorization seems to correlate with McGilchrist's right vs. left hemisphere dominant personality styles mentioned in Chapter 3. A recent meta-analysis of 85 controlled experimental trials regarding hypnosis in the treatment of pain confirmed that hypnotic efficacy was strongly influenced by suggestibility levels.[3] Clinically, I find that clients who are motivated to experience hypnosis, usually as a result of nothing else having worked, are able to enter into trance despite having low hypnotizability scores on scales such as Spiegel's mind styles.[4]

Erickson's approach seems more consistent with anthropological and historical studies which suggest that the capacity for trance is innate, common, and beneficial—a foreign concept to our post-enlightenment rational minds. This "otherness" of trance, coupled with the more directive approach of traditional hypnosis, may be why the phenomenon is regarded with such suspicion in some quarters. At the beginning of any textbook or self-help book concerning hypnosis, you will find a section dealing with misconceptions about hypnosis and a disclaimer to the effect that hypnosis is not mind control. It's remarkable that a process for changing mental states has attracted such a stigma—our rather more imaginative pre-enlightenment ancestors would probably have wondered what all the fuss is about. When you view hypnosis as a state of absorption, like getting lost in a movie, or "highway hypnosis," it becomes a much less mysterious, more commonplace phenomenon. Even today, in many traditional societies (e.g., Bali), the ability to alter one's perception of reality through altered states of consciousness is regarded as totally normal (and a kind of magic). In therapy the challenge really is finding what experiences are hypnotic for your client (i.e., absorbing, enjoyable, transformational) and creating the conditions for them to experience that (e.g., via relaxation, curiosity, capacity to separate themselves from their problems, the realization that they have untapped abilities, ability to see symptoms in terms of solutions, receptivity to new possibilities, etc.). Whether or not you have a diploma in hypnosis, if you have any competence as a therapist, you must be using hypnotic patterns of communication of some sort with your clients.

Hypnosis and EMDR

Although hypnosis and EMDR are categorically different interventions, in practice there is much overlap between the two; both approaches aim to deactivate the left hemisphere of the brain, and many EMDR interventions, such as floatback, EMDR check-in, future template, and ego state interventions, owe their existence to hypnosis. EMDR check-in, for example, involves helping patients recognize physiological changes (relaxation, decreased arousal) to facilitate the change process. Hypnosis relies on a similar process wherein recipients are made aware of trance phenomena such as catalepsy to reinforce their awareness that they are in an altered state and have capacities they don't realize. So even if you don't think you know hypnosis, if you are doing EMDR you are using hypnotic strategies. As Kluft notes, "When one works with patients who have a high capacity for trance and dissociation, there is no such thing as conducting a treatment without hypnosis. Even if the therapist makes scrupulous efforts to avoid inducing heterohypnosis ... the patient's auto-hypnotic proclivities and the frequency of spontaneous trance phenomena inevitably create a hypnotic ambience."[5] While

Kluft's remarks were referring to severely dissociated persons, there would be few chronic pain sufferers who have not experienced some trance/dissociative phenomena such as absorption, amnesia, depersonalization, and compartmentalization.

There are also significant advantages to integrating hypnosis into EMDR, including for purposes of ego-strengthening[6], titrating work with dissociative individuals[7] and accessing unconscious memories or blocked information (exploratory hypnosis)[8], and resourcing (EMDR check-in as trance ratification). For example, in Chapter 9 you saw how to create resources by creating mental associations based on physical changes following BLS (trance ratification). Even a simple EMDR check-in aimed at helping the client notice changes following BLS is harnessing this fundamental hypnotic process. Patients often enter a trance-like state following EMDR reprocessing (van der Kolk's hypnopompic state), marked by relaxation, increased capacity for free association, distancing effects, altered mind-body connection, etc. In EMDR terms this marks a cessation of distress and a readiness to proceed to installation of the positive cognition. However, it also marks a special learning state, a core concept of both hypnosis and EMDR, which can be harnessed to much greater effect than mere installation of the PC. In the moments immediately following EMDR processing, many clients are also in an integrated, present-oriented state of mind and body for the first time in their life. While these learnings are often retained at some unconscious level, explicit hypnotic reinforcement of this state can greatly enhance the patient's altered relationship with their body. ***"So you're sitting in the chair, not thinking about anything, just noticing how empty your mind feels right now, and your awareness of what's happening in your body in this moment in space and time ... nowhere to go and no one to please ... totally present ... and I'd like you to take a moment to really notice what it feels like to feel at home with yourself in your body ... that's right ... mind and body as one ... maybe noticing a warm, soft feeling in the middle of your chest ... or other sensations ... naturally yourself ... and commit this awareness of yourself to memory ... so that in future you can find this sense of connection whenever you need to."***

Both hypnosis and EMDR recognize dissociation as a beneficial phenomenon. In EMDR/traumatology, dissociation is regarded (in part) as an adaptive coping strategy to protect against overwhelming physical or emotional pain. In hypnosis, dissociation is a core element in accessing unconscious resources ("you have a conscious mind and an unconscious mind"). Janet believed that hypnosis and dissociative disorders involved the same underlying mechanisms, particularly a restriction of awareness. See Chapter 2 for a detailed review of trance phenomena in dissociative responses such as avoidance, depersonalization, and compartmentalization. Janet also believed that hypnotizability was a personality trait that increased the propensity to dissociate in individuals exposed to trauma.[9] Spiegel has suggested that dissociative phenomena such as fugue and depersonalization actually represent spontaneous mobilization of hypnotic phenomena. Sadler and Woody (2010)[10] feel that dissociation in hypnosis represents a deliberate disconnect between executive control and lower functions—relinquishing higher order control in favor of lower order autonomic nervous system functioning. However, the sense of disconnection associated with trance and dissociation is different: in trance it's voluntary and present awareness remains accessible, while with dissociation there is a more involuntary and profound sense of "not being present."

Although the popular media often portrays hypnosis as some kind of miraculous cure, in most cases the outcomes of hypnosis are more modest (albeit still significant). As Patterson (2010)[11] notes, "Erickson viewed eliminating all pain through hypnosis as an untenable, unrealistic goal in most circumstances." He preferred trying to replace or change a pain sensation rather than trying to eliminate pain altogether. Erickson also preferred indirect suggestions because he felt they gave the client more opportunity to access their own resources. However, direct suggestions can obviously be helpful for many clients who just may not immediately recall the carefree freedom of floating in warm water or feeling their muscles relaxing in the sun. Although most chronic pain clients are in a state of perpetual discomfort, if their pain is within tolerable levels, they should be able to concentrate sufficiently to engage in the hypnotic process.

When to utilize hypnosis?

Hypnosis should be introduced when the patient is not ready for EMDR or when processing is stuck. Bill O'Hanlon, one of the co-founders of solution oriented psychotherapy, recommends trying hypnosis after other treatments have failed. This would be the case if the client's pain does not respond to EMDR satisfactorily. Then you would employ scripted trances as an adjunct or instead of EMDR (see below). There are two conditions where you might employ hypnosis prior to EMDR: 1) for purposes of accessing target material when the client cannot remember, and 2) for stabilization/resourcing where the client is hyper- or hypo-aroused. The former involves asking the client a series of accessing questions while they are in trance aimed at bringing forward whatever trauma or blocking belief is maintaining their pain. This can then be processed hypnotically or with EMDR (see "Accessing target material" below). The latter applies to clients with complex trauma and medical histories who are often exhausted and lack the energy necessary for engaging in EMDR processing. Hypnosis affords a gentler, more nourishing intervention which allows the client to slowly learn how to contain unpleasant affect and rebuild confidence and energy levels. This might involve trances aimed at reducing pain and its effects, managing negative emotions associated with pain, resourcing and ego-strengthening (see below).

While some highly skilled hypnotists can create effective trance experiences spontaneously, the widely differing clinical presentations and complexity associated with chronic pain/MUS generally demands structured, layered trance experiences which demand a degree of preparation and organization. Scripted trances are most likely to be required as a kind of resource for patients with persistent pain, usually patients who have a significant medical history. Trance is best preceded by an induction, a kind of relaxation process wherein the therapist orients the patient to the possibility of trance and new learning. For most people, three to five minutes should be more than sufficient—it also doesn't hurt to sprinkle in additional suggestions for relaxation and deepening during the active suggestion phase. Below you will find a sample naturalistic induction, some basic imagery for general pain, a script for neuropathic pain, and a script for managing emotional distress associated with pain. All of these scripts are presented as templates with which you are invited to add, subtract, or modify according to the individual needs of your patients.

Naturalistic induction

... Okay so just take a moment to get comfortable ... and take in a few deep, relaxing breaths ... and start to orient yourself to the idea of going inward for a while ... and leaving your everyday cares and thoughts behind ... just taking some time ... to see what you can learn about feeling different ... while you're sitting in the chair, listening to my voice, noticing your reactions to what I say ... and any physical changes you might notice ... or not notice ... because whatever you notice is just fine ... whether you notice that your breathing has changed ... or one limb feels heavier than the other ... and maybe noticing your eyelids feeling heavy ... you can let them close if you like ... allowing the body to relax the mind ... to relax with it ... without realizing how much more comfortable you can become ... noticing and not noticing ... even those feelings ... can start to recede into the distance ... as your mind goes elsewhere ... like when you step out of a forest (or building) into a wide open space, and there are so many different paths open to you ... new ways of thinking ... new ways of feeling ... new things to explore ... and you can take whatever direction is most comfortable for you now ... finding a different perspective ... where you can notice any changes in how you are feeling ... or not feeling ... no need to pay attention to anything that's not important to you right now ... other than learning how much more relaxed you can feel ... without even trying ... no need to fight your mind ... which is always aware of those sensations there for you ... so much easier to feel more and more relaxed with every breath you take ... because it's so much easier to let your body rest comfortably ... without you having to think about it ... nothing to worry ... nothing to bother ... and one part of your mind can hear and understand everything I say ... while another part of your mind can drift off somewhere else ... because you have a conscious mind and an unconscious mind ... and it is the nature of the conscious mind that it can drift ... from here to there ... and to nowhere in particular ... while your unconscious mind, the part of your mind that is infinitely more powerful ... can respond to what I am saying in a way that is most beneficial for you right now ... because you've known all along how much easier it is to learn something new when you're relaxed ... and I wonder how that special part of your mind is going to allow you to feel more relaxed ... because the mind's greatest ability is the freedom ... to go wherever imagination wills it ... and some people like the freedom of having their minds float through space and through time ... others like to drift back in time to the comfort ... of a very special soothing place ... that's prominent in their memory ... and is vivid in their senses ... while others prefer to allow their mind to become absorbed in a particular stream of thought ... that's curiously relevant to this situation now ... remembering something they had forgotten they knew ... out of all the learnings ... that will be most helpful ... in your own time and your own comfortable way ... or just paying close attention to what I am about to say ... about something that could be most helpful for your healing/feeling better ... [go to selected suggestion, from those included in this text or sourced elsewhere].

[Closure—Following the suggestion, close the session by reminding the client that they will continue to feel better and they will continue to experience new learnings and changes.]

So take a moment to reflect on whatever you have learned today ... pleased about whatever you have accomplished ... and can continue to learn ... because each time that you listen to this recording or each time that you sit quietly with your eyes closed ... your unconscious mind can bring you new gifts of awareness and comfort

... and your ability to feel different ... and then when you are ready ... in your own comfortable time ... you can return to wakeful awareness ... as much as is right for you now ...

Healing light

Light is a powerful and natural form of energy that both illuminates and gives life. You can access the healing power of light to help you feel better. (If you haven't already) take a quiet moment now to relax ... and imagine a healing light that can flood your body with a **warm, healing energy ... that relaxes and soothes any physical or emotional discomfort** ...

And you can do this easily if you remember how your body responds to the sun's light from past experiences of feeling the sun's rays on your body ... remembering the feelings of relaxation you experienced as you felt **your muscles softening ... as that warm, gentle energy penetrates your skin ... in just the right amount ... and relaxes the muscles ... everything softening ...**

The warm, healing light of the warm, soft sun ... a star beyond that reaches out and provides that **warm, soft light ... that can penetrate the organs of your body and stimulate the muscles and tissues to relax and soothe the discomfort ...**

And you know that light is a form of energy which can originate not just from the sun ... but from any object, including living beings ... meaning light can come from within you. So imagine that healing light ... coming from within or without ... **penetrating your skin and the tissues and muscles of your body ... and wrapping itself around the hurt ... and bathing it in a warm, healing energy ... calming the excitation ... soothing the nerve activity that maintains your pain ... relaxing the muscles ... feeling them loosening ... everything relaxing ... softer ... smoother** ... so smooth and clear that it disappears when you look for it ... and what appears instead is an absence of discomfort and in its place feelings of relaxation, comfort, and relief ... as you feel everything softening, looser ... **more and more relaxed ... more and more comfortable ... without even having to make any effort ...**

[Closure] And you can continue to enjoy the feelings of relief that you have been experiencing ... and learning about the power of your mind to generate the relief you need ... and every time you think of this you will feel more relief and relaxation more easily ...

Water

Water is one of the most basic and naturally healing elements—one which you can access to stimulate relief from your pain and discomfort. All you have to do is to remember the feeling of floating in warm water and feeling your muscles relax as you notice that wherever the water touches your body, you find **your body becoming more and more relaxed, more and more comfortable. Any discomfort is being washed away**. The water is comforting both your skin and deeper down into your body ... **as that heat gently penetrates the tissues of your body ... softer ... looser ... everything easing.** Like that woman whose psoriasis was healed after she took a bath in one of those natural thermal pools in Iceland, something about that unique combination of warm water with its special chemical that stimulated the healing capabilities of her nervous system ... supporting her body in just the right way.

Everyone has had the experience of gently floating in a pool of warm water, or a bath of some kind ... feeling their muscles relax as that heat penetrates and softens, floating in that warm, buoyant water ... feeling your weight supported ... **weightless state. Remembering or imagining the feeling of that warm water enveloping your body, supporting your limbs and torso. No need to make any effort to do anything ... floating ... effortlessly ... a peaceful, quiet place ... a feeling of security** ... a feeling that you know deep within yourself ... and as you float there, you can be suspended from your everyday cares and worries ... just taking time out ... nowhere to go and no one to please ... **as your mind is becoming quieter as your body feels the warmth penetrating your muscles and tissues ... washing away any tension or discomfort ... cleaning things out ... purifying mind, body, and spirit ... weightlessly supported by that warm, healing water ... feeling your stress and tension drifting away** ... the way waves drift ... from one place to another ... further and further away ...

As that warm water stimulates other changes that happen without you realizing it ... changes in your circulation ... your blood pressure ... reducing any inflammation

... everything ... relaxing, feeling more able to be comfortable in your body refreshed, or more able to sleep.

[Closure] And know that you can return here at any time, just by taking the time to rest your mind and give your body what it needs. Imagining or remembering what it feels like to float in that healing pool of water ... and relax the body and relax the mind with it ... and the more you do that the more your body will learn to feel comfortable.

You might also suggest that your client take a hot bath occasionally, perhaps with bath salts, and a lighted candle and soft music, to create the experience and reinforce the sensations of relaxing in hot water. Taking a nice hot bath is one of the more enjoyable forms of self-care!

Neuropathic pain script

Neuropathic pain is caused by damage or injury to the nerves that transfer information between the brain and the body and is a feature of many chronic pain disorders. Scientists have discovered that the peripheral nerves that connect our limbs and organs to the central nervous system have an astonishing ability to regenerate themselves, rather like neuroplasticity.

Now you are going to learn something interesting about how your mind can allow things to happen for you by accessing that part of your nervous system that takes care of your breathing, your temperature, AND your body's natural ability to repair and regrow injured nerves. Your mind is a very powerful friend to you and it can serve you in a variety of different ways. Just as neuroplasticity gives you the ability to change your brain by changing your thoughts and feelings, communicating with your nervous system can also help change things for the better.

Neuropathic pain comes from damaged nerve cells not being able to communicate normally—but nerve cells can regrow after injury. There are two special cells that are responsible for cell regrowth and communication: Schwann cells and fibroblasts. Fibroblasts are ameba-shaped cells that help with cell connectivity. Picture that ... Schwann cells are hollow, tube-like cells that stimulate cell repair and communication. Picture that ...

Normally these cells do their job automatically, but when there is injury, they need a little help to "wake up". Imagine mentally sending a signal to your (ameba-shaped) fibroblast cells to activate (sleeve-shaped) Schwann cells to guide the regrowth of axons across the injury site, and stimulate more normal nerve activity. And then seeing the axons regrowing and those nerve cells repairing themselves and communicating more normally.

And just keep imagining that **the Schwann cells activated by the fibroblasts continue to work on repairing and improving the communication between the injured cells that have been maintaining your neuropathic pain. And imagine that as they do that, the abnormal activity can gradually decrease ... reducing down ... as your nerves regrow and learn to fire more normally** ... like faulty wiring that works better after you replace the insulation. Because there is really no need for those cells to stay in that excited state ... **it's time to heal now ... so you can feel less discomfort and more comfort ...** as you continue to imagine those **cells repairing themselves and communicating more normally with each other ... everything quieting down ... softer and quieter ... as those nerve impulses become quieter and quieter ... as your mind and your body work together now to harness your body's natural healing capabilities ... naturally and effortlessly ...**

[Closure] And every time that you think of this process, your mind's ability to activate your natural healing capacities can grow in new and interesting ways ... as you remember that healing cycle: **fibroblasts activating the Schwann cells—stimulating regrowth healing and communication—stimulating calmness and relief.**

Fear reduction

This trance is designed to help reduce fear of pain, a natural but pain exacerbating emotional response. The key to managing fear is safety, understanding, being able to draw on past learnings, taking action, and maintaining an attitude of self-compassion.

After induction:

I know that you have been struggling with this problem for a while ... and that fear has been getting in the way ...

And I want you to give yourself a little rest now ... while I talk to you about many things ... which you won't find in any book ... because these things you already know deep within yourself ... just waiting to be uncovered ... which you will find most helpful ...

So even though that discomfort might seem uncontrollable, if you can learn to control your FEAR, you can lose a certain amount of discomfort ...

And I am going to show you several ways how you can achieve this ...

And with each new thing I tell you ... you will find yourself feeling less and less fearful and more and more aware of your capabilities ... to cope calmly and confidently ...

Now the first thing you need is safety ...

A safe place where you feel protected, something ... somewhere ... you can do it in your mind now ... where the scenery is just to your liking, a natural environment where you can relax and just BE ... where there are plants and animals and water and sky, something in the air that is oh so rare, not quite sure what that is but finding that it gives you a feeling of being right there, noticing a very pleasant smell ... a particular perfume ... as you rest in that place ... noticing some very soothing music ... a distant choir singing something about sleeping in heavenly peace ... all you really know is that being in that place gives you a tremendous feeling of peace and safety ... because this is just the RIGHT place for you ... to find a refuge from the world ... and as you rest safely there, you can consider this problem ... calmly and clearly ...

It's true that although it's unpleasant, a little fear is a natural response to pain ...

It's your body's way of letting you know there's danger ahead ... and what to do ...

Fear tells you what things to avoid ... as well as stimulating your fight-flight response—a state of preparedness to help you survive.

So fear is really your friend.

The question is, "How much fear do you really need?"

As Marie Curie, the discoverer of radioactivity, said, "Nothing in life is to be feared, it is only to be understood. And the more you understand, the less FEAR you will have."

So you have got to ask yourself, what is fear's purpose? What can you learn from it?

I wonder what your fear might have to say if we asked it, "What are you trying to tell me?"

And see what comes ... and it doesn't matter whether your receive that answer now or later ...

The important thing is that as you begin to understand ... what the purpose of your fear is ... you can ask that other part of your mind to give you what you need to feel less fear ... something to make you feel strong and safe ... just letting that come to you now ... a little feeling that starts somewhere in your body ... and gradually expands out ...

And everybody has experienced pain as a child and learned to fear it. And everybody knows something about managing fear, through avoidance, learning coping skills, taking action, and then learning to face their fears.

As a child you feared the dark, until you learned that darkness is just an absence of light ... not a hiding place for monsters ...

And infants fear falling over, but somehow you learned to walk and ride a bicycle ... by getting on that bike ... and falling off ... and getting back on again ... until you eventually found your CENTER of BALANCE ...

You didn't let fear stop you ... because courage is not the absence of fear—you could be fearful AND brave.

Taking action stimulates feelings of power and control ... and you have done this many, many times ...

Realizing what action you need to take NOW ... even if that is simply to do NOTHING ... other than to look at things in a slightly different way ...

While your subconscious mind ... that part that controls all your bodily systems ...

That knows how to feel pain and how to not feel pain ... by releasing its own natural painkillers ...

Can work together with your conscious mind now ...

To think of something that could neutralize that fear and discomfort ...

Your own pain antidote that has all the right qualities to shrink, smooth, soften, cool, and dissipate that discomfort there ...

Just letting that come to you however it comes ...

And as you discover that, you will feel less and less afraid ... and more and more relaxed ... as you learn that you have all the resources and knowledge you need ... because, as **you probably know, the thing about fear is that although you feel it NOW, fear really comes from a learned reaction to something scary from your PAST, which is now influencing how you see your FUTURE ...**

And even then sometimes pain is unpredictable ... like the weather ... which is always changing ... unpleasant one moment and calm and quiet the next ... without anyone really knowing how or why ...

Just like your body ... because everything that happens in your body is part of your body's natural systems of balance ...

Scientists have discovered that chronic pain sufferers are better able to survive threats in the wild ... because of their hyperalert nervous system ...

Like your immune system ... which acts to protect you from infections ... but sometimes becomes too active ...

And calming an overactive immune system is not so hard ... you just have to relax and release the tension ... by creating the right conditions ...

Like that man whose psoriasis was cured by bathing in one of those thermal pools in Iceland ... immersing himself in that warm water ... relaxing the muscles

... feeling that warmth penetrating his body ... and letting his body respond to that unique combination of warmth, water, and natural minerals ... so that three hours after he emerged from the water, his skin was completely healed ...

All you have to do is immerse yourself in the right conditions for healing to occur ... taking a bath in the waters of your own healing needs ... working with your own healing team ... Dr. Quiet, Dr. Diet, and Dr. Merryman ... to give to yourself all the physical, mental, and emotional resources that you need ... everything in balance ...

And the more you surround yourself with those healing conditions, the more you will realize that ... fear can be tamed ... once you understand its purpose and what to do about it ...

And maybe there you will find the greatest antidote to fear ... a force that brings happiness, contentment, peace, and joy ... and that force is LOVE ...

Love that melts all fear and tension, love that overwhelms all discomfort and suffering with its warm healing energy ...

Taking that love for yourself now ... because the love you make is equal to the love that you take ... to the part of you that needs it most ...

Accepting that part—with loving kindness and compassion ...

Because love is not a feeling, love is as love does—it's an action you take toward yourself.

Accepting that vulnerable needy part ... giving that part of yourself the support it needs ...

And feeling the fear melting away ... as you clear away any remaining obstacles to your self-healing ...

... You are going to be okay ... you can survive ... you are stronger than you think ...

And in future fear will come less, and when it does come you will understand its purpose and be able to find what you need ...

To take whatever action is necessary to resolve that fear ... and feel more and more safe and secure ...

Based on everything you have learned about overcoming fear ... and balancing your needs ... which will continue ...

Just taking a moment to check that there is nothing else that you need to give yourself ...

And then when you are ready, you can return to normal consciousness, pleased about what you have learned about managing fear ...

And the changes you have begun to experience.

Exploratory hypnosis

Chronic pain expert and hypnotherapist Dabney Ewin feels that chronic pain can be overcome by addressing unresolved stress reactions associated with the onset of pain.[12] Ewin notes that chronic pain often commences under three stressful conditions: 1) mental disorientation, 2) threat of injury or death, and 3) acute pain. The pain sufferer may be unaware of the contribution of these factors to their pain due to dissociation or amnesia. Consistent with trauma-based approaches, Dabney feels that if just one of these factors can be identified and addressed, the pain can be ameliorated, if not reversed. The following process uses trance and ideomotor signals to help a client access and release unconscious trauma that may be maintaining their pain. Ideomotor signals (nodding or moving a finger) are simply designed to help the client communicate simple yes-no answers without talking so as not to disrupt their trance experience.

1. Induce trance using a relaxation process or the naturalistic induction process (three to seven minutes). Include some sort of statement to the effect that the purpose of this process is to help access any old memories or trauma that might be maintaining the pain and that there is no right or wrong here; we are just trying to help you to access a hidden part of your mind that might know something that might be able to help you feel better.

2. I am going to ask you some questions with yes-no answers. You can just nod your head for "yes" and shake your head for "no." (You can substitute moving different fingers but in this age of working via Zoom I find getting the client to move their head a more easily visible way of communicating.) Note: If the client gives a "no" response you stop the questions and ask the client why they don't feel able to proceed and what they need now. Do not resume the process until you have dealt with whatever issue the client raises.
3. Are you ready to find out if there is anything in your subconscious mind that might be maintaining your pain? Y/N
4. Does your subconscious mind know whether your problems are related to some past event? Y/N
5. Are you ready on a conscious level to know or remember what that event was? Y/N
6. Can you direct your conscious mind to that time? Y/N
7. (If "yes") So just take a moment to see what was happening and let me know (by nodding or signaling with your finger) when you feel ready to continue ... Y/N
8. Great. And are you ready to resolve this problem with EMDR or hypnosis? Y/N
9. (If "yes") Great, so just take a moment now to find whatever it is you need to resolve that issue and let that in ... and let whatever needs to happen ... until you can let it go ... and take all the time you need ... and when you are done just let me know by signaling in the usual way ... Y/N
10. Great, well done. Now I'd just like you to take a moment to check if it feels like there are any other issues or memories that might be connected to your present problems that still need to be addressed? Y/N
11. If "yes," repeat step 9.
12. If "no": Great. So, is there any reason for these symptoms to persist? Y/N
13. If "yes," explore/repeat step 9.

    NB: If hypnosis is not working, check if client would prefer EMDR.
14. If "no": Great. So just take a few moments to review what you have learned and absorb those new learnings as deeply as possible, so that when you return to normal consciousness in a few moments' time, you will bring with you those new learnings which will help you continue to feel better now and in the future.

Mary, a 25-year-old female fibromyalgia sufferer, had few memories of her childhood and no conscious memories of any trauma associated with her pain, which had developed in her late teens. However, she could recall having recurring nightmares as a child and she had struggled with sleeping problems and fatigue since her early teens. Mary was a very willing and motivated subject for hypnosis, as after seeing dozens of doctors and allied health professionals, she was willing to try anything to get to the bottom of what was causing her pain. Using the above process, she recalled some trauma involving her father, which we were then able to process with EMDR. Following several months of treatment incorporating some additional hypnosis and ego state work, Mary's fibromyalgia was largely resolved, and her energy levels and confidence increased dramatically.

Summary

In this chapter you have been introduced to the how, what, and when of using hypnosis to address unconscious factors that might be maintaining pain, guided imagery to address pain as a symptom, neuropathic pain and somatic aspects, and resource creation and installation. In most cases hypnotic interventions will need to be used on a daily basis as part of the client's ongoing pain management. Recordings of live hypnotic sessions (incorporating a variety of suggestions) should be provided and listened to regularly. My *Overcoming Pain* app incorporates recordings of some of the scripts in this chapter, plus additional ones. Many more scripts are available from the books and audio page of my website (https://overcomingpain.com/emdr-music-books-store/).

An excellent text for clients wishing to learn self-hypnosis is Bruce Eimer's *Hypnotize Yourself Out of Pain Now!* For therapists, Eimer also runs hypnosis courses for treating pain: https://hypnosisce.com/hypnosis-courses/hypnosis-for-pain/

For a quick and easy introduction to hypnosis I also like the work of Karl Smith who is the principal of the UK Hypnosis Academy.

13

Adjunctive Strategies and Treatments

In addition to being an integrated approach, EMDR treatment of chronic pain/MUS is usually associated with other external treatment inputs, including medical and allied health such as medication, physiotherapy, exercise, diet, etc. Self-care in the form of attention to social relationships, sleep, diet, and spirituality are all necessary in supporting the individual with impaired health toward healing. Self-care rests on having an attitude that "I am worth it," which is not always how chronic pain sufferers feel about themselves. Beliefs about self-worth should be addressed (through EMDR, hypnosis, or other ego-strengthening strategies) prior to addressing external self-care inputs. Making the commitment to ensuring one has adequate rest, nutrition, and emotional and spiritual well-being comes much more naturally when the individual feels that they deserve to have their needs met.

Where chronic pain is associated with injury or illness, and is persistent, psychological treatment often occurs alongside other therapeutic inputs, some provided by external sources (e.g., physician, physiotherapist), and some self-directed (e.g., managing sleep, exercise, diet). The therapeutic parameters should not be limited to processing pain-related trauma and/or other adjunctive strategies but should include attention to multidisciplinary health-related external inputs.

- Has the patient had all appropriate tests and investigations?
- How satisfied are they with the medical treatment they are receiving?
- How confident do they feel to engage other allied health providers (e.g., naturopath, dietician) where appropriate?
- How much responsibility are they willing to take for managing lifestyle issues such as exercise, diet, and sleep, to support health and healing?
- What life goals sustain them?
- How resilient are they?
- How able are they to feel positive emotions such as joy?
- How able are they to find the "silver lining" in negative circumstances?

Sleep

Sleep is a basic human need, necessary for physical and emotional functioning. Good sleep is not a luxury—it is necessary for physical rejuvenation, immune functioning, mood, and thinking. Restful sleep facilitates:

- The production of serotonin and other mood-enhancing chemicals
- The production of growth hormones
- Immune functioning
- Memory consolidation and learning
- Increased supply of oxygen and nutrients to damaged cells and muscles (via increased blood flow)
- Increased production of prolactin (an anti-inflammatory)
- Decreased levels of stress hormones such as cortisol

There is extensive evidence that poor sleep impairs healing.[1] Research regarding the benefits of improved sleep for healing is mixed,[2] but it's hard to imagine that a good night's sleep doesn't help. One study found that good sleep predicted a two-fold remission rate from widespread chronic pain.[3]

Human sleep is a complex, multi-staged process involving two basic types of sleep: rapid eye movement (REM) sleep and non-REM (NREM) sleep. Sleep begins with a gradual descent through drowsiness, light sleep, and eventually into deep sleep. These first four stages (NREM) are the most restful and involve decreased heart rate, body temperature, and brain activity. NREM occurs during the first third to half of the night and is the most restorative type of sleep. The amount of NREM sleep a person needs increases when they are sleep-deprived. REM sleep involves increased brain activity and increased physiological activity, including rapid eye movements. REM sleep is also thought to be necessary for memory consolidation. REM sleep occurs cyclically throughout the night, alternating with NREM sleep about every 80–100 minutes. Most people sleep about seven hours, **two of which will be in REM sleep.**

The sleep cycle is determined by an innate 24-hour body "clock" known as a circadian rhythm. The term comes from the Latin *circa* or "about" and "dia" which means "day": it literally means "about a day". Circadian rhythms are affected by the amount of light the body receives. At night the body produces certain hormones, in response to darkness, which trigger sleep. In the morning, sunlight stimulates wakefulness. Circadian rhythms can be disrupted by stress, jet lag, shift work, and even being woken up by an alarm clock. The sleep cycle is also partly determined by your body's own inbuilt homeostasis mechanisms. For example, the more time that has elapsed since someone last slept, the sleepier they will feel. Figure 13.1 shows the 24-hour circadian rhythm, including the proportion of time spent sleeping each day.

Chronic pain can disrupt the normal sleep cycle in the form of trouble falling asleep, night waking, non-restful sleep, and irregular sleeping patterns. Disturbed sleep can exacerbate pain. Physiological studies of chronic back pain sufferers show they have an arousal disturbance in their brain waves so that they awaken feeling unrefreshed.[4] Lack of sleep is known to be associated with decreased immune functioning, decreased ability to metabolise glucose (blood sugar), decreased cognitive abilities, and even decreased emotional intelligence.[5] One group of researchers found that sleep-deprived people exhibited decreased self-regard, independence, capacity for empathy, and impulse control, and found it harder to relate to others. Sleeping problems, particularly with stage four NREM sleep, have also been found to induce musculo-skeletal pain.[6]

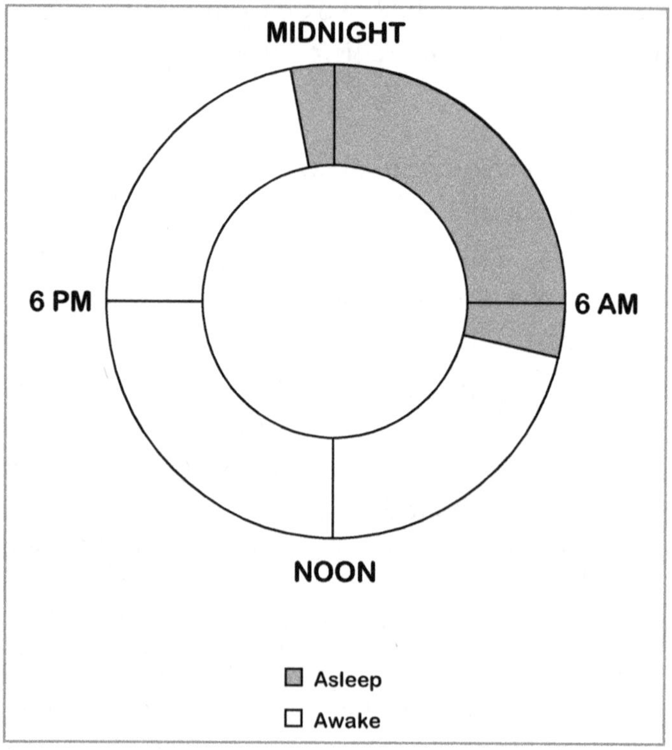

Figure 13.1 The circadian sleep cycle

Sleep management

Sleeping problems have been identified as the #1 contributor to somatic problems in PTSD sufferers. Learning how to sleep well again can greatly reduce the impact and severity of chronic pain.[7] The Talmud (an ancient Jewish text) lists sleep as one of the most important activities for healing a sick person.[8] There are many strategies for facilitating normal sleep, including sleep hygiene, hypnosis, and "free-sleeping." Sleep hygiene simply means making sure that the client has a comfortable mattress, a quiet dark room, etc. Self-hypnosis involves the use of a hypnotic trance to induce sleep. Learning self-hypnosis has many benefits—it helps develop concentration, mindfulness, and relaxation skills. In terms of using self-hypnosis to facilitate sleep, one of the simplest, easiest trance inductions is "Mrs. Erickson's Induction," developed by Elizabeth Erickson, wife of Milton Erickson. This induction utilizes the senses to create a trance-inducing sensory feedback loop. It is very effective.

Mrs. Erickson's Induction

- Begin by making yourself comfortable and finding something to focus on. For example, one corner of a door frame, a light switch, etc. Then, maintaining your focus on that spot try and notice 4 things about that object or spot and mentally feed them back to yourself.

  For example, "Right now I can see the light switch is white, right now I can see the shadow at the edge of the switch, right now I can see the switch is a square shape, right now I can see the switch is in the off position ..."

- Next, try and notice all the things you can hear. Make 4 statements to yourself about that.

  For example, "Right now I hear ... the sound of the air-conditioner," "Right now I hear ... the sound of the clock ticking," "Right now I hear ... voices in the next room," "Right now I hear ... cars passing by outside."

- You must use the phrase "Right now I notice ..." before each item. These words help create the mental separation from experience which is one of the essential elements of the hypnotic state.

- Next, try and notice all the things you can feel physically. One at a time, repeat mentally to yourself, "Right now I notice [details]," e.g., the feeling of my hand on my lap, etc. Repeat this process 4 times.

- Next, go back to the start and repeat the process, starting with the visual stimuli you focused on originally, but this time you only have to find 3 things (e.g., "Right now I notice ... [x 3 things you notice about the spot you are focusing on]" and then hearing, "Right now I can hear ... [x 3 things you can hear]," and things you can feel, "Right now I notice ... [x 3 things you can feel]."

- Then repeat the process again, but this time you only have to find 2 things. Then repeat the process again, looking for one thing. Note: you will probably run out of different things to see, hear, or feel, in which case you are allowed to repeat something you used earlier. But *try* to find something different—you may be surprised at how much more you can notice that at first seems obvious.

- At some point your eyes will feel tired. Close them and continue making statements about your ongoing experience although the visual representations you may be most aware of with your eyes closed will probably be from your imagination. You can carry on with these internal descriptions just as effectively, finding increasingly finer descriptions within your sensory experience. What you are creating is a biofeedback loop.

Another strategy for facilitating sleep is to guide clients in the use of auditory bilateral stimulation to alleviate physical and mental stress that might be inhibiting sleep. This application of BLS is another benefit of self-use which many people appreciate. It often starts in the therapy session when the clients reports feeling drowsy after BLS. If you feel this is a client who can safely utilize BLS, simply instruct the client to play auditory BLS when they go to bed and allow the sounds to disrupt their painful thoughts and feelings in the same way they did in the session. Add that when they start to feel sleepy or like they have had enough, they can just turn off their equipment and allow nature to takes its course. This application of BLS is simply harnessing two of its most well-known effects: decreased ability to think and relaxation effect. A free BLS audio can be accessed via my *Sleep Restore* app (Android and IOS).

Getting restful sleep is another aspect of sleep that you can improve. Once we are asleep the real work of sleep begins, physical and mental replenishment of the mind and body. The following hypnotic script will help retrain your client's nervous system toward a more normal sleep cycle. As with all the hypnotic scripts in this text, a recording should be made with the patient, perhaps interspersed with some personal suggestions, which they can replay as necessary. Patients often return saying they heard things when they replayed the recording that they didn't hear the first time, and that the benefits of listening to such recordings accumulate over time.

Improving quality of sleep trance

[Preamble] Good restful sleep is a process which involves your nervous system transitioning through several different states necessary for physical and mental replenishment: Relax, Rest and Restore. Sleep begins by transitioning from normal wakefulness to a state of deep relaxation, followed by a period of physical rest, followed by a brief period of intense activity as your brain sorts through what it needs to keep and what not before restoring you back to an integrated state of mind and body. Your nervous system goes through this cycle several times, during sleep. Sometimes stress and pain can disrupt the body's ability to do this, like a washing machine with faulty software. So today we're going to give your nervous system a little reset to help it give you the restful sleep you need and deserve.

Sleep is as much a journey as a destination ... and like any journey it involves different stages ... relax, rest, restore, and repeat ... several times every sleep cycle.

Tonight you're going to retrain your nervous system to go through a full sleep cycle including all the necessary stages of rest and repair that will enable you to awaken feeling refreshed and relaxed ... starting by getting as relaxed as possible ... by taking a few slow deep breaths ... in your own time ... and your own comfortable way ... that's it ... as you focus on my words ... getting comfortable ... as comfortable as it is possible for you right now ... which means focusing on whatever can help you be more comfortable and ignoring everything else ... taking that first step toward sleep ... such a small step that you hardly notice that your breathing has slowed down ... and your heartbeat ... and your muscles becoming looser and maybe your eyelids feel a bit heavy ... and your thoughts slowing down too ... and even your brain waves are slowing down ... entering the theta range ... as your conscious mind and your unconscious mind start to work together a little more separately ... as one part of your mind can hear what I am saying while another part of your mind can drift off someplace else ... drift, dream away ... where letting go allows the soft drifting downward ... where your mind can respond however it wants to ... in whatever way it needs to ... to help you find what you need to sleep naturally and effectively ... and know that whatever happens is just your nervous system doing what it needs to do ...

... and if there is anything missing that you need to know to help you relax and let go in the way that you need to, you can take a moment to find that for yourself now ... just letting it come to you however it comes to you ... so that you can enter the next stage of sleep ...

[1 minute]

Now entering the next stage of non-REM sleep, a slightly deeper stage where you will rest a bit longer but can still awaken easily if necessary for any reason. Now you can notice your heartbeat and breathing slow down even further, and your body temperature dropping a little ... as your mind and body become even more relaxed ... and your thoughts slowing down even more ... as your brain activity changes too ... into sleep spindles and K-complexes that signal that your conscious mind is entering a more synchronized state ... meaning that the physical changes you have been experiencing are coupled with changes in your brain ... like a kind of inner resonance ... everything working together ... as your whole nervous system transitions from one state to another ... getting ready for the next, deepest stage of sleep ...

... and if there is anything missing that you need to know to help you relax even more and enter that synchronized stage of sleep you can take a moment to find that for yourself now ... just letting it come to you however it comes to you ... finding what you need to enter this stage of sleep ...

[1 minute]

In this final deepest stage of non-REM sleep, your heartbeat and breathing are at their slowest rate ... your body is fully relaxed ... your muscles are soft and loose ... your conscious mind is asleep and your whole nervous system is engaged in allowing you to derive the benefits of sleep ... everything is working together for you now ... your brain waves have entered a slow and deep delta frequency as your nervous system makes the changes associated with transitioning into a deep sleep. What Shakespeare meant when he described sleep as "nature's great second course, chief nourisher in life's feast." Your nervous system also conducts important health promoting tasks such as tissue repair and growth, cell regeneration, and strengthening of your immune system in this stage ...

... and if there is anything missing that you need to know to help you enter this most restful stage of sleep you can take a moment to find that for yourself now ... just letting it come to you however it comes to you ... finding what you need to enter this stage of sleep ...

[1 minute]

And now that your body has had some rest, you are ready to enter REM sleep—the "dreaming" stage of sleep where your brain completes the mental work of sleep—integrating new learnings with what you already know and discarding what's not necessary. In REM sleep your nervous system enters a state of increased arousal as your sensing and thinking minds work together to bring together everything you need to resolve any trauma or conflict that might be bothering you. In this stage of sleep your breathing and heart rate will be increased, which your conscious and unconscious minds can know is completely normal ... nothing to be worried about. Drift, dream away ... and in this dreaming state you will have a special dream—one that will help you find the solution to a problem you have been struggling with—like how Einstein discovered the theory of relativity after he dreamed he was skiing down a hill and he noticed that the faster he went, the more the stars changed position relative to each other. So although the dream will seem strange, at some deeper level your unconscious mind will know what you need to do ... to cope with that challenging situation. Even scary dreams can be helpful—it's all just part of your nervous system processing mental and emotional information and it will result in new learning without your conscious mind understanding how it happened.

And you will notice that after you awaken from a full sleep cycle you will be less fearful and more energetic and more confident and more able to solve problems. All you have to do is drift, dream away for a while and trust that your unconscious mind will take care of things. And I wonder what messages might come in your dreams? What surprising new ideas or possibilities you might discover that will help with your healing? Because we've all had the experience of being surprised by some new insight ... that changes everything ...

... and if there is anything missing that you need to know to help you enter the dreaming state of sleep you can take a moment to find that for yourself now ... just letting it come to you however it comes to you ... finding what you need to have your dreams ...

[1 minute]

And then you can return to the beginning and start the whole Relax, Rest and Restore cycle again. And the more that you do this the more able you will be to pass through each stage of sleep normally and safely, trusting that your nervous system can find everything it needs to allow you to pass through all the stages of sleep safely and thoroughly, allowing you to enjoy all the physical and mental benefits of sleep that each stage has to offer. After which you will awaken feeling rested and ready to face the challenges of life in the best way possible for you.

So take a moment now to prepare your nervous system for taking all the necessary steps to enjoy a good sound sleep where your mind and body can experience the full cycle of relaxing, resting and restoration ... Relax, Rest, Restore ... that's it. As you continue to drift down toward deeper relaxation and sleep, which will give you the physical and mental rest and restoration you need ... until it's time to awaken, feeling rested and ready to face life.

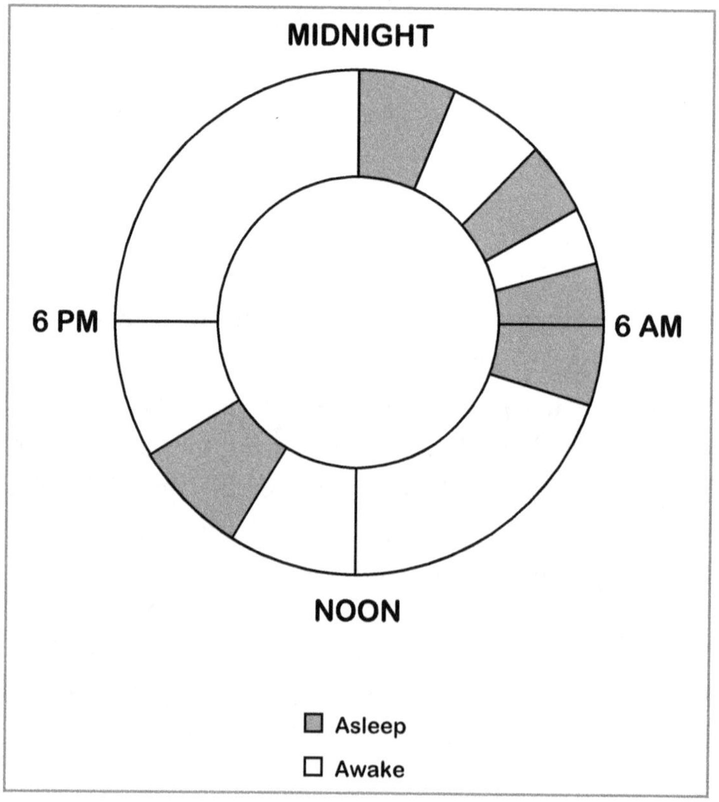

Figure 13.2 Free-sleeping

Another strategy for managing sleep is to just accept that normal sleep is not possible and sleep where and when one can. "Free-sleeping," as it's known, means giving up on the idea of normal sleep and adapting to a fragmented, changeable sleep pattern. Free-sleeping is based on "poly-phasic" sleeping, used by solo yachtsmen who can only sleep in 45-minute chunks because that's how long it takes for a ship to reach them from over the horizon. People suffering from sleeping problems mainly just want to get back to sleeping normally. But for a person affected by chronic pain who may be cycling between episodes of pain and less or no pain, they are living with an ongoing threat. It is not hard to imagine that their nervous system finds it hard to shut down in the way that is necessary for normal sleep. It's rather like trying to fall asleep in a bear cave! Free-sleeping offers a way to get more sleep over any given 24-hour cycle, just not in a normal way.

Free-sleeping begins by changing the way you (and your client) think about sleep, and the relationship between sleep, waking, and activity. Sleep becomes the priority, which can be entered into at any convenient time of day or night, anywhere (the couch, the kitchen floor, whenever your body's sleep button is activated, wherever it happens). Life has to fit around this, which is the opposite of how most people think about sleep. This may seem like a crime if you were raised in a culture which regards napping as a sign of laziness—but what about the fact that you are only getting three or four hours' sleep out of 24? Where's the balance? Yes, but won't the client then learn bad sleeping habits? Arguably bad sleeping habits are better than none—a rested person copes better with pain than a tired one. See the "Free-sleeping tip sheet" in the Client Resources section at the rear of this book.

Exercise

Another adjunctive treatment strategy is exercise. Most chronic pain sufferers have reduced their physical activity in order to avoid aggravating their pain. Or they may simply not exercise because they are too busy doing other things. Not exercising causes a number of problems, including physical deconditioning, reinforced feelings of helplessness, decreased mental functioning, and neuronal atrophy. Human beings need to move. It is through movement that we accomplish the basic tasks of life: working, loving, and playing. Regular physical activity stimulates cardiorespiratory and muscular endurance, flexibility, reduced body fat, improved physical function, and decreased depression and anxiety. Exercise also decreases the risk of chronic conditions such as coronary heart disease, diabetes, obesity, hypertension, stroke, colorectal cancer, breast cancer, and osteoporosis. Regular physical activity is also known to help reverse brain activity associated with stress, illness, and pain.[9, 10]

Exercise also builds stress resistance. In the 2008 best-selling book about exercise and the brain, *Spark*, Harvard psychiatrist John Ratey describes how physical exercise can supercharge (provide a "spark" to) mental circuits to neutralize stress, sharpen thinking, lift mood, and so on.[11] Ratey describes how physical activity increases levels of tryptophan in the bloodstream and thus serotonin in the brain. It also balances dopamine, norepinephrine, and synaptic mediators such as BDNF. Whereas neurotransmitters such as serotonin and dopamine enhance mood and energy levels, BDNF actually helps build and maintain the infrastructure of cell circuitry. Not surprisingly, most treatments for depression, including antidepressants and ECT, act to boost BDNF levels in the hippocampus. MRI studies of people undergoing exercise regimes found that the capillary volume in the memory area of the hippocampus (an area of the brain which is susceptible to damage by stress) increased by 30%. Exercise also turns on the genes that produce GABA, which puts the brakes on excessive cellular activity associated with stress. Regular exercise also stimulates the production of IGF-1 (insulin growth factor), which increases neuroplasticity and neurogenesis in the hippocampus.

Exercise and pain

Exercise has also been found to reduce stress and pain. In one famous study in 1999, researchers at Duke University found that exercise was just as effective as Zoloft in alleviating depression.[12] The exercise group was assigned to supervised walking or jogging, at 70–85% of aerobic capacity, for 30 minutes (not including a 10-minute warm-up, and a 5-minute cooldown), three times a week. Around half of the people who exercised overcame their depression completely, a similar proportion to those taking medication. The researchers concluded that exercise is just as effective as anti-depressants for treating depression. A survey of 1,800 women who suffer from PMS pain found that at least half of them use exercise to alleviate the symptoms of PMS. In addition to decreased pain, the women who exercised regularly also had better concentration and mood. Another study found that exercise in waist-high warm water decreased pain and improved health-related quality of life and strength in the lower extremities in women with fibromyalgia.

The benefits of exercise vary according to what type of pain the client has. Exercise therapy seems to be slightly effective at decreasing pain and improving function in adults with chronic low back pain, particularly in health-care patients. With acute low back pain, exercise therapy is as effective as either no treatment or other conservative treatments.[13] Patients with complex medical conditions who exercised needed fewer medical consultations.

Why exercise?

Regular exercise of some kind is a vital treatment ingredient for most chronic pain sufferers. Clients need to be educated about the wide range of benefits that accrue from exercise, in addition to the obvious physical benefits. Exercise has mental and emotional benefits which are as important, if not more so, than its physical effects. Many people find the notion that exercise will benefit their brain functioning even more appealing than its effects on their physical well-being. Below is a brief summary of the benefits of exercise:

Neurological:

- Increased dopamine, serotonin, BDNF and GABA
- Increased brain resources
- Rerouting of brain circuits
- Enhanced brain functioning

Psychological:

- Distraction
- Learning different outcomes
- Increased self-confidence
- Increased social support

Physiological:

- Increased blood flow
- Reduced muscle tension
- Increased strength, flexibility, range of movement

In terms of the amount of exercise necessary, health experts recommend that adults engage in at least 30 minutes of moderate physical activity five days a week. This may not always be possible for persons severely affected by chronic pain, but some activity should be attempted. There are different levels of exercise, from low intensity (walking), to moderate intensity (jogging), to high intensity (running). Walking is an easy, effective way to start exercising. Aerobic exercise ideally requires four 30–60 minute sessions per week. Aerobic exercise of this intensity will burn fat and stimulate the structural changes in the brain discussed above. Weights or strengthening exercises such as tennis, dancing, or running are good. Exercise which involves complex motor movements, such as dance or martial arts, seems to benefit both body and brain. Yoga, Pilates, Tai Chi and martial arts are all good for balance and flexibility. Obviously the amount and type of exercise needs to be appropriate to the client's physical condition and they should consult a physical therapist for advice.

Pleasure and pain

Another well-known strategy is encouraging pain clients to engage in activities which stimulate pleasurable emotions. Chronic pain sufferers have often forgotten how to enjoy themselves as a result of avoiding activities which might exacerbate their pain and/or depression. Either way, they have no positive emotional inputs with which to counteract the effects of their pain. Somehow their capacity to absorb positive affect needs to be reactivated. The power of *experiencing* something enjoyable as a way of alleviating pain was dramatically illustrated in a recent research study in which participants were asked to rate their pain while viewing either pleasant or unpleasant pictures (pain was induced by having participants hold their arm in freezing water). The participants who viewed the pleasant pictures reported experiencing less pain than those who viewed the unpleasant pictures.[14] Pain can also be reduced by seeing or remembering pleasant events, including movies, pictures, music, and even reading pleasant statements. A legendary example of this comes from the story of the "African Violet Lady" of Milwaukee.

Mary was a lonely, depressed old woman after the death of her husband some years earlier. One day she received a visit from legendary hypnotherapist Dr. Milton Erickson, after a call from a concerned relative. As he entered the house, Erickson noticed that all the window shades were down so that hardly a chink of light came in. He also learned that Mary was a Christian and that she used to like growing cuttings from African violets. Taking advantage of Mary's religious beliefs, Erickson suggested that it would be the Christian thing to do to give cuttings of violets to people in the community who were sick or bereaved. Somehow Mary liked this idea and by the time she died 10 years later, she had become famous as the "African Violet Lady" of Milwaukee. As a result of this activity, Mary ended her life feeling fulfilled and happy. Several hundred people attended her funeral.

As Mary's story demonstrates, the most beneficial activities are those that give life meaning. But any activity which gives pleasure can create an emotional antidote to pain. Emotional numbness and alexithymia can make it difficult to extract emotion from normally enjoyable activities. Clients may also have to overcome feelings of apathy or lack of motivation, but they should be reassured that if they make the effort they will feel better. For example, Helen was depressed after she had been seriously injured in an assault. Although she really didn't feel like going out, she had bought her mother tickets to see a concert for her birthday. Right up until they were about to go Helen wanted to cancel, but she couldn't let her mother down and so she reluctantly went. To Helen's surprise, once she got to the theater she actually enjoyed herself and for a few hours she forgot about all her troubles. Helen realized that if she had given in to her depression she would have missed out on a much-needed enjoyable experience. The point is that for clients to overcome negative feelings, they sometimes also have to consciously ignore them. In addition to providing a sensory-emotional buffer against pain, engaging in meaningful pleasurable activities helps reduce the negative neuroplastic effects of stress and pain (see "Engaging in enjoyable absorbing activities" in the Client Resources section).

Resilience

Resilience is the ability to overcome adversity. Resilience means having the ability to respond flexibly to negative circumstances and move on. Resilience is a body-based state that involves a healthy nervous system which can manage energy effectively. People who cope by getting highly stressed are not resilient. Neither are people who cope by switching off emotionally. Resilience expert Dr. Richard Davidson defines resilience as,

> *"... the maintenance of high levels of positive affect and well-being in the face of adversity. It is not that resilient individuals never experience negative affect, but rather that the negative affect does not persist ..."*[15]

Resilience is helpful for coping with ongoing adverse circumstances, such as chronic illness or pain. A key quality of resilience is flexibility: the ability to move relatively freely between high energy states (stress) and low energy states (relaxation).

Resilience is a kind of energy which fuels endurance, persistence, creative problem-solving, and the ability to learn from almost any experience. Why aren't paraplegic people more depressed? Because they are not paraplegic full time; they do other things.

How to increase resilience

Clients who feel overwhelmed by their problems may benefit from resilience-enhancing activities. We have already looked at resource development and future templates as ways of helping clients cope with pain. Building resilience means developing even deeper reserves of stress tolerance and functioning despite the pain. Resilience can also be enhanced by other internal and external resources, including having supportive relationships, having goals, having a sense of humor, and mental flexibility.

Feeling supported means having access to emotionally close others to share and draw strength from. Developmental expert Daniel Siegel has suggested that intimate relationships are necessary for the development of neural networks responsible for emotional regulation, memory, and information processing. Secure attachments are thought to be necessary for the balanced development of the left and right hemispheres of the brain, which mediates the ability to relate emotionally to one's self and others. Secure attachments also allow the balanced development of the sympathetic and parasympathetic nervous systems—the ability to balance arousal with self-soothing (high energy vs. low energy states).[16]

As discussed in Chapter 2, the feeling that comes from sharing and having one's feelings understood by another is called *attunement*. Attunement can help alleviate pain. Researchers have discovered certain neurons that fire as a result of just *watching* someone else in pain—so-called mirror neurons. The discovery of mirror neurons means that our brain doesn't just react because we see someone in pain—it also recreates what's going on in their mind, enabling us to feel their pain, and vice-versa. This would seem to be the basis for the beneficial effects of shared affect and feeling understood in alleviating pain.

It is no accident that expressing feelings helps. Expressing emotions involves *both* the left and right sides of the brain, leading to greater integration between mental and emotional aspects of experience.[17] Expressing feelings seems to stimulate the whole brain, bringing the nervous system "online" to better process negative sensory-emotional experiences. For more information about how to help clients express their feelings about their pain, see the "How to talk about pain" handout in the Client Resources section.

The need for goals

Milton Erickson believed that one of the best prescriptions for overcoming adversity was having a real goal—in the near future.[18] Erickson was right: goal-directed behavior builds purpose and mastery. Setting goals is a top-down strategy involving increased activation of the left prefrontal cortex.[19] Having goals also stimulates the areas of the brain involved in recovery from negative emotions and the generation of positive emotions. Chronic pain sufferers often feel unable to achieve their goals because of decreased physical functioning. The answer is to find something they can succeed at within the limitations of their condition.

As a child, Milton Erickson was diagnosed with poliomyelitis. Soon after being diagnosed, the family doctor came to the house and Erickson overheard him telling his mother, "The boy will be dead by morning." Erickson recalls, "Being a normal kid, I resented that." When his mother came back into the bedroom, Erickson said nothing about what he'd overheard, but instead asked her to move a large chest of drawers away from where it was blocking the window. Then he asked her to move it back. He kept this up for some time, asking his mother to move the chest back and forth, until he was finally satisfied. Erickson's exasperated mother thought he was delirious, but wanted to humor what she thought were her dying son's last wishes. Erickson, however, had decided that he was "damned if I wasn't going to see the sunset" before he supposedly died. Erickson's strategy of keeping his mother busy until *after* sunset kept his mind off his condition and helped him survive. Three days later Erickson emerged from a coma and went on to live a long and very productive life.

Having a goal gives the client a reason to keep going during difficult times. Goals should be specific—wanting to be happy is not a viable goal, but wanting to learn the guitar or educate one's children is. Goals should also be personally meaningful. Goals are an external expression of your clients' deepest wishes. Everyone wants something; everyone is betting their life on something—you just have to find out what. Some experts recommend writing goals down to make them more real.

Knowing how to turn a problem into a strength

Another strategy for overcoming adversity is knowing how to turn a problem into a strength. At some point in the life of any problem, clients have to be able to look back on it and feel that they learned something from it. This is not to say that suffering is good, merely that being able to perceive some kind of benefit transforms suffering into something beneficial. Turning problems into strengths is more than just being able to find something positive in a negative situation; it's about processing what's happened, absorbing change, and moving on. Stephen King turned to writing horror stories to cope with his night terrors. James A. Michener wrote *Tales of the South Pacific* out of his wartime experiences. Michener also famously said, "Mankind was destined to live on the edge of disaster. We are mankind because we survive. We do it in a half-arsed way but we do it." [20]

Milton Erickson turned the paralysis associated with his polio into a resource by utilizing his time as a bedridden invalid to study human behavior.

Erickson's polio left him confined to his bed, virtually only able to move his eyelids. During this time Erickson occupied his mind by studying human behavior. He learned to tell when his sister's "no" really meant "yes." He learned how to tell what a person was feeling by changes in their breathing. He hypnotized his sisters and told them to undress in preparation for a medical examination just to see what they would do (they refused). When he had to learn how to walk again, he observed what it felt like to locate and recognize the signals from the various parts of his body. From this he learned what it must feel like when a child learns to walk, and how easily adults forget what they have learned. Erickson used this knowledge of basic life processes in his hypnotic inductions—he could hypnotize someone by talking about a tomato plant. Erickson became one of the most influential hypnotherapists of the 20th century. Erickson also learned how to use self-hypnosis to manage his lifelong post-polio pain. One of his favorite sayings was that life's difficulties are merely necessary roughage.

As Milton Erickson's story demonstrates, turning a problem into a strength requires mental flexibility and effort. But even the most adverse circumstances can always be turned into something useful. Clients need to be encouraged that despite its devastating effects on life functioning, chronic pain can also stimulate us to review our priorities, focus more on our own health and well-being, and develop other aspects of our personalities.

Getting better takes time

Unlike EMDR treatment of simple trauma, healing pain takes time. Clients (and therapists) can become frustrated because they are not seeing the results they expect. When this happens it can be helpful to think of healing pain as like baking a cake. Once you have assembled all the right ingredients (which can take time) and put them in the oven, you have to WAIT while that cake bakes. Don't give up because the cake doesn't bake in the time you expect it to. I had a client who suddenly stopped coming to therapy after he had been seeing me for a few months. Although he had been diligently applying all the strategies I had shared with him, together with many he had discovered himself, there had been little change in his pain levels. I assumed he had finally given up, but gave him a call to check what was happening. To my surprise and delight he told me that his pain had slowly started easing off to a much less distressing level. He had reduced his medication intake and reported that the pain no longer occupied center stage in his life. When I asked him how this happened he simply replied, "It just felt like everything I had learned finally came together." So it's important to be patient and keep practicing those pain and stress management strategies as long as necessary. When clients express despair about how long it's taking to feel better, I give them a copy of my "Pain management recipe" to remind them getting better takes time (see Client Resources section).

14

22 Things I Wish I'd Known Before I Started Working with Chronic Pain

Here are my 22 key learnings from treating chronic pain sufferers. If I had known these things when I started this work 30 years ago, I would have been a much more effective therapist and a much less stressed one. These points are the distillation of everything in this book and will give you all the fundamentals for working with this population. If you are ever trapped in a log cabin in the middle of winter and have to use the pages of this book to keep warm, burn the pages of this chapter last.

1. **Chronic pain involves a lot more than nociception.**

   Although physical discomfort (nociception) is what first comes to mind when we think of chronic pain, it's really a syndrome involving nociception, fatigue, anxiety, injury/disease, traumatic stress, brain processes, disability, identity changes, and hereditary and environmental factors. Even then there are traumas that still go unrecognized: recipients of multiple surgeries are more than twice as likely to develop PTSD, as are women diagnosed with breast cancer, etc. Simply treating chronic pain as just a maladaptive outgrowth of acute pain is an inadequate way of perceiving this problem and one that effectively closes down acknowledging the various other contributing factors.

2. **How addicted Western civilization is to the idea that pain for which there is no obvious medical explanation is invalid.**

   The ancient Greeks saw disease as a mind-body problem and treated it with a combination of surgery, herbs, and holistic interventions such as rest, diet, and prayer. With the rise of the scientific method in the 19th and 20th centuries, pain came to be viewed primarily in terms of its role as a warning sign of injury. By the late 20th century the limitations of this view could no longer be ignored and pain was officially redefined as "an unpleasant sensory and emotional experience associated with, or resembling that associated with, actual or potential tissue damage." Despite this, and the fact that over 50% of visits to general physicians are for medically unexplained pain, most of us continue to view pain in terms of its signal value. Doctors continue to tell sufferers it's all in their head, physical therapists continue to tell sufferers "no pain, no gain," and sufferers continue to disbelieve their own bodies and wonder if they are crazy. The idea that pain could, at least in part, be a legitimate symptom of unresolved emotional stress seems to be too threatening a possibility, as though this were the path to madness (or hysteria). Challenging this view of pain and opening clients to acceptance that pain may have other meanings is the key to effective psychological treatment of chronic pain.

3. **How much discrimination chronic pain sufferers experience.**

   Because their pain does not fit the generally accepted view, chronic pain sufferers are subject to a lot of discrimination and invalidated. This adds to their suffering, makes them doubt their felt reality, and prevents them taking the necessary steps to help themselves. For survivors of abuse or neglect, it is also a repeat of the invalidation they experienced previously, in effect blaming them for what is happening. As May et al. (2019) has observed,

   > *"The disparity between expressed symptoms, pathological signs and perceived disability in CLBP has led to the moral character of the sufferer forming a constant subtext to medical discourse about the condition."*

In fact, the true incidence of malingering in chronic pain sufferers is very low.

The invalidation becomes institutionalized when an insurance provider is involved and sufferers are questioned and forced to defend their symptoms. As van der Kolk has written,

> *"When the issue of causation (blame and responsibility) becomes the main focus, one is inevitably confronted with man's inhumanity to man, carelessness and callousness, abrogation of responsibility, manipulation and failure to protect."*

So one of the most useful things you can do for a chronic pain sufferer is to validate their feelings.

4. **How much trauma chronic pain sufferers have endured prior to developing pain.**

   As trauma therapists we expect to find traumatic antecedents to our clients' problems: physical or sexual abuse, life-threatening accidents, attachment problems, and emotional neglect. Chronic pain sufferers do not mostly come complaining about these things; they come complaining about pain, misunderstood medical problems, disability, losses, disrupted relationships, etc. These stressors afford an easier, more obvious focus of attention than those earlier adversities and they deserve attention. The challenge is to treat these issues with the respect they deserve while recognizing that the client is very likely suffering from the effects of earlier unrecognized trauma or neglect which must eventually be addressed.

5. **The story of the symptom is not the full story.**

   Regardless of how, when, or where the pain started, the true final causes of the pain are often more than the injury, accident, or illness that triggered the pain (see below). In contrast to the more visible medical aspects of pain, many of the psychological drivers of pain remain unknown to the sufferer due to lack of awareness, denial, or dissociation. The uncovering of that story is an essential part of the treatment and the key to healing. So if you are going to work with chronic pain, training in trauma-informed approaches is essential.

6. **Chronic pain sufferers experience dissociative symptoms.**

To the extent that chronic pain is an expression of unprocessed physical and emotional stress, regardless of any associated injury or illness, it is a kind of somatization. The key process in somatization is dissociation, a disconnection between sensory and mental aspects of experience. Dissociation can manifest in different ways. Pain is, to some extent, the client's body saying what the sufferer cannot say or even know about. Other dissociative symptoms include absorption, amnesia, and depersonalization. Chronic pain sufferers who are experiencing severe emotional distress and isolation are more likely to rely on dissociation that those with higher subjective levels of pain per se. Pain is also dissociative in and of itself. As Canadian hypnotherapist Marlene Hunter has noted, "Pain is a dissociative experience—it separates us from what's going on around us." These symptoms reflect the need for interventions such as distraction, mindfulness, focusing on positive affective experiences, emotional regulation, and ego enhancing.

7. **The role of brain functioning—chronic pain as a kind of memory.**

In addition to understanding the contribution of trauma, the other major trend of the last 20 years is the recognition of the role of the brain in chronic pain. Apkarian has described chronic pain as "a neuro-degenerative disorder." The trauma-informed approach teaches us that present symptoms can be a manifestation of past trauma, maintained by central sensitization and kindling. As Scaer describes it,

> *"... a traumatic event whose completion is truncated by lack of spontaneous resolution of a freeze/immobility response ... is associated with a complex set of somatic pathologic events ... kindling is intrinsic to the self-perpetuation of this pathologic process, driven by internal cues derived from unresolved procedural memory of threat, and enhanced by endorphinergic mechanisms inherent to both the initial response to threat, and subsequent freeze/dissociation."*

Whether the traumatic event was a car accident or years of developmental abuse, the subsequent changes to brain structure and functioning and the central nervous system are the key to understanding and unlocking chronic pain. Because pain is a procedural memory, the precipitating circumstances are often forgotten or disconnected from the current symptoms.

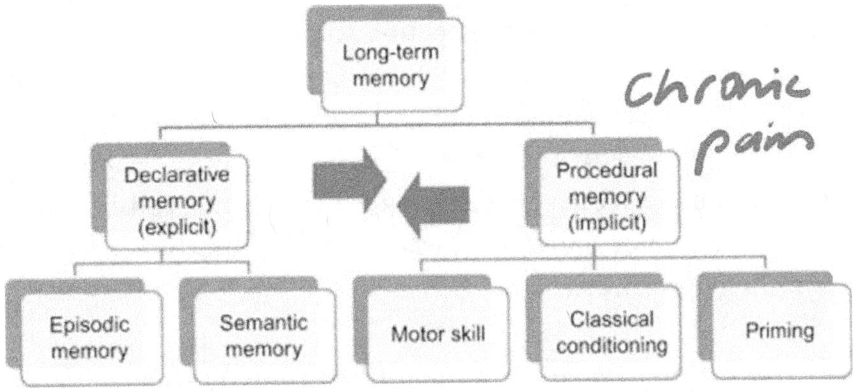

8. **There is (nearly) always a psychological component to chronic pain.**

Many (though not all) chronic pain sufferers are fixated on seeking a medical explanation or solution to their pain, not unreasonably if they have suffered serious illness or injury and deficient medical treatment. Regardless of what injuries or illnesses the client has been diagnosed with, there is nearly always a significant psychological component to chronic pain. When you consider the high likelihood that chronic pain sufferers have endured previous trauma, together with the effects of their illness and pain, this is not surprising. At the risk of repeating myself, the challenge is to shift the focus from medical concerns, once these needs have been reasonably adequately satisfied, and create a safe space within which to uncover the psychological factors that are contributing to the pain (e.g., "I deserve to suffer," "It's not safe to not have pain," etc.). Unlike some kinds of physical damage, psychological factors are changeable. Never suggest that pain is all psychological because it isn't, and even if it was, this is something the client has to discover for themselves.

9. **People have different constitutions.**

Charcot believed that somatization (or hysteria) was caused by a combination of environmental stressors and hereditary disposition. His successor Pierre Janet believed that human beings have an innate amount of latent psychic energy (force) that can be activated (manifest) to accomplish tasks of living. Tension is the capacity to utilize that energy. Janet believed that some of us have more force (energy reserves) than others. For example, he viewed Napoleon as a force "millionaire" because of his capacity to accomplish numerous tasks over a sustained period. In contrast, many of Janet's hysteria patients had lower reserves of that kind of energy. Individuals with lower reserves of force are more susceptible to psychological and health problems (agitation) because of an imbalance between energy and force, and excessive depletion of force. A person with low reserves of force might develop tinnitus following sustained stress, while a person with high levels might be completely unaffected. When treating chronic pain sufferers, each client's innate energy levels, constitution, and tolerance for adversity should be individually evaluated, beneath the veneer of coping, achieving, appearing normal, etc.

10. **Genetic factors may also be an unquantified contributing factor.**

Twin studies indicate that about half the risk of developing chronic pain can be attributed to genetic factors. Heritability estimates range from 30–70% for most pain conditions. Having a genetic predisposition doesn't mean someone will develop pain, but it does mean that the risk is increased, particularly following severe stress and/or illness. When environmental stress and genetics interact to produce illness, genes actually get altered—a process known as epigenetics. It's worth sharing this information with clients who may feel weak or ashamed for having pain.

11. **Chronic pain has survival value.**

From a survival perspective, chronic pain has traditionally been viewed as having no value since it is no longer telling the organism anything that is new. The pain has already done its job of alerting the organism to the fact that there is injury and, assuming treatment has been sought, there should be no further need for it. Well, that was the theory. In 2014 researchers from the University of Texas decided to test this popular view of acute vs. chronic pain by inducing central sensitization in squid and seeing what happened. To cut a long story short, the researchers found that the squid in the chronic pain condition were better at avoiding predators than both the healthy and injured no-pain squid. They surmised that the hyper-aware state in the injured non-anesthetized squid must be serving to protect them from the increased risk of death associated with their injury. The researchers concluded that "the propensity to develop chronic pain is an evolutionarily encoded feature of complex neural systems." Chronic pain is rarely meaningless or unnecessary. But once its survival purpose is understood, it can be resolved.

12. **Medication has its place.**

Many chronic pain sufferers are on a cocktail of medications including opiates, antidepressants, hypnotics, mood stabilizers, etc., etc. Drugs can help ameliorate the physical and mental suffering of chronic pain, but they are no substitute for self-management. Before the opioid crisis of recent years, when undertreatment of chronic pain was more widespread, I used to be an advocate of opioids. Now I have a more neutral position: I view them as the pharmacological equivalent of a splint that helps support a broken leg while it's healing, in this case the pain sufferer while they are learning to develop their own coping resources. With the exception of a person with pre-existing addiction problems, it is a mark of desperation that a person would want to take opioids to cope or feel "normal." The natural thing is to want one's independence: to be able to function normally without having to rely on drugs. I view medication usage as an indicator of how much access the client has to their own coping resources, but unless the client is really abusing their medications, I do not involve myself. I trust that my chronic pain clients will naturally reduce their reliance on medication as treatment progresses. I have seen many clients who were initially on high levels of opioids and other medications eventually wean themselves off all medications, without any pressure from myself, because in their own time they concluded these medications were at best doing nothing and at worse robbing them of their senses.

13. **Non-Western approaches.**

Non-Western approaches such as Chinese or Eastern medicine, Ayurvedic medicine, and homeopathy have long offered a more holistic approach to treating disease and illness. For example, according to Ayurvedic medicine, everything is composed of five elements: Space, Air, Fire, Water, and Earth. Disease arises because of imbalance that systematically moves through the following stages:

1. **Accumulation:** In the first stage of the disease, one or more of the five elements begins to accumulate within the body or mind.
2. **Aggravation:** When the imbalanced element moves outside of its normal boundaries, it is believed to have entered the second stage of the disease.
3. **Dissemination:** The wandering elements move throughout the body, in essence, looking for weak points in which to settle.
4. **Localization:** The wandering elements settle in a different part of the body.

5. **Manifestation:** Recognizable symptoms manifest.
6. **Disruption:** A chronic disease condition arises.

Recent discoveries regarding the role of trauma are stimulating theories of pain that are increasingly consistent with these old ideas. For example, the Ayurvedic concept of localization has its parallel with the modern concept of central spreading where pain develops in other areas of the body beyond the site of the original illness or injury. Ayurvedic medicine involves recognizing and reversing early signs of imbalance (in a trauma sufferer this might mean paying more attention to their feelings), and managing illness with mind-body inputs such as increased exposure to nature, supplements, massage, and diet. There are many other approaches which adopt this more systemic, holistic outlook, and seeing pain this way, regardless of the approach adopted, seems to be a common element of the healing journey.

14. Overcoming chronic pain involves a lot more than pain control.

As Fuchs (2009) says, "A psychiatry of the brain has to be systemic ... [that is] one that addresses the physical, emotional and environmental aspects of illness and corresponding dysfunctional patterns of neural activity." Given the sensory, emotional, and cognitive elements that make up chronic pain, overcoming pain involves much more than just pain management, namely:

1. Tame the pain
2. Emotional regulation
3. Trauma processing
4. Uncovering the meaning of your pain
5. Dealing with other stressors
6. Self-care
7. Reintegration

These steps offer a comprehensive, task-oriented approach to overcoming pain and its effects from the most basic physical aspects of pain through to its effects on identity. Your assessment and case-conceptualization will determine the order of proceedings although in most cases therapy involves incremental work and much circling around and moving backward and forward.

15. The ascending and descending analgesic systems.

Human beings are endowed with bottom-up and top-down pain pathways, each of which relies on differed types of neurotransmitters. Both system can be "retooled" to act as analgesic pathways. Bottom-up strategies include sensory inputs such as hot and cold stimulation, topical creams, and of course bilateral stimulation. Top-down strategies include inputs such as imagery, mindful attention, and accessing memories of comfort. Most chronic pain clients will benefit from employing a combination of top-down and bottom-up interventions. The point is that human beings have an in-built capacity for controlling pain and that there are many, many strategies which can be harnessed so long as the client is willing to take responsibility for overcoming their pain.

16. The client must want to get better.

No one wants to be in pain, but human beings are complex and there may be parts of the client's personality that need the pain as a substitute for other unmet needs. Beyond the signal value of acute pain, people need pain for many, usually unconscious, reasons. An adult survivor of abuse might subconsciously "need" their pain as evidence of their deserving to be punished, or fear of negative consequences of feeling well (where being in pain is part of a state of heightened alertness). A female survivor of trauma and neglect, with a very logical approach to life, couldn't understand why she still hurt despite doing everything right in terms of managing her pain. After further exploration of her subconscious (under hypnosis) it emerged that there was a part of her that believed that she deserved to suffer. Once we found out what survival need this part was serving, coupled with some ego strengthening, her levels of emotional distress decreased and although her pain did not cease, she started to have fewer flare-ups and to generally feel less overwhelmed.

17. Eye movement desensitization and reprocessing (EMDR).

EMDR is indicated as a treatment for chronic pain for many reasons:

1. The method's efficacy with psychological trauma, one of the most significant contributing psychological factors (McWilliams et al., 2003; Fishbain et al., 2017).
2. The method's ability to ameliorate physiological aspects of traumatic memories (Elofsson et al., 2007).

3. The method's ability to rectify maladaptive emotional processing (Tesarz et al., 2019).
4. The method's consistency with neurological mechanisms of pain, including kindling and neuroplasticity (Ray & Zbik, 2002).

EMDR is one of the most direct ways to process trauma-related pain such as whiplash, phantom limb pain, gastro-intestinal problems, fibromyalgia, chronic fatigue pain, etc. As in the treatment of trauma, the key to successful treatment is identifying the right target: that is the issue or memory that is the most fear-laden, the thing that is maintaining the client's current stress/pain levels. In the assessment phase you should consider developmental trauma in addition to more obvious forms of trauma such as physical or sexual abuse.

18. Hypnosis.

Hypnosis is an indispensable adjunct/alternative to EMDR for clients whose pain does not resolve following EMDR or for clients whose pain is treatment resistant. Hypnosis is a learning state, not unlike EMDR, but hypnosis offers a different path for accessing the client's subconscious resources, via direct or indirect suggestion, dissociation, age regression, etc. This is helpful when the client is unable to access traumatic antecedents of their pain through conscious channels such as floatback, affect bridge, etc. There are numerous hypnotic interventions for controlling pain, including glove anesthesia, displacement, light and water imagery, antidote imagery, etc. As a tool for ongoing pain control, recordings of hypnotic sessions can be made and given to clients to help them absorb whatever lessons or skills they need to manage their discomfort. Hypnosis seems to be most helpful for clients whose pain is entrenched and who need more time to transform pain-maintaining patterns of feeling and thinking.

19. Parts/ego state work.

Although we and our clients like to present ourselves as having one identity, one overarching self, most of us are made up of a collection of parts or ego states. These are clumps of feelings, thoughts, and behaviors—usually some variation of parent-child-adult. Ideally our parts work together to help us meet our physical, emotional, and social needs in an appropriate, balanced way. The child part tells us when we are feeling scared or need a hug. The adult part hears that and takes appropriate action. Trauma survivors tend to have overdeveloped survivor parts and limited awareness of their vulnerable parts. In a chronic pain sufferer this might take the form of being overinvested in appearing strong (adult part) at the expense of emotional needs (child part). This means living in a permanent state of alert and eventually leads to exhaustion and ill-health. Parts work is about helping the client develop a healthier relationship between their parts, leading to greater integration and wholeness. Other than a few very uncomplicated cases of post-traumatic pain, I have not encountered many chronic pain sufferers who did not need this kind of help.

20. **Somatic psychology.**

Somatic psychology reminds us of the need to help our clients be present to what they are experiencing in their bodies and allow emotional responses to complete. As van der Kolk says, "The two most important phrases in therapy are 'Notice that' and 'What happens next?' Once you start approaching your body with curiosity rather than with fear, everything shifts." It's so easy to get beguiled by our clients' words and stay in talk-therapy mode. We need to constantly check in with our bodies and those of our clients to ensure that we are working in a grounded space. Of course, this needs to be done sensitively and based on the client's readiness and needs. There are many times when clients need to avoid what they are feeling in their bodies until they have sufficient safety and confidence to encounter their feelings. But so many times when I have been stuck in therapy, just asking to client to notice what is going on in their body has gotten things moving again.

21. **There are limits regarding what the human body can manage.**

Even with the best treatment, complete pain relief may not be possible. People who have suffered pain for many years, whose innate energy (force) is spent, whose immune system is exhausted, may just not have the necessary resources to completely overcome pain. But if they can be assisted to cope better, live without the pain being "center stage," and feel less defined by their pain, then something of value has been achieved. As Carl Rogers used to say,

> *"In my early professional years I was asking the question:* ***How can I treat, or cure, or change this person?*** *Now I would phrase the question in this way:* ***How can I provide a relationship which this person may use for his own personal growth?"***

22. How inspiring helping people who are suffering can be.

The greatest thing you can do as a human being is to sit with someone who is suffering and just be with them. If at the end of the day this is all you can offer, you have given your client something of tremendous value. You have to trust in people's strength, even in the face of tremendous adversity. So many of my clients, after eventually triumphing not so much over their pain as themselves, are able to conclude, "This is the best thing that ever happened to me."

PART THREE

TREATMENT RESOURCES

15

Therapist Resources

- Intake questionnaire
- Pain risk factors questionnaire (PRFQ)
- EMDR pain protocol (short version)
- Pain and comfort words
- Effects of BLS menu
- Dissociative Experiences Scale (DES)
- Somatoform Dissociation Questionnaire (SDQ-20)
- EMDR+ strategies
- EMDR– strategies
- Healing traumatic stress app series
- Online training

These resources can be photocopied and used as treatment aids. Digital versions can be downloaded from the "Self help" page of www.overcomingpain.com.

Intake questionnaire

Thank you for giving me the opportunity to assist you. In order to help me understand your needs and to make our first meeting as productive as possible, please complete this questionnaire as much or as little as you feel comfortable.

NAME:____DOB:__________

Phone:___________________________Email: __________________________

Address:_________________________________Insurance claim details?__________

1. What is the best thing about you?

____

2. What is your proudest achievement?

____

3. What is your favorite place to relax and feel safe?

____

4. What is your favorite color?

____

5. How do you most like to spend YOUR time?

____

6. What gives your life meaning (if different to 5)?

____

7. What problem are you seeking help for (e.g., anxiety, depression, chronic pain) and how is it affecting you (e.g., trouble sleeping, can't relax, avoiding social situations, can't work, etc.)? How long have you struggled with this problem? What made you decide to seek help now?

____

8. Background, e.g., I am the second of three children. My parents divorced x years ago and I was raised by my mother. Include any other major life stresses, trauma, or health problems (e.g., father always criticized, bullied at school, viral illnesses, hospitalizations, etc.).

____

9. Any physical symptoms or complaints not already mentioned (e.g., headaches, insomnia, back pain)?

____

10. Treatment and outcomes—previous (how many other doctors, psychologists you have seen, with what results), e.g., my GP has prescribed antidepressants but I didn't like the side effects.

____

11. What would you like to get out of treatment?

____

12. Anything else you would like me to know about you?

____

Pain risk factors questionnaire

The pain risk factors questionnaire was developed to assess the likely contribution of known physical and non-physical risk factors for chronic pain. Responses to this questionnaire can be used to help guide treatment planning.

		True	Not True
1	I have suffered an accident, illness or injury		
2	I have chronic pain		
3	As a child I didn't have anyone to turn to for help or even if I did I kept my feelings to myself		
4	I never felt safe		
5	There was conflict or violence at home		
6	One of my parents had a mental illness/drug or alcohol problems/committed suicide/died		
7	My family life was very unstable		
8	I was physically and/or sexually abused		
9	I have suffered or am facing threatening circumstances over which I feel I have no control		
10	If I have a problem, the only person I can rely on is myself		
11	I have trouble sleeping		
12	I often feel tired and lacking in energy		
13	I find it hard to relax		
14	I don't know what's going on inside me		
15	I have feelings I can't quite identify		
16	Sometimes I feel like my body is disconnected from my mind		
17	I feel like a failure		
18	I worry all the time about whether my problems will ever end		
19	Sometimes I have disturbing memories or dreams about the past		
20	I often feel "super alert," or watchful, or on guard		

Scoring

The 20 items are divided into seven sections. Each set of two or three questions assesses a different type or effect of stress. To assess the client's risk factor exposure, give them one point for each "true" response in the scoring key below. Write the total number of true responses for each risk factor in the right-hand column of the scoring key. For example, if the client answered "true" to two items in questions 1–5, their score for "Emotional neglect" would be "2." If the client answered "not true" to all questions 6–10, their score for "Trauma" would be "0," and so on.

Q	SCORING KEY	Total
1–2	Physical injury or illness	
3–5	Emotional neglect	
6–8	Childhood trauma	
9–10	Safety and support	
11–13	Increased physiological arousal	
14–16	Emotional disconnection	
17–18	Negative thinking/"catastrophizing"	
19–20	Post-traumatic stress disorder	
	Total	

Once the client has completed scoring the questionnaire, evaluate their pain risk factors as follows:

1. A score of one or more for any individual risk factor means the client is affected by that pain risk factor.
2. If the total score was over three, the client has suffered moderate but significant stress.
3. If the total score was over five, the client has likely suffered severe stress and exposure to pain risk factors.

Treatment planning

The next step is to use the results from the questionnaire to plan the client's treatment. This is best done by making a case conceptualization around the seven tasks from least to most urgent.

- Injury and illness (questions 1–2)
  If the client scored one or more on this risk factor, they have been exposed to one of the leading risk factors for chronic pain and treatment will need to proceed with some mindfulness of the impact and progress of the injury. Particular attention may need to be paid to the diagnosis, medical treatments, and outcomes.
- Emotional neglect/childhood trauma (questions 3–8)
  If the client scored one or more for either of these risk factors, they have been exposed to leading non-medical risk factors for chronic pain. Treatment is likely to need to incorporate emotional skills training, ego work, and self-care skills training.
- Safety and support (questions 9–10)
  If the client scored one or more for this risk factor, they have insufficient safety and support. Treatment is likely to need to incorporate safe place installation and development of psychological support structures. These needs can be addressed within the first three tasks of pain management (below).
- Increased physiological arousal (questions 11–13)
  If the client scored one or more for this risk factor, it is likely that they are suffering from the effects of increased physiological arousal and they will need to learn how to de-arouse themselves. Treatment is likely to need to incorporate self-awareness training, self-soothing with BLS, relaxation training, and self-care work. These issues are addressed in the first three of the seven tasks of pain management.
- Emotional disconnection (questions 14–16)
  If the client scored one or more for this risk factor, it is likely that emotional disconnection is contributing to their pain. Treatment will need to incorporate elements of awareness and emotional self-regulation training.
- Negative thinking/"catastrophizing" (questions 17–18)
  If the client scored one or more for this risk factor, negative attitudes and thinking patterns are likely to be exacerbating their pain. Treatment should incorporate cognitive restructuring. The development and installation of a positive cognition and more positive attitudes and beliefs will be essential. This issue is usually addressed in the trauma processing, dealing with other stressors and uncovering meaning of the pain tasks.

- Post-traumatic stress disorder (questions 19–20)
  If the client scored one or more for this risk factor, it is likely that symptoms of post-traumatic stress are exacerbating their pain. Treatment will need to focus on reprocessing the trauma, safety and support, and emotional skills training for coping with any residual anxiety and/or pain. PTSD is obviously addressed in task 2, trauma processing.

The treatment planning chart (below) can be used to summarize the goals and directions of treatment, based on the above results. There is also a blank column at the end which can be used for any additional elements of treatment not mentioned here. In general, treatment should attend to these elements in the order in which they are listed. For example, most experts recommend attending to safety and support before commencing trauma work. However, it's also recognized that in practice, therapy is not so black and white and there will inevitably be some degree of overlap in how and when the therapist addresses each of these treatment elements.

Treatment element ➔ Risk factor ➔	Tame the pain	Trauma processing	Emotional regulation	Self-care	Uncovering the meaning of pain	Dealing with other stressors	Reintregration	
Injury or illness								
Emotional neglect								
Childhood trauma								
Safety and support								
Increased physiological arousal								
Emotional disconnection								
Negative thinking								
Post-traumatic stress disorder								
Total								

Additional notes ______________________________

EMDR pain protocol (short version)

Target

Develop target based on whether pain is trauma-related or not.

a) **Traumatic Pain**

"When you think of the incident that led to your pain, what picture do you get?"

____

b) **Non-Traumatic Pain**

"Can you describe the pain in terms of how it feels physically?" (suggest size, color, etc., if client needs help describing their pain)

____

"Is there an image that goes with that?" or *"When you describe your pain that way, what does it feel like? What does it remind you of?"*

____

Negative cognition

"What does the pain (or memory) make you believe about yourself?"

____

Positive cognition

"When you bring up that picture or incident, or when you think of your pain, what would you like to believe about yourself, instead?"

____

VoC

Elicit a Validity of Cognition.

"When you think of the pain, how true do those words____ [clinician repeats the positive cognition] feel to you now on a scale of 1–7, where 1 feels completely false and 7 feels totally true?"

1	2	3	4	5	6	7
(completely false)						(completely true)

Emotions

Elicit the emotions.

"When you think of the pain and those words_____ [clinician states the negative cognition], what emotion do you get now?" Note, if pain is the main presenting problem, you may skip this question.

____

SUDs

Elicit the SUDs.

"On a scale of 0 to 10, where 0 is no pain (or distress) or neutral and 10 is the worst you can imagine, how bad does your pain feel right now?"

0	1	2	3	4	5	6	7	8	9	10
(no disturbance)										(highest disturbance)

Sensation/location

Elicit the sensation/location. If you have already done this (e.g., when you asked the client to describe their pain earlier), you may go straight to desensitization.

"Where do you feel it [the pain] in your body?"

___

Desensitization

"Now I'd like you to focus on the pain (or memory) the way you've just described it, and those words [NC], listen to the bilateral tones and just let whatever happens happen." Commence BLS (preferably continuous audio and do not cease BLS when checking in with client until after you notice a change or you feel like it's been long enough for something to have happened).

Say, ***"What do you notice now?"***

___

If the client reports a positive difference, say,

"That's fine, just go with that."

Continue BLS, reviewing the client's experience at appropriate periods without ceasing BLS until a relatively stable level of improvement is achieved.

When the pain is gone or the changes have plateaued, review SUDs and VoC.

Say, ***"On a scale of 0 to 10, where 0 is no disturbance or neutral and 10 is the highest disturbance you can imagine, how bad does it feel now?"***

0	1	2	3	4	5	6	7	8	9	10
(no pain)										**(highest pain)**

"Does it feel like you can achieve any further improvement?"

___

If the SUDs is 0, either strengthen it with an additional set of BLS or go to installation phase. If the pain (or distress) is still a SUDs of more than 0 ask,

"What prevents the number from being a 0?"

____

"Go with that." Discuss whatever response is given and ask the client whether or not they would like to continue working.

Pause and ask the client what they notice now. If they report feeling better ask,

"Do you want to continue?" If the client answers "yes," restimulate until the pain has resolved fully or the changes plateau and return to VoC. If "no," go to installation phase (either creating antidote imagery if client has residual pain, or normal installation if pain is satisfactorily resolved).

Installation (antidote imagery)

1. Imagery based on sensory changes

"What's there now where the pain was before? Can you describe those feelings of comfort (e.g., soft, loose, natural, etc.)?"

"Is there an image that goes with those feelings?"

"What do those feelings remind you of? What do they feel like (e.g., a pool of water, a wet towel, etc.)?"

____

"Now think of a word that goes with that image and go with that."

Restimulate.

"How does ____[repeat the PC] sound?"

____

"Do those words still fit, or is there another positive statement that feels better?"

____

If the client accepts the original positive cognition, the clinician should ask for a VoC rating to see if it has improved:

"Think of the pain (or memory), and hold it together with the words ________________

________________________ ***[repeat the PC]."***

Do a long set of BLS to see if there is more processing to be done.

Finish up by instructing client to practice BLS and activating and thinking of their healing imagery as often as they can when they are in pain.

2. Imaginal healing imagery

"Think of something that could take the pain away or make it better; don't worry about whether it seems realistic or not, just let your imagination run wild."

____

Commence BLS while the client is still searching for an answer to the question. Cease BLS after 30–45 seconds and ask, ***"What did you get?"*** or ***"What came up?"***

____

"How does that make you feel?"

____

Assuming it's something positive, instruct the client to ***"think of that"*** and restimulate with BLS.

If the client can't think of anything, advise them this is just an imaginal exercise and it doesn't have to be realistic. But do not accept answers like "an injection" or "an operation"—these are not sufficiently client-based.

Once the client has focused on the healing image + BLS a couple of times with it either holding or strengthening, ask,

"Is there a word that goes with how you feel when you think of that image?"

____

Resume BLS until the client reports a stable link between the image and the trigger word and instruct the client to practice thinking of their healing imagery as often as they can when they are in pain and to try and find or add a new detail each time they do it so it becomes richer and stronger.

Installation phase

VoC

If you skipped the VoC in the set-up, say, ***"So, if I ask you to think of the changes that have happened here, what belief do you have about your ability to manage the pain now?"***

If you did obtain a VoC in the set-up phase, say, ***"When you think of the pain now, how true do those words____ [clinician repeats the positive cognition] feel to you now on a scale of 1–7, where 1 feels completely false and 7 feels totally true?"***

1 2 3 4 5 6 7

Sometimes the original VoC is no longer a good fit. Ask, ***"Is there another positive statement or cognition that fits better now? If so, what would it be?"***

____

Instruct the client to ***"just think of your pain now and that thought and just notice ..."***

Perform eight slow bilateral eye movements. Check again.

"So how does that feel now?"

____

Body scan

"So if I ask you to think of your original pain (or distress) now, how does it feel in your body?"

____

You should have already done this but if any significant discomfort is still reported, restimulate with BLS or create antidote resources if you haven't already.

"Okay, do you have any idea about what's stopping the pain from changing?"

____

When the client reports no pain or it is apparent that the client cannot improve any further,

"Close your eyes and keep in mind the original memory/image and the positive cognition. Then bring your attention to the different parts of your body, starting with your head and working downward. Any place you find any tension, tightness, or unusual sensation, tell me."

____

Closure

"Now that you are feeling better you are probably wondering how long the effects will last. Experience suggests that these changes can last anywhere from a few hours to being permanent. Even if the pain comes back, it is often weaker because of the way EMDR affects memory. The most important thing is to just have an open mind and pay attention to what you are feeling in the present. Many people find that EMDR helps them feel more in touch with their feelings and this can lead to increased self-care and reduced stress and pain flare-ups.

"You can also use the antidote imagery we created or bilateral stimulation by yourself to control your pain. I am going to give you a recording of this sound. Whenever you need relief from pain (or stress, or even insomnia) just play this app/audio download/CD, etc. (whatever applies), and concentrate on the negative feelings you want relief from, just like you did here today. The more you practice, the more you will succeed. Of course, if your pain persists beyond what you feel you can cope with, you should always seek medical help."

Pain and comfort words

Targeting phase (pain words)

"Pain can be hard to describe. On the left is a list of words commonly used to describe pain. Which words best describe your pain?"

Desensitization-installation (pain and comfort words)

"It can also be hard to find the words to describe how it feels when the pain changes or goes away. On the right is a list of words people often use to describe what happens when they feel better. Which words best describe how it feels now where the pain was before?"

[These words should be shown to clients who report "nothing" following BLS or have difficulty describing what they feel.]

Pain Words	**Comfort Words**
Hot	Cool
Gnawing	Warm
Sharp	Dull
Aching	Draining
Hard	Soft
Tight	Loose
Heavy	Light
Burning	Ebbing
Pulsing	Flowing
Pressure	Tingling
Stinging	Shrinking
Growing	Easing
Pounding	Relaxed
Stabbing	Melting
Stiff	Disappearing
Spreading	

Effects of bilateral stimulation menu

Because of sensory numbing, lack of emotional awareness, and the relative "smallness" of sensory effects, clients may not be able to recognize important sensory effects of BLS. In the treatment of chronic pain, the EMDR therapist should take an active role in helping the client recognize and label sensory changes following BLS, including suggesting possibilities in an open-ended way.

Below is a menu of possibilities.

Physical:

- Decreased tension
- Decreased agitation
- Decreased heart rate
- Decreased breathing rate
- Decreased physical discomfort/pain
- Relaxation
- Feeling drowsy
- Feeling energized

Mental:

- Decreased anxiety
- Decreased worry
- Decreased thinking/mental activity
- Decreased emotional distress
- Decreased vividness of mental images
- More distant perspective on problem

Dissociative Experiences Scale (DES)

Serenity Programme™ - www.serene.me.uk - Dissociative Experiences Scale (DES)

Dissociative Experiences Scale (DES)

Identifier [ ] Date [ ]

This questionnaire consists of 28 questions about experiences that you may have in your daily life. We are interested in how often you have these experiences. It is important, however, that your answers show how often these experiences happen to you when you are not under the influence of alcohol or drugs. To answer the questions, please determine to what degree the experience described in the question applies to you and select the number to show what percentage of the time you have the experience. 100% means 'always', 0% means 'never' with 10% increments in between. This assessment is not intended to be a diagnosis. If you are concerned about your results in any way, please speak with a qualified health professional.

Never 0% | 10% | 20% | 30% | 40% | 50% | 60% | 70% | 80% | 90% | 100% Always

1	Some people have the experience of driving a car and suddenly realizing that they don't remember what has happened during all or part of the trip. Select a number to show what percentage of the time this happens to you	0%
2	Some people find that sometimes they are listening to someone talk and they suddenly realize that they did not hear all or part of what was said. Select a number to show what percentage of the time this happens to you	0%
3	Some people have the experience of finding themselves in a place and having no idea how they got there. Select a number to show what percentage of the time this happens to you	0%
4	Some people have the experience of finding themselves dressed in clothes that they don't remember putting on. Select a number to show what percentage of the time this happens to you	0%
5	Some people have the experience of finding new things among their belongings that they do not remember buying. Select a number to show what percentage of the time this happens to you	0%
6	Some people sometimes find that they are approached by people that they do not know who call them by another name or insist that they have met them before. Select a number to show what percentage of the time this happens to you	0%

Serenity Programme™ - www.serene.me.uk - Dissociative Experiences Scale (DES)

7	Some people sometimes have the experience of feeling as though they are standing next to themselves or watching themselves do something as if they were looking at another person. Select a number to show what percentage of the time this happens to you	0%
8	Some people are told that they sometimes do not recognize friends or family members. Select a number to show what percentage of the time this happens to you	0%
9	Some people find that they have no memory for some important events in their lives (for example, a wedding or graduation). Select a number to show what percentage of the time this happens to you	0%
10	Some people have the experience of being accused of lying when they do not think that they have lied. Select a number to show what percentage of the time this happens to you	0%
11	Some people have the experience of looking in a mirror and not recognizing themselves. Select a number to show what percentage of the time this happens to you	0%
12	Some people sometimes have the experience of feeling that other people, objects, and the world around them are not real. Select a number to show what percentage of the time this happens to you	0%
13	Some people sometimes have the experience of feeling that their body does not belong to them. Select a number to show what percentage of the time this happens to you	0%
14	Some people have the experience of sometimes remembering a past event so vividly that they feel as if they were reliving that event. Select a number to show what percentage of the time this happens to you	0%
15	Some people have the experience of not being sure whether things that they remember happening really did happen or whether they just dreamed them. Select a number to show what percentage of the time this happens to you	0%
16	Some people have the experience of being in a familiar place but finding it strange and unfamiliar. Select a number to show what percentage of the time this happens to you	0%
17	Some people find that when they are watching television or a movie they become so absorbed in the story that they are unaware of other events happening around them. Select a number to show what percentage of the time this happens to you	0%

Serenity Programme™ - www.serene.me.uk - Dissociative Experiences Scale (DES)

18	Some people sometimes find that they become so involved in a fantasy or daydream that it feels as though it were really happening to them. Select a number to show what percentage of the time this happens to you	0%
19	Some people find that they are sometimes able to ignore pain. Select a number to show what percentage of the time this happens to you	0%
20	Some people find that they sometimes sit staring off into space, thinking of nothing, and are not aware of the passage of time. Select a number to show what percentage of the time this happens to you	0%
21	Some people sometimes find that when they are alone they talk out loud to themselves. Select a number to show what percentage of the time this happens to you	0%
22	Some people find that in one situation they may act so differently compared with another situation that they feel almost as if they were different people. Select a number to show what percentage of the time this happens to you	0%
23	Some people sometimes find that in certain situations they are able to do things with amazing ease and spontaneity that would usually be difficult for them (for example, sports, work, social situations, etc.). Select a number to show what percentage of the time this happens to you	0%
24	Some people sometimes find that they cannot remember whether they have done something or have just thought about doing that thing (for example, not knowing whether they have just mailed a letter or have just thought about mailing it). Select a number to show what percentage of the time this happens to you	0%
25	Some people find evidence that they have done things that they do not remember doing. Select a number to show what percentage of the time this happens to you	0%
26	Some people sometimes find writings, drawings, or notes among their belongings that they must have done but cannot remember doing. Select a number to show what percentage of the time this happens to you	0%
27	Some people find that they sometimes hear voices inside their head that tell them to do things or comment on things that they are doing. Select a number to show what percentage of the time this happens to you	0%
28	Some people sometimes feel as if they are looking at the world through a fog so that people or objects appear far away or unclear. Select a number to show what percentage of the time this happens to you	0%

Serenity Programme™ - www.serene.me.uk - Dissociative Experiences Scale (DES)

Print Form   Clear Form   Mean DES Score   0

The Dissociative Experiences Scale (DES) is a simple questionnaire widely used to screen for dissociative symptoms. Tests such as the DES provide a quick screening method so that the more time-consuming structured clinical interview (SCID-D) can be used for those people with high DES scores.

The higher the DES score, the more likely it is that the person has a dissociative disorder. The DES is not a diagnostic instrument; it is designed for screening only. High scores on the DES do not show that a person has a dissociative disorder; they only suggest that clinical assessment for dissociation may be warranted. Different studies suggest different cut-off scores for the DES, but a score of more than 45 suggests a high likelihood of a dissociative disorder alongside a reduced likelihood of a 'false positive'.

Privacy - please note - this form does not transmit any information about you or your assessment scores. If you wish to keep your results, either print this document or save this file locally to your computer. If you click 'save' before closing, your results will be saved in this document. These results are intended as a guide to your health and are presented for educational purposes only. They are not intended to be a clinical diagnosis. If you are concerned in any way about your health, please consult with a qualified health professional.

Bernstein EM, Putnam FW (1986). "Development, reliability, and validity of a dissociation scale". J. Nerv. Ment. Dis. 174 (12): 727–35.

Frischholz, E.J. et al The dissociative experiences scale: further replication and validation. Dissociation, Vol. III, September 1990.

The Somatoform Dissociation Questionnaire (SDQ-20)[1]

The 20-item Somatoform Dissociation Questionnaire (Nijenhuis et al., 1996) evaluates the severity of somatoform dissociation. The SDQ-20 items were derived from a pool of 75 items describing clinically observed somatoform dissociative symptoms that in clinical settings had appeared upon activation of particular dissociative parts of the personality and that could not be medically explained. The items pertain to both negative (e.g., analgesia) and positive dissociative phenomena (e.g., site-specific pain).

Each individual item asks about the frequency that a particular somatoform dissociative symptom is experienced using a 5-point Likert scale, ranging from "1 = this applies to me NOT AT ALL" to "5 = this applies to me EXTREMELY." The respondent is also asked to indicate whether a physician has connected the symptom or bodily experience with a physical disease. In clinical practice the relevant item score can be adjusted to "1" when physical disease is indicated, the medical diagnosis has been checked with the physician who assigned it, and this diagnosis seems valid. The SDQ-20 score, which may range from 20 to 100, is obtained by the sum of the individual item scores.

The SDQ-20 discriminates between dissociative identity disorder, dissociative disorder NOS (not otherwise specified), somatoform disorders, and other psychiatric diagnostic categories. Scores over 30 are significant for the presence of somatoform dissociation. In studies using this scale, most patients with DID scored over 50, most of those with DDNOS scored over 40, and most of those with somatoform disorders scored over 30.

SDQ-20

This questionnaire asks about different physical symptoms or body experiences, which you may have had either briefly or for a longer time. Please indicate to what extent these experiences apply to you *in the past year*. For each statement, please circle the number in the first column that best applies to YOU.

The possibilities are:

1 = this applies to me NOT AT ALL

1. From "The Scoring and Interpretation of the SDQ-20 and SDQ-5" (Nijenhuis, 2010).

2 = this applies to me A LITTLE

3 = this applies to me MODERATELY

4 = this applies to me QUITE A BIT

5 = this applies to me EXTREMELY

If a symptom or experience applies to you, please indicate whether a physician has connected it with a *physical disease*. Indicate this by circling the word YES or NO in the column "Is the physical cause known?" If you circle YES, please write the physical cause (if you know it) on the line.

Example:

Sometimes	**Extent to which the symptom or experience applies to you**	**Is the physical cause known?**
My teeth chatter	1 2 3 4 5	NO YES, namely__________
I have cramps in my calves	1 2 3 4 5	NO YES, namely__________

If you have circled a 1 in the first column (i.e., This applies to me NOT AT ALL), you do NOT have to respond to the question about whether the physical cause is known. On the other hand, if you circle 2, 3, 4, or 5, you MUST circle NO or YES in the "Is the physical cause known?" column.

Please do not skip any of the 20 questions. Thank you for your cooperation.

Here are the questions:

1 = this applies to me NOT AT ALL

2 = this applies to me A LITTLE

3 = this applies to me MODERATELY

4 = this applies to me QUITE A BIT

5 = this applies to me EXTREMELY

	Sometimes	Extent to which the symptom or experience applies to you	Is the physical cause known?	
1.	I have trouble urinating	1 2 3 4 5	NO	YES, namely ________________
2.	I dislike tastes that I usually like (women: at times *other than* during pregnancy or monthly periods)	1 2 3 4 5	NO	YES, namely ________________
3.	I hear sounds from nearby as if they were coming from far away	1 2 3 4 5	NO	YES, namely ________________
4.	I have pain while urinating	1 2 3 4 5	NO	YES, namely ________________
5.	My body, or a part of it, feels numb	1 2 3 4 5	NO	YES, namely ________________
6.	People and things look bigger than usual	1 2 3 4 5	NO	YES, namely ________________
7.	I have an attack that resembles an epileptic seizure	1 2 3 4 5	NO	YES, namely ________________
8.	My body, or a part of it, is insensitive to pain	1 2 3 4 5	NO	YES, namely ________________
9.	I dislike smells I usually like	1 2 3 4 5	NO	YES, namely ________________
10.	I feel pain in my genitals (at times *other than* sexual intercourse)	1 2 3 4 5	NO	YES, namely ________________
11.	I cannot hear for a while (as if I am deaf)	1 2 3 4 5	NO	YES, namely ________________
12.	I cannot see for a while (as if I am blind)	1 2 3 4 5	NO	YES, namely ________________
13.	I see things around me differently than usual (for example, as if looking through a tunnel, or merely seeing part of an object)	1 2 3 4 5	NO	YES, namely ________________
14.	I am able to smell much *better* or *worse* (even though I do not have a cold)	1 2 3 4 5	NO	YES, namely ________________

15.	It is as if my body, or part of it, has disappeared	1	2	3	4	5	NO	YES, namely ______________
16.	I cannot swallow, or can only swallow with great difficulty	1	2	3	4	5	NO	YES, namely ______________
17.	I cannot sleep for nights on end, but remain very active during the day	1	2	3	4	5	NO	YES, namely ______________
18.	I cannot speak (or only with great effort) or I can only whisper	1	2	3	4	5	NO	YES, namely ______________
19.	I am paralyzed for a while	1	2	3	4	5	NO	YES, namely ______________
20.	I grow stiff for a while	1	2	3	4	5	NO	YES, namely ______________

Adjunctive strategies for pain control (EMDR+)

These are for clients who are responsive to EMDR but have ongoing pain, and are receptive to the use of strategies incorporating focused attention, mindfulness-based strategies, memory, and guided imagery to help manage their pain.

Antidote imagery

So just take a moment to focus in on your body ... as much as you comfortably can right now ... and notice your pain ... noticing where you feel it in your body ... and what it really feels like ... is it hot ... or cold? If it had a color, what color would it be? Is it hard or soft? Constant or fluctuating? What shape is it? And any other sensory or mental qualities that you might want to be aware of. And once you have allowed yourself to explore your pain as fully as possible and you have a distinct sense of it ... what does it remind you of ... what is the pain/discomfort like? Let an image of that form in your mind ... and then put that image aside for a moment and think of something else ... something that could take it away or make it feel better ... the opposite of what you just got. So if your pain was hot, something cool, if it was stabbing, something dull, the opposite ... and notice what comes to mind ... and how that feels ... and then imagine laying that over the top of your pain, and feeling that antidote resource overtaking your pain.

Positive memory

Take a moment to get comfortable ... as comfortable as you can at this moment ... just letting your body relax a bit ... and take three deep breaths ... with each breath letting yourself feel more and more relaxed ... that's right ... and now think back to a time or a place where you felt safe and well ... a place where you could just be yourself ... without having to make any effort or care or worry ... somewhere quiet and peaceful ... a place where you could rest without having to make any effort at all ... before all the craziness began ... when life had a more natural rhythm ...which we all need from time to time ... and you can go back to that place ... which is always there in the recesses of your mind and notice how the memory of that place makes you feel in your body right now ... and just notice that ... a place where there is nothing you have to do, no one to face ... just peace and quiet ... and is there a word that summarizes how the memory of that place makes you feel? ... And whenever you are feeling stress or discomfort, or you need a break, just take a moment and close your eyes and think of that place ... and that word ... and you will feel better.

Hypno-mindfulness

Take a moment to relax and get as comfortable as you can at this moment. And as you relax you may notice ... how difficult it is to not be aware ... of that discomfort ... and that's right ... because pain can be hard to ignore and sometimes necessary ... so you don't need to fight your mind ... which is always aware of those feelings there for you ... or resist those feelings ... so much easier instead ... to just accept those feelings for what they are ... just observing them ... like scenery from a train ... passing by in front of you ... and as you observe those feelings you might even begin to wonder what it really is about them that is so unpleasant ... they are what they are ... neither good nor bad. Just a part of life ... like the seasons ... where all present experience, even unpleasant things ... eventually become part of the flow of past, present, and future, as that scenery passes by in front of you and recedes into the distance ...

Breathing away the pain

a) Focus on your breathing. And take three deep breaths.

b) Notice how your chest expands with each in-breath, and contracts with each out-breath ... and how it tenses up when you breathe in and how it relaxes when you breathe out.

c) Imagine that with every in-breath you are breathing in comfort ... and that with every out-breath you are breathing out discomfort ... so that with every breath you take, you can experience a little more comfort ... and a little less discomfort ...

d) And with every breath you take, you can imagine that comfort spreading through your body, as those molecules of oxygen travel through the walls of your lungs into your bloodstream ... taking that comfort to the rest of your body.

e) So, you can control your pain as naturally as breathing ... in, comfort ... out, pain and with every breath you take ... you can feel that comfort spreading ...

Containing the pain with pendulation

Notice the part of your body where the pain is.
Let your attention be drawn to that part of you.
What does it feel like?
What are its qualities? Is it hard ... or soft? Throbbing ... or steady? Hot ... or cold? If the pain had a color, what color would it be?
What emotions does it trigger?
If you can, let an image of your pain form in your mind.
Now, if you can, give your whole pain experience a name.
Now put that aside and see if you can notice a part of your body where there is no pain.
A part that feels absent of tension or discomfort.
A part that feels comfortable ... okay ...
And notice what that feels like.
What are its qualities? Is it soft or smooth? Throbbing ... or steady? Is it hot ... or cold? If the comfort had a color, what color would it be?
What emotions does it trigger?
If you can, let an image of your comfort form in your mind.
Now, if you can, give your whole comfort experience a name.
Now put that aside and let your attention go back to the pain, and notice again how that feels ...
The sensations ... the feelings ... the image ...
And notice whether it feels the same as before, or slightly different?
And if so, how?
Now put that aside and let your attention go back to the comfort, and notice again how that feels ...
The sensations ... the feelings ... the image ...
And notice whether it feels the same as before, or slightly different?
And if so, how?
And as you switch your attention backward and forward between the pain and the comfort, you can learn that you can control your pain, just by focusing your attention.

Acknowledgment: Peter Levine.

Adjunctive strategies for pain control (EMDR–)

For clients who don't respond to EMDR because of cognitive style, pain levels too high, concentration problems, etc. These strategies are more cognitive but not mentally demanding (e.g., they don't require a great deal of concentration, imagination, or ability to revivify memories).

Easy everyday mindfulness

(A brief unstructured mindfulness strategy for people who can't concentrate for long or dislike formal mindfulness approaches)

Try to uncouple your attention from your normal inner stream of consciousness (default mode network) and focus on your current external surroundings. For example, where am I? What do I see around me? What do I hear around me? What smells do I notice? What external physical sensory stimulation do I notice? The aim is to get out of your head and into other aspects of your sensory reality. Why? Because you are hurting inside, but outside your body are pleasant or at least neutral stimuli that can alter how you are feeling simply by paying attention to them. For example, you are sitting in a chair of your living room, hurting and noticing that discomfort. But you can also notice that sunlight is pouring through an open window and there is a faint smell of primrose, and the sound of birds singing. A good shortcut into this is to regularly stop and ask yourself, "Where am I and what am I doing?" Again the idea is to become more connected to your present sensory reality and less divided between your sensory reality and your mind, as summarized in the Buddhist saying, "When you're chopping wood—chop wood."

Distraction

Distraction is simply moving your attention away from your pain, with a minimum of concentration or mental effort. You can do this consciously, as when you deliberately focus your attention on something else, or involuntarily as when your attention is captured by a song or something in your environment and you forget about your pain. Obviously, if you can use distraction consciously, you can derive more benefit from this commonest of pain management strategies. As Chuck Close says, "I like a certain amount of distraction—it keeps me from being anxious, it keeps things at a little bit more of an arm's length."

Engaging in enjoyable absorbing activities

Focus on activities that absorb your attention and take your mind away from the discomfort, so that the discomfort becomes less center stage. Even the most stressed, traumatized person encounters moments where a song, an exchange with a friend, or an interesting activity diverts their attention from their suffering. In that moment they are free. As one chronic pain sufferer put it, "When you're building the models, you don't think about it [the pain] ... it's like a pain blocker. Little things like that are the things that are getting me through." What sorts of activities interest you such that you lose awareness of other things when you are doing them? Hint: They will reflect your primary emotional style, whether you are a seeker (someone who most enjoys finding new things, e.g., collecting cars, playing *Pokémon Go*,) a carer (someone who most enjoys looking after people or animals), or a player (someone who can enjoy activities that have no real purpose, e.g., knitting, listening to music, gardening, playing golf). So, what activities enable you to forget yourself?

Contralateral stimulation

(Using touch to activate competitive neuroplasticity to alleviate unilateral pain)

The brain processes pain contralaterally in the somatosensory cortex (SC) (e.g., pain on the right side gets processed in the left side of the SC and vice-versa). What happens on one side of the SC affects what happens on the other side and you can use this process to change pain perception and memories. Now get someone (your therapist or a relative or friend) to touch or hold the non-painful limb in the same location as the pain in the painful limb, in such a way that it creates a counter stimulus to the pain. So, if the pain is in the outside left elbow, you would apply touch to the outside right elbow. Once you have located the exact location on the opposite limb (e.g., outside area of right elbow), apply gentle but firm pressure to that area sufficiently to create a not unpleasant counterstimulus to the painful sensations. The toucher should ask the pain sufferer, "Is this the right spot?" "Is this too hard/soft?" Once you have got a suitably noticeable overriding touch, hold that touch for a few minutes, inquiring every minute or two if it's still okay and later "and what are you noticing now?" You may also ask the recipient to "notice any changes in the pain" while you do this.

Quite often the pain sufferer will report significant relief and even total cessation of the pain. At the least they will report that it feels different. Reinforce their experience by telling them that they are learning to feel different and these effects will last for some time, and that the more they do this, the more they can retrain their brain and change their pain memories.

Note: For best results it's ideal to get a friend or relative to apply the touch rather than the pain sufferer themselves.

Exercise/movement

Decreased activity and immobility are common responses to chronic pain and trauma, whether as a result of fear of aggravating the pain or the freeze response (in PTSD). But inactivity inhibits your body's natural balance and can actually exacerbate pain, stress, and depression. Movement stimulates your natural healing capabilities, including:

- Increased serotonin, dopamine
- Improved mood
- Reduced anxiety and depression
- Improved cardiovascular functioning
- Increased BDNF (a substance that helps maintain brain functioning)
- Increased IGF-1, a hormone that promotes cell growth and repair

Amplification of positive emotion

Whatever you do and however long you do it for, even if only briefly, try and notice whatever physical, mental, or emotional changes you experience (e.g., decreased tension, relaxation, decreased awareness of discomfort, interest, joy) and practice noticing those changes more and more each and every time you engage in that activity. It's the difference between walking around with blinkers on and walking around with your eyes open. With your eyes open you are more open to being positively influenced by what you see, hear, and feel in life and this will change how you experience and cope with your problems. As Spinoza said, "The more capable the body is of being affected in many ways ... the more capable of thinking is the mind." Noticing and paying attention to what you experience takes effort and practice, but it is the key to learning to feel better and think differently.

Healing traumatic stress app series

Sleep Restore

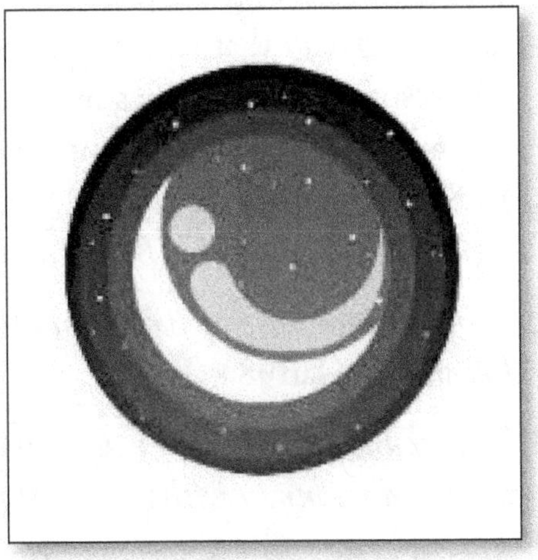

Uniquely designed for sufferers of stress-related insomnia, this app harnesses the power of bilateral stimulation (BLS) to turn off tension and worry and restore normal sleep functioning. BLS is a treatment element of EMDR therapy, a psychological treatment method that harnesses your brain's ability to process sensory information to deactivate the physical and mental distress which inhibits sleep. The resulting normalization of brain activity creates the conditions for sleep to happen, naturally and effortlessly. BLS has been found to stimulate increased delta wave activity, which is associated with restful sleep. If you suffer from insomnia related to PTSD, medical problems, or just general stress and anxiety, this app is for you. 20 sessions of guided meditations, music, nature sounds, and BLS.

"I have been using this app for two months and it really works. I particularly like 'The Night Watchman' and 'Waiting for Morning'—I haven't actually heard the end of either of them." **–Simon**

Overcoming Pain

25 sessions of guided meditations incorporating bilateral stimulation, focused attention, and mental and sensory-based pain control strategies. Designed to complement the strategies described in this book by providing convenient real-world guided meditations and strategies. Three playlists are designed to address the sensory-emotional components of chronic pain: Mental Healing Strategies, Sensory Healing Strategies, and Stress Management.

"So grateful. Helped me reduce most of my pain, get off pain-killers and get back to work. Great for anyone who wants to get off the 'hamster wheel' of life with pain." **–TH**

"Incredibly beneficial ... helped a lot [for my spinal surgery pain and insomnia] ... I am continuing to use this app." **–PainResource.com**

Anxiety Release—Based on EMDR

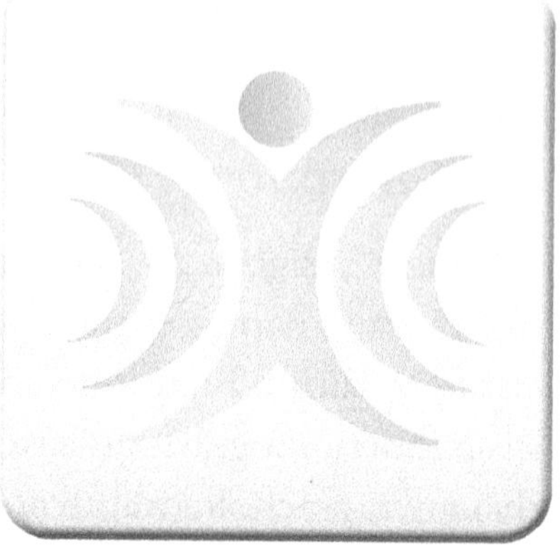

Seven sessions of guided focused attention plus bilateral stimulation. Designed to alleviate the physical and mental overactivity that maintains anxiety. The app version of this resource incorporates brain imagery designed to help enhance responsivity. Pain sufferers also report finding the BLS on this resource helpful, as documented by a recent report in the *Journal of Behavioral Medicine.*

"The freedom this app has given me from my anxiety is unbelievable." **–Gaff98**

"Life changing. After listening to the app I am somehow able to control my breathing, ease my chest pain and reconnect with reality. It feels like magic." **–Ellen Maree**

Available from the Apple App Store, Apple iTunes, and Google Play.

Calm & Confident—Based on EMDR

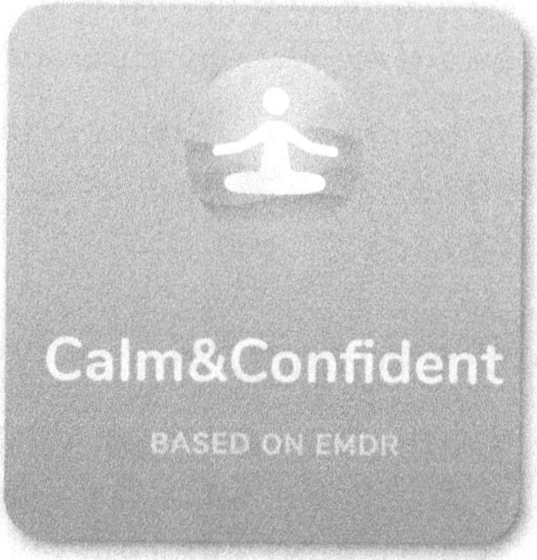

Comprised of 10 guided meditations that incorporate auditory, visual, and mental prompts, *Calm and Confident* is designed to stimulate increased self-awareness, self-acceptance, and emotional regulation. One of the central sessions is a 19-minute guided sensory-emotional experience called "Calm and Confident" which incorporates focused attention, sensory stimulation, and relaxation to stimulate reconnection with positive self resources. Another session entitled "Healing Anxiety" addresses the role that childhood emotional deficits play in maintaining stress. Other sessions stimulate increased self-awareness, emotional regulation, and security. Simply stated, the app teaches users how to communicate more effectively with their nervous system to unlearn stressful patterns of being and adopt a more confident sense of self.

"This app is amazing. The first time I heard it I felt so upbeat. Subsequent plays have been similarly positive. Over the course of a few weeks of listening I have found some long lost confidence which has helped me to start to deal with a person in my life who regularly undermined my confidence. Long may its effect last." **–Sharri**

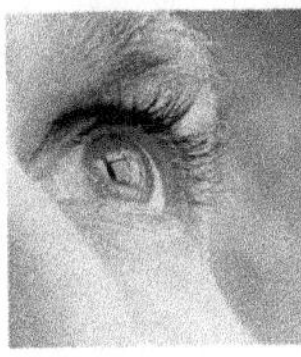

Online Training

Over 12 hours of teaching, incorporating numerous video demonstrations of Mark's work and the opportunity to see, hear, and feel how it's done

For online training in EMDR treatment of chronic pain/MUS visit:
https://overcomingpain.com/workshops/

EMDR treatment of chronic pain/MUS
10 EMDRIA credits

- Introduction (a brief history of pain)
- EMDR pain protocol
- 8 key differences between the standard trauma protocol and EMDR pain protocol(s)
- Case conceptualization patterns, themes, and pitfalls
- Safety issues associated with pain and MUS
- Normal dissociative phenomena in chronic pain clients
- Personality factors and pain
- Obtaining client-centered targets for reprocessing
- Maximizing somatic effects of BLS
- Why a SUDs of "0" is not the end of processing
- Identifying and developing resources
- EMDR treatment of medical vs. medically unexplained pain
- Some common stuck points and how to address them
- Adjunctive strategies for complex cases

EMDR and hypnosis in the treatment of chronic pain/MUS
5.5 EMDRIA credits

- EMDR and hypnosis
- What is hypnosis
- Trauma, dissociation, trance, and pain, how to utilize natural trances to ameliorate pain
- Similarities and differences between EMDR and hypnosis
- Double binds and pain
- 8 ways in which hypnosis can enhance EMDR
- 5 ways hypnosis can be used as an adjunct to EMDR
- How, when, and where to apply hypnotic strategies in EMDR
- Formal and informal trance work
- Hypnotic aspects of ego state work

"An amazing training–such a perspective shift."
Paula

"Lots of learning, lots of reflecting, lots of 'how to'."
Sangita

16

Client Resources

- Mark Grant's chronic pain fact sheet
- Normal emotional stages and reactions to pain
- Understanding feelings exercise
- Basic relaxation/meditation script
- Mark Grant's pain management recipe
- How to talk about pain
- Free-sleeping tip sheet
- Further reading

Digital versions can be downloaded from www.overcomingpain.com.

Mark Grant's chronic pain fact sheet

Despite the amazing advances of modern medicine, chronic pain continues to be one of the most misunderstood and poorly treated health problems. Here are a few facts that will help you navigate the confusion and understand what you need to do to help yourself.

1. **Chronic pain is not like normal pain.**

   Chronic pain is different to what we think of as normal pain—pain caused by injury. Although it usually (though not always) starts with injury, chronic pain is maintained by many hidden causal factors, including biochemical changes, changes in brain activity, genetic predisposition, prior stress, and psychological factors just to name a few. That's why it does not show up on x-rays, scans, or other medical tests, and that's why it does not respond to treatments that are normally effective for normal pain, like rest, medication, physiotherapy, etc.

2. **Chronic pain is often associated with substandard medical care.**

   Medicos get it wrong between 25% and 50% of the time with chronic pain sufferers—diagnosing someone who has a real illness as suffering from a conversion disorder, especially if you are a woman. Female chronic pain sufferers are also more likely to be prescribed inadequate pain medication. Generally speaking, chronic pain sufferers are more likely to have experienced delayed access to medical treatment, diagnostic failures, substandard treatment, and to be blamed for their problems. These delays allow the pain to persist longer than it should and make it all the more difficult to reverse once the right treatment mix is finally found. The final treatment mix is likely to include a lot more than what your doctor prescribed.

3. **Your doctor will (not) take care of everything.**

   More than for any other condition, chronic pain sufferers should not just trust their doctor to take care of things. Most medical schools offer little or no education in pain medicine. At best your physician will offer you medication, and a referral to a physical therapist and/or a specialist, and maybe a psychologist. Overcoming chronic pain requires a lot more than that. You should adopt a proactive approach to managing your own treatment and recovery, asking questions, getting a second opinion, learning about your condition, investigating alternative treatment strategies, making lifestyle changes, and taking responsibility for your own health and well-being.

4. **Just because they can't find a cause doesn't mean you are crazy.**

   Modern medicine is based on being able to identify a biological cause for pain and illness. In the 19th century there was a trend to label patients (especially women) with medically unexplained pain as crazy (they called it hysteria) because they didn't have the technology we have today. Despite increased scientific understanding of chronic pain, some professionals (and members of the public) still view unexplained pain in this "either ... you must have something wrong with you—or ... you must be crazy" way. You might even feel this way from time to time too—chronic pain can certainly make you feel like you are going crazy. But you are just suffering from a complex interacting set of physical, neurological, and biochemical reactions for which there is no simple cause or cure. It is lazy and unscientific to think of chronic pain sufferers as being weak or having a mental illness, and you are not being fair to yourself if you see yourself this way.

5. **It really is all in your mind.**

   On the other hand ... if anyone ever tells you it's all in your head, they are right, sort of. Although chronic pain starts in your body and feels like it's coming from your body, it's actually coming from your mind. That's because your brain doesn't just passively receive signals from your body, it also generates sensory experience. Different parts of your brain do different things. Only two of the nine areas of the brain involved in chronic pain are responsible for processing sensory signals from your body ("physical" pain). The other seven actually deal with emotional processing! The fact that chronic pain has such a significant emotional component is good news: you can't change a prolapsed disc, or damaged nerves, but you can change how it affects you.

6. **It's not your fault.**

   Although it can feel unfair and you may wonder what you did to deserve such suffering, you are not really being punished for past misdeeds. Chronic pain develops as a result of a combination of past and present factors, including genetic predisposition, which is responsible for about 30% of chronic pain, physical or sexual abuse in childhood, emotional neglect, lack of safety, etc. Although you may have survived, surviving comes at a cost. Chronic, severe stress causes a lot of "wear and tear" on the human nervous system which is not immediately apparent, but over the long term weakens your body's ability to withstand later injury and illness. Trauma therapists refer to this as "the body keeps the score." When a stressed body suffers even a mild injury, it has no reserves to fight inflammation and injury, leading to chronic pain. See my book *Change Your Brain, Change Your Pain* for more information about how the effects of severe stress lead to chronic pain.

7. **You are not alone.**

   Although you might feel like you are the only one experiencing it, chronic pain is quite common, affecting up to one in five adults, women at least twice as much as men. But because it's so misunderstood, because of the way we view pain, having chronic pain can make you feel very alone and isolated. It's really important to find someone who makes you feel validated and understood, such as fellow sufferers (via online support groups) or mental health professionals who specialize in chronic pain and trauma.

Normal emotional stages and reactions to pain

Chronic pain is a long-term problem which triggers different feelings at different times. This is a summary of the main emotional responses to pain and what they mean. The more you understand your feelings, the less stressed you will feel and the better able to cope you will be.

Emotion	Thought	Behavior
1. Denial	"It's probably nothing serious." "I'll be alright."	Ignore the pain. Keep going as though nothing has happened. Not seeking medical help. Not following medical advice/treatment.
2. Fear/Anxiety	"Something's wrong." "What's going to happen?" "Will I be able to cope?"	Rest/seek medical help. Worry/preoccupation. Avoidance.
3. Depression	"What is the use?" "It's hopeless." "I'm weak/inadequate." "Why bother?"	Reduced participation in physical activities, even enjoyable ones. Social withdrawal. Sleeping problems.
4. Anger	"It's not fair." "Why me?" "Nobody cares."	Impulsive or compulsive behaviors. Aggressive behavior. "Overreacting" to things. Self-destructive behavior (e.g., abusing drugs or alcohol).
5. Shame	"I'm bad." "I'm unlovable." "I'm worthless." "I'm a failure."	Social withdrawal. Decreased confidence and assertiveness. Self-destructive behavior (e.g., abusing drugs or alcohol).
6. Acceptance	"What has happened has happened." "It's not my fault." "I deserve help." "It is up to me." "I can cope."	Being less focused on the past. Having more realistic expectations of self. Maintaining appropriate levels of physical activity. Using medication more appropriately. Reduced mental and emotional stress. Increased feelings of peace and calmness.

Understanding feelings

Feelings are part of your normal response to events. Sometimes they can become part of the problem. Knowing what your feelings mean and how to react to them can reduce the contribution of negative feelings to pain and improve coping.

1. **Think about your pain** whether physical or emotional.
2. **Notice** how your pain makes you *feel*. Notice what physical sensations those feelings involve. **Don't react or judge, just notice.**
3. Try and **stay tuned to what's happening in your body in the present moment.**
4. Next, **label the feelings.** What emotion do those body sensations signify? (e.g., Fear? Anger? Anxiety? Depression? Terror?)

   ____

5. Now, going from a sensing mode to a more analytical mode, try and **interpret what your feelings signify about yourself** and your ability to cope with your pain. (Hint: Feeling afraid might mean feeling unsure about your ability to cope. Feeling angry might mean feeling victimized. Feeling depressed probably means feeling hopeless.)

   ____

6. Try and **make an "I-statement"** out of that realization, such as "I feel vulnerable/punished/helpless [choose one]."

   ____

7. Try and **maintain a neutral, detached observer stance** in relation to your thoughts (don't judge your judging). **Accept your feelings and thoughts** as though they were just neutral pieces of information.
8. Decide on an appropriate course of action.

   E.g.: Feeling afraid—take action to increase your sense of safety.
   Feeling anxious—take action to increase preparedness for future threats.
   Feeling angry—take action to protect your rights.
   Feeling depressed—acknowledge fatigue, re-evaluate past coping strategies.

Basic relaxation/meditation script

1. Assume a comfortable position.
2. Begin by attending to whatever physical sensations you notice in your body.
3. Try and "just notice" whatever is happening in your body in a detached way without thinking about it or analyzing it too much.
4. JUST NOTICE whatever you're feeling ...
5. Avoid analyzing, thinking, or problem-solving. If you catch yourself doing this, just bring your attention back to just noticing whatever is going on.
6. Notice your breathing, the gradual rise and fall of your chest with each breath.
7. Notice how your chest expands with each in-breath and deflates with each out-breath. You may notice that there is a slight feeling of tension with each in-breath, and a feeling of relief with each out-breath.
8. As you focus on your breathing, you might like to think about how NATURAL breathing is, how CONNECTED breathing makes you feel with your body and the rhythm of life. You might also enjoy the realization that breathing happens AUTOMATICALLY, without you having to make any special effort.
9. As you continue to focus on your breathing, you may also notice the rate of your breathing slowing down, as your mind becomes more detached from your everyday consciousness.
10. If any other thoughts or feelings intrude into your awareness of yourself, just notice them and let them go by.
11. Notice any changes about how you are feeling, including your awareness of what you are feeling. If nothing seems different, that's fine too.
12. Just keep breathing and keep noticing. Whatever you feel or notice, just observe it and let it go.
13. Continue doing this for 15 to 20 minutes.
14. At the end of that time, give yourself a few moments to gradually reorient yourself.
15. If you have been able to maintain your attention on your breath reasonably consistently, you should notice mild feelings of detachment and lightness; some people notice other sensations, such as tingling or numbness. Whether you do or not, regular practice of this technique will help you learn how to experience your pain differently, in ways you might never have imagined.

Mark Grant's pain management recipe 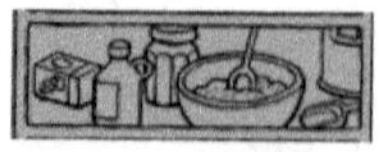

Overcoming chronic pain involves many elements, like baking a cake. First you have to find all the right ingredients, mix them together under ideal conditions, and then wait (baking a cake takes time). The waiting part can be hard because you never know quite when that cake is going to rise, but if you have the right mix of ingredients (below), practice them regularly, and maintain hope and patience, you will eventually feel better.[1]

1. **Find safety (the 3 S's).**

   Find somewhere, someone, or something (3 x Ss) to hold on to that makes you feel secure. It must be something/somewhere/someone that stimulates a state of unconditional safety and well-being in you, through the very sensory reactions it stimulates. An idyllic natural place you have visited, a trusted friend or mentor, a hot pool, etc. And then practice imagining yourself there and how being there makes you feel as an antidote to your pain and stress.

2. **Accept the pain.**

   Although unpleasant and sometimes inexplicable, pain is an unavoidable part of life. You cannot get rid of the pain any more than you can get rid of yourself. Accepting the pain means being open to those unpleasant feelings, and really engaging with them. There is a saying in science that just observing something changes it. Accepting the pain also means letting go of the desire to control it. But when you do this, the pain will reveal its secrets to you and start to change. This takes real courage.

3. **Understand the pain.**

   Acceptance leads to understanding; what unmet need is this pain alerting you to? What is its hidden message or purpose? (To warn, punish, or protect?) Based on your answer to this question, what do you need to be able to live with less pain? After initially finding it hard to answer this question, Donna finally realized that there was an old and deep part of her personality that believed she deserved to be punished. In the unsafe world of her childhood this was about being invisible so as not to attract negative attention. Once she was able to let go of this attitude (with the help of a therapist), her stress levels decreased, her self-care improved, and her pain slowly started to decrease.

4. **Heal any unresolved emotional trauma.**

   If there are any unresolved intensely painful memories that you have not dealt with, now is the time to address them. Otherwise they will continue to exacerbate your pain through raised levels of physical tension, emotional distress, and decreased ability to get your needs met. A trauma therapist with EMDR training can help here.

5. **Stabilize your feelings.**

   Chronic pain is 80% emotion. Practice managing negative feelings such as anger, shame, anxiety, and depression through emotional regulation strategies such as breath awareness, accepting and acting on feelings, expressing feelings vs. holding them in, letting go of negative emotions such as anger or shame (forgiving yourself and others), and engaging in activities which stimulate joy, peace, and hope. The more in control you feel of your emotions, the more in control you will feel generally. The author's *Anxiety Release* and *Sleep Restore* apps can help with this.

6. **Learn how to manage the pain.**

   You don't have to suffer or learn to live with it. Learn how to harness the power of your mind to manage chronic pain using self-hypnosis, self-use of BLS, meditation, distraction, engaging in enjoyable activities, and other self-management strategies. The author's *Change Your Brain, Change Your Pain* book and his *Overcoming Pain* app can help with this.

7. **Avoid stress.**

   Go through your contacts list and delete all negative relationships, people, and circumstances from your life (including members of your family if necessary!). You simply cannot afford to be tolerating any toxic relationships or carrying people who are "dead weight" in your life. All your energy must be directed toward your well-being. It's not selfish—it's survival. The author's *Calm and Confident* app will help you with this.

8. **Develop an attitude of self-compassion.**

   Stop judging yourself and start loving yourself. This means accepting your physical limitations (including grieving lost capabilities), adopting an attitude of tolerance and kindness toward yourself, living life at your pace, and ensuring you get adequate rest and nutrition. You must be there for yourself in life—no one else will be.

9. **Do something.**

   No matter how helpless and hopeless you feel, setting goals and taking action (however little) will help restore your sense of control. Depending on your personality, it could be collecting stamps, caring for a pet, learning a new skill, etc.

10. **Reinvent yourself.**

    The Chinese symbol for crisis also means opportunity. Surviving pain means you will need to find new ways of finding joy, purpose, and meaning, and possibly new things based on your changed physical capabilities. This will require internal mental adjustments and alterations in your sense of self/identity (e.g., "I am okay even if I can't do everything I think others expect"). Change can be scary, but like pain it too is inevitable.

11. **Give it time.**

    Unlearning painful patterns of feeling takes time, like learning to ride a bike in reverse. While it is natural to want to know, "How long before I feel better?" this too is actually part of your old controlling self. Maintain hope and trust that your subconscious mind will respond to your efforts in its own time.

How to talk about pain

Sharing our hurt with others is one of the most powerful ways of overcoming pain and stress. Even if it doesn't take the pain away, just expressing our feelings can relieve tension and make adversity easier to bear. Talking about pain can be difficult: the person with pain may not want to burden their family and friends; family and friends may not know what to say. Either way, not talking about pain only makes things worse, so here are some guidelines for how to talk about pain.

For the chronic pain sufferer:

1. *Tell someone how you are feeling.* Having chronic pain can make you feel guilty, anxious, and depressed; these are normal feelings which must be acknowledged and expressed. Not expressing your feelings often leads to a build-up of frustration, depression, and anger. Expressing your feelings relieves tension and improves coping. Obviously you should be careful about whom you tell and how: your feelings are personal and you do not want them to be mistreated by sharing them with the wrong person.

2. *Finding the words.* Sometimes it's hard to find the right words to describe pain and stress. If you are not accustomed to expressing your feelings, you may need to learn more words to describe how you are feeling. Some emotional intelligence websites or books have lists of feeling words, but this won't show you how to connect the words with the feelings. A better technique is to observe people you know who are good at expressing themselves, or watch dramas or foreign movies. Being able to name what you are feeling is powerful: it leads to mastery over feelings.

3. *Know what you want.* Try to be conscious of what you want out of expressing your feelings. It is human to need to share our pain—to feel that someone else understands us. Remember, though, that perfect understanding between two human beings is rare—particularly when it comes to suffering. The important thing is that even if the person you express yourself to doesn't completely understand you, you have at least expressed yourself.

4. *Find the right balance.* Naturally, you don't need (or want) to talk about your pain all the time—that would be too depressing. The trick is to express your feelings enough to feel supported and not alone. This can be challenging, even for a good communicator; however, once you have built up an empathic relationship, there will be many times when you won't need to say anything—just a look is often enough to convey how you are feeling.

5. *Be patient.* Because pain is invisible, well people around you will sometimes "forget" that you are in pain and expect things of you that you cannot manage. Understand that it's hard for others to be mindful of your needs all the time and that you will have to remind them of your condition from time to time.

For family members:

1. *Learn to listen.* Listening is one of the most helpful things you can do for a person in pain. Listening involves more than just hearing what is being said—a good listener listens with their heart too. Notice where the words resonate in your own body—this will give you a direct, non-verbal connection with the person in pain.
2. Listening is hard. It may not feel like you are doing anything, but by being a good listener you create a space for the pain sufferer's feelings—sometimes a space that they are unable to give themselves. Listening is thus a very powerful communication tool.
3. *Pay attention.* Listening is a full-brain activity—you can't listen properly while you are doing something else. To listen properly, you must focus your attention completely on the person you are communicating with, listening with your whole heart and mind. Don't feign interest if your attention is really on something else; better to ask them to wait until you are finished with what you are doing.
4. *Have an open mind.* Don't assume you know what the chronic pain sufferer in your life feels or is going through. Their reality is probably very different to yours. Avoid judging—in general, people do not go around pretending they are in pain to get sympathy—research shows that exaggerating or malingering are actually rare. Remember: "Pain is **whatever the experiencing person says it is, whenever the experiencing person says it happens."**
5. *Demonstrate that you understand—or are at least trying.* Repeating and summarizing what is said is a good way of showing that you are trying to understand. Just a simple "that sounds pretty frustrating" shows the other person that you have listened and are in tune with their feelings.
6. *Only ever offer advice when asked.* It's tempting to offer advice and solutions to people with chronic pain—you want to help, and offering advice can seem like a practical thing to do. Although well-intentioned, this often just gets in the way of good listening and empathy when this is most needed. If they really need you to tell them how to manage their pain they will ask.
7. *Be patient.* Communicating with a chronic pain sufferer can be challenging at times. They may not always tell you directly what they are feeling or want. They may be irritable, changeable, and contradictory. Remember that they are going through a very stressful experience and that it is probably not you that they are really angry with most of the time.

Free-sleeping tip sheet

Many people with chronic illness, pain, or severe stress are exhausted from lack of sleep and find it impossible to achieve a normal sleep routine. In that case it may be best to accept that you are just not going to get a solid eight hours' sleep a night and instead of trying to make your body conform to a normal sleep routine, allow your body to dictate when and how long you sleep. Thus instead of one x eight-hour block of sleep every 24 hours, you might have three x two- to three-hour blocks of sleep at say, midnight, dawn, and noon. This method enables you to get more sleep over the course of 24 hours, just not at the normal times. Obviously your sleep has to fit around your daytime obligations, but wherever possible you should try and fit these around your body's sleep schedule rather than the other way around. Trying to force yourself to fall asleep when your body is not ready will just make you feel more stressed. In time, when your pain has healed, your sleep should return to normal. In the meantime, try the following:

1. Change the way you think about sleep. Make sleep a priority. Instead of fitting sleep into your busy schedule, fit your schedule around your sleep. Know that sleep is one of the most important elements for overcoming stress and pain.
2. Learn to think of sleep as something natural that you can do anytime, anywhere, instead of just at night in bed.
3. Learn to recognize the signals that your body is ready for sleep and act on them. Don't put off going to bed once you realize you are feeling sleepy.
4. Learn to sleep anywhere, anytime. Bed is nice, but if you find it easier to fall asleep on your favorite easy chair or couch, sleep there.
5. Before sleep, try and engage yourself in mildly stimulating but relaxing activities (e.g., knitting, reading, watching a boring movie).
6. Try not to worry about whether or not you are going to fall asleep—it only makes you less likely to fall asleep.
7. Understand that your sleeping pattern will vary so long as you are affected by severe stress or pain. This is normal and the best thing is to just take it "a day at a time."

Further reading

Stress, trauma and pain

Barsky, A.J. (1989). Somatoform disorders. In H.I. Kaplan & B.J. Sadock (Eds.), *Comprehensive textbook of psychiatry*, Vol. 1 (5th ed., pp. 1009–1027). Williams & Wilkins. Baltimore.

Scaer, Robert (2001). *The body bears the burden: Trauma, dissociation and disease.* The Hawthorne Press.

Goodwin, Jean, & Attias, Reina (1999). *Splintered reflections: Images of the body in trauma.* Basic Books.

Felitti V.J., Anda R.F., Nordenberg D., et al. (1998). Relationship of childhood abuse and household dysfunction to many of the leading causes of death in adults. The Adverse Childhood Experiences (ACE) Study. *American Journal of Preventative Medicine*, May, 14(4), 245–58.

Treatment

Blakeslee, Sandra, & Blakeslee, Matthew (2007). *The body has a mind of its own: How body maps in your brain help you do (almost) everything better.* Random House.

Eimer, Bruce (1998). *Pain management psychotherapy: A practical guide.* John Wiley & Sons, Inc. New York.

Eimer, Bruce (2008). *Hypnotize yourself out of pain now!* Crown House Publishing Ltd. UK.

Grant, Mark (2009). *Change your brain, change your pain.* Mark Grant. www.overcoming-pain.com

Grant, Mark (2014a). The use of an app to manage carpal tunnel syndrome. *OA Behavioural Medicine,* Mar 20, 2(1), 3.

Grant, Mark (2014b). Eye movement desensitization reprocessing treatment of chronic pain. *OA Musculoskeletal Medicine,* Aug 17, 2(2), 17.

Haley, Jay (1993). *Uncommon therapy: The psychiatric techniques of Milton H. Erickson.* WW Norton & Company. New York.

Jensen, Mark (2011). *Hypnosis for chronic pain management.* Oxford University Press. New York.

Parnell, Laurel (2008). *Tapping in: A step-by-step guide to activating your healing resources through bilateral stimulation.* Sounds True. Denver.

Ratey, John (2008). *Spark: The revolutionary new science of exercise and the brain.* Little Brown & Co. New York.

EMDR in the treatment of pain research summary

de Roos, C.J., Veenstra, A.C., den Hollander-Gijsman, M.E., van der Wee, N.J.A., de Jongh, A., Zitman, F.G., & van Rood, Y.R. (2010). Eye movement desensitization and reprocessing (EMDR) for chronic phantom limb pain (PLP): A preliminary study of 10 cases. *Pain Res Management*, Mar–April, 15(2), 65–71.

Grant, M. (2000). EMDR: a new treatment for trauma and chronic pain. *Complimentary Therapies in Nursing & Midwifery*, 6(2), 91–94. Harcourt.

Grant, M. & Threlfo, C. (2002). EMDR in the treatment of chronic pain. *Journal of Clinical Psychology*, 58(12), 1505–1520.

Hassard, A. (1993). Investigation of eye movement desensitization and reprocessing in pain clinic patients. *Behavioral and Cognitive Psychotherapy Journal*, 23(2), 177–185.

Hekmat, H., Groth, S. & Rogers, D. (1994). Pain ameliorating effects of eye movement desensitization. *Journal of Behavior Therapy and Experimental Psychiatry*, 25, 121–130.

Mazzola, A., Calcagno, M.L., Goicochea, M.T., et al., (2009). EMDR in the treatment of chronic pain. *Journal of EMDR Practice and Research*, 3(2), 66–79.

McCann, D.L. (1992) Posttraumatic stress disorder due to devastating burns overcome by a single session of eye movement desensitization. *Journal of Behavior Therapy and Experimental Psychiatry*, 23, 319–323.

Ray, P., & Page, A.C. (2002). A single session of hypnosis and eye movement desensitisation and reprocessing (EMDR) in the treatment of chronic pain. *Australian Journal of Clinical and Experimental Hypnosis*, 30(2), 170–178.

Schneider, J., Hofmann, A., Rost, C., Shapiro, F. (2006). EMDR and phantom limb pain: Theoretical implications, case study and treatment guidelines. *Journal of EMDR Practice & Research* 1(1), 31–45.

Wilson S.A., Tinker, R., Becker, L.A., Hofman, A. & Cole, J. (2000 September). *EMDR treatment of phantom limb pain with brain imaging (MEG)*. Paper presented at the annual meeting of the EMDR Association, Toronto, Canada.

Appendices

How does EMDR work?

In EMDR clients are asked to describe and quantify their complaints and to describe the memory from which they wish to obtain relief. This involves asking them how the problem makes them feel and rating their level of distress on a SUDs of 0 to 10 where 0 = no distress and 10 = the worst distress they could possibly imagine. They are then asked to isolate a single picture that represents either the worst aspect of the event or an early memory that relates to the trauma. Then they are asked to state what they think about themselves in relation to the traumatic memory ("What words about your self best go with that picture?"). Finally, they are asked to state how they would like to feel about themselves when they think of that memory in future and rate how true that feels to them now on a scale of 0 to 7 where 0 = not true and 7 = very true.

During the desensitization phase of treatment clients are instructed to visualize the traumatic scene, recall the negative self-statement and associated emotional distress, and attend to a bilateral stimulation (finger movements, tapping, or auditory clicks). Clients are instructed to "just notice" and "let whatever happens happen". After each set, they are asked to take a deep breath and report on whatever feelings or sensations they now notice. Clients often report feeling significantly better, if somewhat confused by the reduction in the previously distressing thoughts and feelings. If asked to think of it again, they often report feeling much less bothered by the problem and make comments like: "It seems further away" or "It doesn't seem as important anymore." If another memory or feeling emerges, the process is repeated from the point just prior to commencing the bilateral stimulation ("Okay, so just notice that ..."). When the problem has been reduced to a SUD of 1 or 0, the client is asked to think of the positive cognition and rate their belief in that on a scale of 1 to 7.

Recipients of EMDR usually report feeling more relaxed, less distressed, and more able to distinguish between real and imagined threats. These affective changes are the key to EMDR's efficacy with chronic pain. For example, Jenny, a chronic fatigue sufferer, lived in fear of the next pain flare-up and how she was going to cope. The anxiety that she felt about her pain caused tension, which added to her pain. Intellectually Jenny "knew" that she was a strong person, but emotionally she didn't feel it. After EMDR treatment, which involved learning to soothe her pain using a combination of dual attention stimulus and healing imagery, Jenny felt more confident in her ability to cope, which made her feel less anxious and less vulnerable to pain flare-ups.

There is a lot of curiosity about how EMDR works, perhaps because of its unorthodox methodology. It's not a bad thing that people, both professionals and non-professionals, want to understand more about how their mind works and how treatments like EMDR harness mental abilities. Although we still don't fully know, regardless, it is incumbent upon the therapist to have some idea about why they do what they do, and to be able to offer some explanation to their clients. EMDR was initially thought to be a kind of operant conditioning procedure, akin to traditional desensitization. However, this is no longer thought to be the case since EMDR relies on much shorter amounts of exposure than traditional exposure and seems to work much more quickly. Others believe that EMDR works by activating the orienting reflex (OR). The OR is an innate response to new or novel stimuli from the environment (exogenous attention). The OR is thought to have an evolutionary basis in that it seems to facilitate scanning for danger. If danger is detected, the OR is triggered, stimulating an increase in physiological arousal. But if no danger is detected, as with bilateral stimulation, the OR is followed by a decrease in physiological arousal. This would facilitate the processing of physical and emotional pain. In a review of the effects of bilateral stimulation of interhemispheric communication, Propper and Christman (2008)[10] concluded that EMDR increases communication between the left and right hemispheres. It is known that this is aided by increased feelings of calmness. This is also consistent with the improved memory consolidation and recall that follows EMDR treatment of traumatic memories. Harvard psychiatrist Robert Stickgold has suggested that EMDR is activating a biochemical process normally associated with REM sleep, when information processing occurs.

Some experts believe that bilateral stimulation/dual attention stimulus works by promoting a sense of detachment from the problem, similar to that produced by meditation. Consistent with this, a recent review by Australian researcher Chris Lee found that the main treatment effect of EMDR is indeed a distancing effect. My own (ongoing unpublished) research involving 20 clients with various diagnoses, all involving some level of physiological distress (e.g., chronic pain, GAD (generalized anxiety disorder), PTSD), found that most clients reported an immediate decrease in negative thoughts and feelings associated with their condition following their first experience with dual attention/bilateral stimulation process. Many also reported feelings of drowsiness and increased well-being. All reported the distancing effect (feeling that the problem seemed further away). These effects lasted anywhere from 24 hours to over a week. Recipients also often reported that when the effect wore off, their experience of the problem was different to how they usually experience it. With further treatment, these effects were generally associated with significant improvement and enduring increased feelings of efficacy and control. Dual attention/bilateral stimulation clearly shoulders much of the weight of the changes associated with EMDR and it deserves to be a subject of research on its own. In terms of how it works, I like the OR account, and usually incorporate this with sensory processing when explaining EMDR to clients.

Research review

Currently there are six randomized controlled clinical trials that demonstrate the efficacy of EMDR in various pain conditions. Tesarz et al. (2019)[4] concluded these studies showed a good to very good efficacy of EMDR in the treatment of chronic pain. They add that EMDR in the treatment of chronic pain may require a greater variety of goals and more flexibility in protocol application than the treatment of post-traumatic stress disorder. They also note that additional larger studies are needed to overcome methodological problems of existing studies and to clarify what modifications to the protocol need to be made for different presentations. Based on the Australian National Health and Medical Research Council, which vets new treatments, EMDR meets the criteria for a level-2 treatment (moderate evidence levels), where 1 signifies excellent and 5 signifies no evidence. However, as with EMDR as a treatment for PTSD, it will take time for professional awareness regarding the efficacy to EMDR as a treatment for pain to develop.[5–8] It does appear that the effects of EMDR are strongest where pain is trauma-related. These studies indicate that recipients of EMDR benefit in terms of both reduced emotional distress and reduced physical discomfort. For example, Barry, a chronic low back pain sufferer, felt depressed and anxious about his pain and its effects on his life. Although medication helped to some degree, he hated how it made him feel and it didn't help with the stress of having to change his working life. EMDR helped Barry learn how to control his pain naturally (using bilateral stimulation) and feel less negative about his decreased physical functioning. This also helped Barry feel less negative about himself.

In conclusion it can be said that EMDR is an evidence-based treatment for chronic pain, but that treatment needs to be tailored to the individual client and, of course, results may vary.

References

Introduction

1. Elofsson, U.O., von Schèele, B., Theorell, T., Söndergaard, H.P. (2008). Physiological correlates of eye movement desensitization and reprocessing. *Journal of Anxiety Disorders,* 2008 May, *22*(4), 622–34. doi: 10.1016/j.janxdis.2007.05.012. Epub 2007 Jun 3. PMID: 17604948

2. Tesarz, J., Wicking, M., Bernardy, K., & Seidler, G.H. (2019). EMDR therapy's efficacy in the treatment of pain. *Journal of EMDR Practice and Research, 13*(4), 337–344. https://doi.org/10.1891/1933-3196.13.4.337

3. Ettensohn, M. (2013). How I learned to stop worrying and love the word "patient." *Sacramento Valley Psychologist.* Retrieved from http://sacramentovalleypsychologist.com/page-1776093#section5

Chapter One

1. van der Kolk, Bessel, A., & van der Hart, Onno (1989). Pierre Janet and the breakdown of adaptation in psychological trauma, *American Journal of Psychiatry, 146*(12), 1530–1540.

2. Dyde, Sean (2015). Cullen, a cautionary tale. *Medical History, 59*(2), 222–240.

3. Davies, K.A., Macfarlane, G.J., McBeth, J., Morriss, R., Dickens, C. (2009). Insecure attachment style is associated with chronic widespread pain. *Pain*, 2009 Jun, *143*(3), 200–205. doi: 10.1016/j.pain.2009.02.013. Epub 2009 Apr 2. PMID: 19345016; PMCID: PMC2806947

4. Freud, S. (1962). On the psychical mechanism of hysterical phenomena: A lecture. In J. Strachey (Ed. and trans.), *The standard edition of the complete psychological works of Sigmund Freud* (Vol. 3, pp. 25–39). Hogarth Press. London. (Original work published 1893.)

5. Dyde, Sean (2015). Cullen, a cautionary tale. *Medical History, 59*(2), 222–240.

6. Dyde, Sean (2015). Cullen, a cautionary tale. *Medical History, 59*(2), 222–240.

7. van der Kolk, Bessel, A., & van der Hart, Onno (1989). Pierre Janet and the breakdown of adaptation in psychological trauma, *American Journal of Psychiatry, 146*(12), 1530–1540.

8. Melzack, R. (1965). Pain mechanisms, a new theory. *Science, 150*(3699), 971–151.

9. Nicholas, Michael (1996). The pain self-efficacy questionnaire: Taking pain into account. *Pain – 1996 An updated review* (Refresher course syllabus) (JN Campbell editor). IASP. USA.

10. Gatchel, R.J., Polatin, P.B., & Mayer, T.G. (1995). The dominant role of psychosocial risk factors in the development of chronic low back pain disability. *Spine, 20*(24), 2702–2709.

11. Williams, A.C.C., Fisher, E., Hearn, L., Eccleston, C. (2020). Psychological therapies for the management of chronic pain (excluding headache) in adults. *Cochrane Database of Systematic Reviews*, 2020 August 12, *8*(8), CD007407. doi: 10.1002/14651858.CD007407.pub4. PMID: 32794606; PMCID: PMC7437545

12. Felitti, V.J., Anda, R.F., Nordenberg, D., et al. Relationship of childhood abuse and household dysfunction to many of the leading causes of death in adults. The Adverse Childhood Experiences (ACE) Study. *American Journal of Preventative Medicine,* 1998 May, *14*(4), 245–258; Dionne, C.E. (2005). Psychological distress confirmed as predictor of long-term back-related functional limitations in primary care settings. *Journal of Clinical Epidemiology, 58*(7), 714–718; Sansone, Randy A., Pole, M., Dakroub, H., & Butler, M. (2006). Childhood trauma, borderline personality symptomatology and psychosocial and pain disorders in adulthood. *Psychosomatics, 47*(2), 158–162; Cohen, S. (2005). Keynote presentation at the Eight International Congress of Behavioral medicine: The Pittsburg common cold studies: Psychosocial predictors of susceptibility in respiratory infectious illness. *International Journal of Behavioral Medicine, 12*(3), 123–31.

13. Felitti, V.J., Anda, R.F., Nordenberg, D., et al. Relationship of childhood abuse and household dysfunction to many of the leading causes of death in adults. The Adverse Childhood Experiences (ACE) Study. *American Journal of Preventative Medicine,* 1998 May, *14*(4), 245–258.

14. Harris, N. (2019). Part 1: Proposed new classifications and nomenclatures for chronic pain. Reflections. *RGA Newsletter, Vol. 47,* 2–8. Downloaded from https://www.rgare.com/knowledge-center/media/articles/part-i-proposed-new-classifications-and-nomenclatures-for-chronic-pain on July 15, 2021.

15. van der Linden, R., Bolt, T., Veen M. (2022). "If it can't be coded, it doesn't exist." A historical-philosophical analysis of the new ICD-11 classification of chronic pain. *Studies in History and Philosophy of Science, 94,* 121–132.

Chapter Two

1. Sansone, R.A., Pole, M., Dakroub, H., & Butler, M. (2006). Childhood trauma, borderline personality symptomatology and psychophysiological and pain disorders in adulthood. *Psychosomatics,* 2006 Mar–April, *47*(2), 158–162; Rubin, J.J. (2005). Psychosomatic pain: New insights and management strategies. *Southern Medical Journal,* 2005 Nov, *98*(11), 1099–1110; Roberts, S.J. (1996). The sequelae of childhood sexual abuse: A primary care focus for adult female survivors. *The Nurse Practitoner,* 1996 Dec, *21*(12 Pt 1), 42, 45, 49–52; Gamsa, A. (1994). The role of psychological factors in chronic pain. II. A critical appraisal. *Pain, 57,* 17–29.

2. Geisser, M.E., Roth, R.S., Bachman, J.E., & Eckert, T.A. (1996). The relationship between symptoms of post-traumatic stress disorder and pain, affective disturbance and disability among patients with accident and non-accident related pain. *Pain,* Aug, *66*(2–3), 207–214. (See also 28.)

3. Rapkin, A.J., Kames, L.D., Darke, L.L., Stampfler, F.M., & Naliboff, B.D., (1990). History of physical and sexual abuse in women with chronic pelvic pain. *Obstetrics & Gynecology,* 1990, *76,* 92–96; Goldberg, R.T., & Goldstein, R. (2000). A comparison of chronic pain patients and controls on traumatic events in childhood. *Disability & Rehabilitation: An International Multidisciplinary Journal,* Nov 2000, *22*(17), 756–763; Linton, S.J. (1997). A population-based study of the relationship between sexual abuse and back pain: Establishing a link. *Pain, 73,* 47–53; Otis, John D., Keane, Terence M., & Kerns, Robert D. (2003). An examination of the relationship between chronic pain and post-traumatic stress disorder. *Journal of Rehabilitation Research & Development,*

September/October 2003, 40(5), 397–406; National Center for PTSD Fact Sheet. Based on: Ronald C. Kessler et al., Posttraumatic stress disorder in the National Comorbidity Survey. *Archives of General Psychiatry,* December 1995, *52*(12), 1048–1060.

4. Walz, Garry R., & Bleuer, Jeanne C. (2013). *When treatment becomes trauma: Defining, preventing and transforming medical trauma*. Paper based on a program presented at the 2013 American Counseling Association Conference. Cincinnati, OH. VISTAS online, article 73.

5. Baker, D.G., Mendenhall, C.L., Simbartl, L.A., Magan, L.K., & Steinberg, J.L. (1997). Relationship between posttraumatic stress disorder and self-reported physical symptoms in Persian Gulf War veterans. *Archives of Internal Medicine,* 1997, Oct 13, *157*(18), 2076–2078; Arguelles, L.M., Afari, N., Buchwald, D.S., Clauw, D.J., Furner, S., & Goldberg, J. (2006). A twin study of posttraumatic stress disorder symptoms and chronic widespread pain. *Pain,* 2006, May 13, Epub ahead of print. Downloaded July 4, 2006 www.ncbi.nlm.nih.gov/entrez

6. Walker, E.A., Katon, W.J., Roy-Byrne, P.J., Jemelka, R.P., & Russo, J. (1993). Histories of sexual victimization in patients with irritable bowel syndrome or inflammatory bowel disease. *American Journal of Psychiatry, 150*(10), 1502–1506; de Leeuw, Bertoli E., Schmidt, J.E., & Carlson, C.R. (2005). Prevalence of traumatic stressors in patients with temporomandibular disorders. *Journal of Oral Maxillofac Surgery,* Jan, *63*(1), 42–50.

7. de Leeuw, R., Schmidt, J.E., & Carlson, C.R. (2005). Traumatic stressors and posttraumatic stress disorder symptoms in headache patients. *Headache,* 2005 Nov–Dec, *45*(10), 1365–1374; Geisser, M.E., Roth, R.S., Bachman, J.E., & Eckert, T.A. (1996). The relationship between symptoms of post-traumatic stress disorder and pain, affective disturbance and disability among patients with accident and non-accident related pain. *Pain,* Aug, *66*(2–3), 207–214. (See also 28.); Taal, L.A., & Faber, A.W. (1998). Post-traumatic stress, pain and anxiety in adult burn victims. *Burns, 23*(7/8), 545–549; Schwartz, A.C., Bradley, R., Penza, K.M., Sexton, M., Jay, D., Haggard, P.J., Garow, S.J., & Ressler, K.J., (2006). Pain medication use among patients with posttraumatic stress disorder. *Psychosomatics,* 2006 Mar–April, *47*(2), 136–142.

8. Rothenhausler, H.B., Ehrentraut, S., Kapfhammer, H.P., Lang, C., Zachoval, R., Bilzer, M., Schelling, G., & Gerbes, A.L. (2002). Psychiatric and psychosocial outcome of orthotopic liver transplantation. *Psychotherapy Psychosomatic,* 2002 Sep–Oct, *71*(5), 285–297; Schofferman, J., Anderson, D., Hines, R., Smith, G., & Keane, G. (1993).

Childhood psychological trauma and chronic refractory low-back pain. *Clinical Journal of Pain, 9,* 260–265.

9. Felitti, V.J., Anda, R.F., Nordenberg, D., et al. (1998). Relationship of childhood abuse and household dysfunction to many of the leading causes of death in adults. The Adverse Childhood Experiences (ACE) Study. *American Journal of Preventative Medicine,* 1998 May, *14*(4), 245–258; Walker, E.A., Katon, W.J., Roy-Byrne, P.J., Jemelka, R.P., & Russo, J. (1993). Histories of sexual victimization in patients with irritable bowel syndrome or inflammatory bowel disease. *American Journal of Psychiatry, 150*(10), 1502–1506; de Leeuw, R., Schmidt, J.E., & Carlson, C.R. (2005). Traumatic stressors and posttraumatic stress disorder symptoms in headache patients. *Headache,* 2005 Nov–Dec, *45*(10), 1365–1374; Holmes, T., & Rahe, R. (1967). The Social Readjustment Rating Scale. *Journal of Psychosomatic Research, 11*(2), 213–218; Gupta, Madhulika A., Lanius, Ruth A., & van der Kolk, Bessel A. (2005). Psychologic trauma, posttraumatic stress disorder and dermatology. *Dermatologic Clinics, 23,* 645–649; Seng, J.S., Graham-Bermann, S.A., Clark, M.K., McCarthy, A.M., & Ronis, D.L. (2005). Posttraumatic stress disorder and physical comorbidity among female children and adolescents: Results from service-use data. *Pediatrics,* 2005 Dec, *116*(6), 767–776.

10. van der Kolk, Bessel, A., & van der Hart, Onno (1989). Pierre Janet and the breakdown of adaptation in psychological trauma, *American Journal of Psychiatry, 146*(12), 1530–1540.

11. Schnurr, Paula P., & Green, Bonnie L. (2003). A context for understanding the physical health consequences of exposure to extreme stress. In Paula P. Schnurr & Bonnie L. Green, *Trauma and health: Physical health consequences of exposure to extreme stress* (pp. 3–10). American Psychological Association, Washington. USA.

12. Child abuse: A history. Downloaded from https://www.encyclopedia.com/reference/encyclopedias-almanacs-transcripts-and-maps/child-abuse-history on October 17, 2023.

13. Delap, L. (2015). *Child welfare, child protection and sexual abuse, 1918—1990.* Retrieved from https://www.historyandpolicy.org/policy-papers/papers/child-welfare-child-protection-and-sexual-abuse-1918-1990 on October 17, 2023.

14. Butler, S. (2019). The impact of advanced capitalism on well-being: An evidence-informed model. *Human Arenas, 2,* 200–227.

15. Tidmarsh, L.V., Harrison, R., Ravindran, D., Matthews, S.L., Finlay, K.A. (2022). The influence of adverse childhood experiences in pain management: Mechanisms, processes, and trauma-informed care. *Frontiers in Pain Research* (Lausanne), 2022 Jun 10, 3:923866. doi: 10.3389/fpain.2022.923866. PMID: 35756908; PMCID: PMC9226323.

16. Meredith, P., Ownsworth, T., Strong, J. (2008). A review of the evidence linking adult attachment theory and chronic pain: Presenting a conceptual model. *Clinical Psychology Review*, 2008 Mar, *28*(3), 407–429. doi: 10.1016/j.cpr.2007.07.009. Epub 2007 Jul 19. PMID: 17719157.

17. Goodwin, Jean, & Attias, Reina, (1999). *Splintered reflections: Images of the body in trauma*. Basic Books.

18. Kluft, R.P. (2009). A clinician's understanding of dissociation: Fragments of an acquaintance. In P.F. Dell & J.A. O'Neil (Eds.), *Dissociation and the dissociative disorders: DSM-V and beyond* (pp. 599–624). Routledge/Taylor & Francis Group.

19. Holmes, E.A., Brown, R.J., Mansell, W., Fearon, R.P., Hunter, E.C., Frasquilho, F., & Oakley, D.A. (2005). Are there two qualitatively distinct forms of dissociation? A review and some clinical implications. *Clinical Psychology Review*, *25*(1), 1–23; van der Hart, O., & Dorahy, M.J. (2009). History of the concept of dissociation. In P.F. Dell & J.A. O'Neil (Eds.), *Dissociation and the dissociative disorders: DSM-V and beyond* (p. 19). Routledge/Taylor & Francis Group.

20. Dell, P.F. (2009). Understanding dissociation. In P.F. Dell & J.A. O'Neil (Eds.), *Dissociation and the dissociative disorders: DSM-V and beyond* (pp. 723–725). Routledge/Taylor & Francis Group.

21. Nijenhuis, E.R.S. (2009). Somatoform dissociation and somatoform dissociative disorders. In P.F. Dell & J.A. O'Neil (Eds.), *Dissociation and the dissociative disorders: DSM-V and beyond* (p. 262). Routledge/Taylor & Francis Group.

22. Shore, A. (2009). Attachment trauma and the developing right brain. In P.F. Dell & J.A. O'Neil (Eds.), *Dissociation and the dissociative disorders: DSM-V and beyond* (pp. 124–125). Routledge/Taylor & Francis Group; Nijenhuis, E.R.S. (2009). Somatoform dissociation and somatoform dissociative disorders. In P.F. Dell & J.A. O'Neil (Eds.), *Dissociation and the dissociative disorders: DSM-V and beyond* (pp. 261). Routledge/Taylor & Francis Group.

23. Dalenberg, Constance J. (2009). The case for the study of "normal" dissociation processes. In P.F. Dell & J.A. O'Neil (Eds.), *Dissociation and the dissociative disorders: DSM-V and beyond* (p. 261). Routledge/Taylor & Francis Group.

24. Dell, P.F. (2009). Understanding dissociation. In P.F. Dell & J.A. O'Neil (Eds.), *Dissociation and the dissociative disorders: DSM-V and beyond* (pp. 742–753). Routledge/Taylor & Francis Group.

25. Dell, P.F. (2009). Understanding dissociation. In P.F. Dell & J.A. O'Neil (Eds.), *Dissociation and the dissociative disorders: DSM-V and beyond* (pp. 724–725). Routledge/Taylor & Francis Group.

26. Dell, P.F. (2009). Understanding dissociation. In P.F. Dell & J.A. O'Neil (Eds.), *Dissociation and the dissociative disorders: DSM-V and beyond* (pp. 777–778). Routledge/Taylor & Francis Group.

27. Nijenhuis, E.R.S. (2009). Somatoform dissociation and somatoform dissociative disorders. In P.F. Dell & J.A. O'Neil (Eds.), *Dissociation and the dissociative disorders: DSM-V and beyond* (p. 269). Routledge/Taylor & Francis Group.

28. Putnam, F.W. (1997). *Dissociation in children and adolescents: A developmental perspective.* Guilford Press; Cardeña, E., & Carlson, E. (2011). Acute stress disorder revisited. *Annual Review of Clinical Psychology, 7*, 245–267.

29. Steele, K., van der Hart, O., & Nijenhuis, E.R.S. (2009). Dissociation versus alterations in consciousness: Related but different concepts. In P.F. Dell & J.A. O'Neill (Eds.), *Dissociation and the dissociative disorders: DSM-V and beyond* (p. 159). Routledge. New York.

30. Rosenthal, H. (2017). 12 things you didn't know about Milton H. Erickson and his daughter Betty. Psychotherapy.net.

31. Steele, K., van der Hart, O., & Nijenhuis, E.R.S. (2009). Dissociation versus alterations in consciousness: Related but different concepts. In P.F. Dell & J.A. O'Neill (Eds.), *Dissociation and the dissociative disorders: DSM-V and beyond* (p. 162). Routledge. New York; Simeon, D. (2009). Neurobiology of depersonalization disorder. In P.F. Dell & J.A. O'Neill (Eds.), *Dissociation and the dissociative disorders: DSM-V and beyond* (p. 369). Routledge. New York.

32. Simeon, D. (2009). Neurobiology of depersonalization disorder. In P.F. Dell & J.A. O'Neill (Eds.), *Dissociation and the dissociative disorders: DSM-V and beyond* (p. 369). Routledge. New York.

33. Tanner, J., Zeffiro, T., Wyss, D., Perron, N., Rufer, M., & Mueller-Pfeiffer, C. (2019). Psychiatric symptom profiles predict functional impairment. *Frontiers in Psychiatry, 10*, 37; Simeon, D. (2009). Neurobiology of depersonalization disorder. In P.F. Dell, & J.A. O'Neill (Eds.), *Dissociation and the dissociative disorders: DSM-V and beyond* (p. 437). Routledge. New York.

34. Duckworth, M.P., Iezzi, T., Archibald, Y., Haertlein, P., & Klinck, A. (2000). Dissociation and posttraumatic stress symptoms in patients with chronic pain. *International Journal of Rehabilitation and Health*, 5(2), 129–139.

35. Dell, P.F. (2009). Understanding dissociation. In P.F. Dell & J.A. O'Neil (Eds.), *Dissociation and the dissociative disorders: DSM-V and beyond* (p. 159). Routledge/Taylor & Francis Group.

36. King, S. (2000). *On writing: A memoir of the craft*. Scribner.

37. Steele, K., van der Hart, O., & Nijenhuis, E.R.S. (2009). Dissociation versus alterations in consciousness: Related but different concepts. In P.F. Dell & J.A. O'Neill (Eds.), *Dissociation and the dissociative disorders: DSM-V and beyond* (p. 157). Routledge. New York.

38. Brown, R.J. (2002). The cognitive psychology of dissociative states. *Cognitive Neuropsychiatry, 7*(3), 221–235. https://doi.org/10.1080/13546800244000085; Cardeña, E. (1994). The domain of dissociation. In S.J. Lynn & J.W. Rhue (Eds.), *Dissociation: Clinical and theoretical perspectives* (pp. 15–31). Guilford Press.

39. Schwartz, R. (2019). *Internal family systems therapy* (2nd edition). Guilford Press.

40. Holmes, E.A., Brown, R.J., Mansell, W., Fearon, R.P., Hunter, E.C., Frasquilho, F., & Oakley, D.A. (2005). Are there two qualitatively distinct forms of dissociation? A review and some clinical implications. *Clinical Psychology Review, 25*(1), 1–23.

41. Nijenhuis, E.R., Spinhoven, P., van Dyck, R., van Der Hart, O., & Vanderlinden, J. (1996). The development and psychometric characteristics of the Somatoform Dissociation Questionnaire (SDQ-20). *Journal of Nervous and Mental Disease*.

42. Scaer, R. (2014). *The body bears the burden* (3rd edition). Routledge.

43. Porges, S.W. (2009). The polyvagal theory: New insights into adaptive reactions of the autonomic nervous system. *Cleveland Clinic Journal of Medicine, 76*(Suppl 2), S86.

44. Michener, J.A. (2007). *The world is my home: A memoir.* Dial Press Trade Paperback.

45. Martins, D.F., Viseux, F.J., Salm, D.C., Ribeiro, A.C.A., da Silva, H.K.L., Seim, L.A., ... & Mazzardo-Martins, L. (2021). The role of the vagus nerve in fibromyalgia syndrome. *Neuroscience & Biobehavioral Reviews, 131*, 1136–1149.

46. Rothschild, B. (2000). *The body remembers.* WW Norton & Company. New York.

47. Spitzer, C., Barnow, S., Völzke, H., John, U., Freyberger, H.J., & Grabe, H.J. (2009). Trauma, posttraumatic stress disorder, and physical illness: Findings from the general population. *Psychosomatic Medicine, 71*(9), 1012–1017.

48. Johnson, C.M., & Makai, G.E. (2018, March). Fibromyalgia and irritable bowel syndrome in female pelvic pain. In *Seminars in Reproductive Medicine, 36*(02), 136–142. Thieme Medical Publishers.

49. Mannino, D.M., Thorn, D., Swensen, A., & Holguin, F. (2008). Prevalence and outcomes of diabetes, hypertension and cardiovascular disease in COPD. *European Respiratory Journal, 32*(4), 962–969.

Chapter Three

1. Apkarian, A.V., Sosa, Y., Sonty, S., Levy, R.M., Harden, R.N., Parrish, T.B., & Gitelman, D.R. (2004). Chronic back pain is associated with decreased prefrontal and thalamic gray matter density. *The Journal of Neuroscience, 24*(46), 10410–10415. https://doi.org/10.1523/jneurosci.2541-04.2004

2. Apkarian, A.V., Sosa, Y., Sonty, S., Levy, R.M., Harden, R.N., Parrish, T.B., & Gitelman, D.R. (2004). Chronic back pain is associated with decreased prefrontal and thalamic gray matter density. *The Journal of Neuroscience, 24*(46), 10410–10415. https://doi.org/10.1523/jneurosci.2541-04.2004

3. Mokhtar, M., Singh, P. (Updated July 24, 2023). Neuroanatomy, Periaqueductal Gray. In: *StatPearls* [Internet]. StatPearls Publishing, Treasure Island (FL). Available from: https://www.ncbi.nlm.nih.gov/books/NBK554391/

4. Basbaum, A.I., Fields, H.L. (1978). Endogenous pain control mechanisms: Review and hypothesis. *Annals of Neurology*, November, *4*(5), 451–62. doi:10.1002/ana.410040511. PMID 216303. S2CID 72620829

5. Wu, D., Wang, S., Stein, J.F., Aziz, T.Z., Green A.L. (2014). Reciprocal interactions between the human thalamus and periaqueductal gray may be important for pain perception. *Experimental Brain Research*, *232*(2), 527–34. doi: 10.1007/s00221-013-3761-4. Epub 2013 Nov 12. PMID: 24217977

6. Kulkarni, B., Bentley, D., Elliott, R.M., Julyan, P.J., Boger, E., Watson, A., Boyle, Y., El-Deredy, W., & Jones, A.K. (2007). Arthritic pain is processed in brain areas concerned with emotions and fear. *Arthritis Rheum*, *56*(4), 1345–1354. https://doi.org/10.1002/art.22460

7. Crook, R.J., Dickson, K., Hanlon, R.T., & Walters, E.T. (2014). Nociceptive sensitization reduces predation risk. *Current Biology*, *24*(10), 1121–1125. https://doi.org/10.1016/j.cub.2014.03.043

8. Cozolino, L. (2017). *The neuroscience of psychotherapy* (3rd edition). WW Norton & Company.

9. Apkarian, A.V., Hashmi, J.A., Baliki, M.N. (2011). Pain and the brain: Specificity and plasticity of the brain in clinical chronic pain. *Pain*. https://journals.lww.com/pain/Citation/2011/03001/Pain_and_the_brain__Specificity_and_plasticity_of.8.aspx; Tajerian, M., Hung, V., Nguyen, H., et al. (2018). The hippocampal extracellular matrix regulates pain and memory after injury. *Molecular Psychiatry*, *23*(12), 2302–2313. https://www.nature.com/articles/s41380-018-0209-z; Smallwood, R., Laird, A., Ramage, A., Parkinson, A., Lewis, J., Clauw, D., et al. (2013). Structural brain anomalies and chronic pain: A quantitative meta-analysis of gray matter volume. *The Journal of Pain*, *14*(7), 663–675.

10. Rauch, S.L., Shin, L.M., & Phelps, E.A. (2006). Neurocircuitry models of posttraumatic stress disorder and extinction: Human neuroimaging research—past, present, and future. *Biological Psychiatry*, *60*(4), 376–382. https://doi.org/10.1016/j.biopsych.2006.06.004

11. Woon, Fu L., & Hedges, Dawson W. (2008). Hippocampal and amygdala volumes in children and adults with childhood maltreatment-related posttraumatic stress disorder: A meta-analysis. *Hippocampus*, *18*(8), 729–736.

12. Teicher, M.H., Samson, J., Tomoda, A., Ashy, M., & Andersen, S. (2006). Neurobiological and behavioral consequences of exposure to childhood traumatic stress. In B.B. Arnetz & R. Ekman, *Stress in health and disease* (pp. 180–195). Wiley-VCH Verlag GmbH & Co. KGaA eBooks. https://doi.org/10.1002/3527609156.ch9

13. Coghill, R., Gilron, I., & Iadarola, M. (2001). Hemispheric lateralization of somatosensory processing. *Journal of Neurophysiology*, *85*(6), 2602–2612; Wasan, A.D., Anderson, N.K., & Giddon, D.B. (2010). Differences in pain, psychological symptoms, and gender distribution among patients with left- vs right-sided chronic spinal pain. *Pain Medicine*, *11*(9), 1373–1380. https://doi.org/10.1111/j.1526-4637.2010.00922.x

14. LeDoux, J. (1998). *The emotional brain*. Simon & Schuster, US.

15. Spitzer, C., Willert, C., Grabe, H.J., Rizos, T., Möller, B., & Freyberger, H.J. (2004). Dissociation, hemispheric asymmetry, and dysfunction of hemispheric interaction: A transcranial magnetic stimulation approach. *Journal of Neuropsychiatry and Clinical Neurosciences*, *16*(2), 163–169. https://doi.org/10.1176/jnp.16.2.163

16. Fisher, J. (2017). *Healing the fragmented selves of trauma survivors*. Routledge.

17. Shore, A. (2023). *Attachment trauma and the developing right brain*. In Martin J. Dorahy, Stephen N. Gold, & John A. O'Neill (Eds.), *Dissociation and dissociative disorders: Past, present, future* (2nd edition). Routledge.

18. Woon, Fu L., & Hedges, Dawson W. (2008). Hippocampal and amygdala volumes in children and adults with childhood maltreatment-related posttraumatic stress disorder: A meta-analysis. *Hippocampus*, *18*(8), 729–736.

19. Teicher, M.H., Samson, J.A., Tomoda, A., Ashy, M., & Andersen, S.L. (2006). Neurobiological and behavioral consequences of exposure to childhood traumatic stress. In B. B. Arnetz & R. Ekman; *Stress in health and disease* (pp. 190–205). Wiley-VCH. Verlag GmbH & Co.

20. Kuchinad, Anil, Schweinhardt, Petra, Seminowicz, David., et.al., (2007) Accelerated brain gray matter loss in fibromyalgia patients: Premature aging of the brain? *The Journal of Neuroscience*, April 11, 2007, *27*(15), 4004–4007.

21. Apkarian, A.V., Thomas, P. Sebastian, Krauss, Beth R., & Szeverenyi, Nikolaus M. (2001). Prefrontal cortical hyperactivity in patients with sympathetically mediated chronic pain. *Neuroscience Letters*, *311*, 193–197.

22. Baliki, Marwan N., Geha Paul Y., Apkarian, A. Vania., & Chialvo, Dante R. (2008). Beyond feeling: Chronic pain hurts the brain, disrupting the default-mode network dynamics. *The Journal of Neuroscience,* February 6, 2008, *28*(6), 1398–1403; References and further reading may be available for this article. To view references and further reading you must purchase this article.

23. Schwoebel, J., Friedman, R., Duda, N., & Coslett, H.B. (2001). Pain and the body schema: Evidence for peripheral effects on mental representations of movement. *Brain,* 2001 Oct, 124 (Pt 10), 2098–104.

24. Apkarian, A.V., Hashmi, J.A., Baliki, M.N. (2011). Pain and the brain: Specificity and plasticity of the brain in clinical chronic pain. *Pain.* https://journals.lww.com/pain/Citation/2011/03001/Pain_and_the_brain__Specificity_and_plasticity_of.8.aspx; Ray, A., & Zbik, A. (2002). Cognitive behavioral therapies and beyond. In Tollison, C. David, Sattherwaite, John R., & Tollison, Joseph W., (Eds.), *Practical pain management* (pp. 189–207). Lippincott Williams & Wilkins, Philadelphia; Rome, H.P., & Rome, J.D. (2000). Limbically augmented pain syndrome (LAPS): Kindling, corticolimbic sensitization, and the convergence of affective and sensory symptoms in chronic pain disorders. *Pain Medicine, 1*(1), 7–23. https://doi.org/10.1046/j.1526-4637.2000.99105.x; Mansour, A.R., et al. (2014). Chronic pain: The role of learning and brain plasticity. *Restorative Neurology and Neuroscience, 32*(1), 129–39; Borsook, D., Moulton, E.A., Schmidt, K.F., & Becerra, L. (2007). Neuroimaging revolutionizes therapeutic approaches to chronic pain. *Molecular Pain, 3,* 1744–25. https://doi.org/10.1186/1744-8069-3-25

25. Borsook, D., Moulton, E.A., Schmidt, K.F., & Becerra, L. (2007). Neuroimaging revolutionizes therapeutic approaches to chronic pain. *Molecular Pain, 3,* 1744–25. https://doi.org/10.1186/1744-8069-3-25

26. Apkarian, A.V., Hashmi, J.A., Baliki, M.N. (2011). Pain and the brain: Specificity and plasticity of the brain in clinical chronic pain. *Pain.* https://journals.lww.com/pain/Citation/2011/03001/Pain_and_the_brain__Specificity_and_plasticity_of.8.aspx

27. Ray, A., & Zbik, A. (2002). Cognitive behavioral therapies and beyond. In Tollison, C. David, Sattherwaite, John R., & Tollison, Joseph W., (Eds.), *Practical pain management* (pp. 189–207). Lippincott Williams & Wilkins, Philadelphia.

28. Rome, H.P., & Rome, J.D. (2000). Limbically augmented pain syndrome (LAPS): Kindling, corticolimbic sensitization, and the convergence of affective and sensory symp-

toms in chronic pain disorders. *Pain Medicine, 1*(1), 7–23. https://doi.org/10.1046/j.1526-4637.2000.99105.x

29. Borsook, D., Youssef, A.M., Simons, L.E., Elman, I., & Eccleston, C. (2018). When pain gets stuck: The evolution of pain chronification and treatment resistance. *Pain, 159*(12), 2421–2436. https://doi.org/10.1097/j.pain.0000000000001401

30. Apkarian, A.V., Hashmi, J.A., Baliki, M.N. (2011). Pain and the brain: Specificity and plasticity of the brain in clinical chronic pain. *Pain.* https://journals.lww.com/pain/Citation/2011/03001/Pain_and_the_brain__Specificity_and_plasticity_of.8.aspx

31. Siegel, D. (2020). *The developing mind* (3rd edition). Guilford Press; van der Kolk. (2015). *The body keeps the score.* Penguin Press; Ogden, P., & Fisher, J. (2015). *Sensorimotor psychotherapy.* WW Norton & Co. Chapters 8, 9 & 11; Schore, A.N. (2022). Right brain-to-right brain psychotherapy: Recent scientific and clinical advances. *Annals of General Psychiatry, 21*(1). https://doi.org/10.1186/s12991-022-00420-3

32. Shapiro, F. (1995). *EMDR: Basic principles, protocols and procedures.* Guilford Press, NY; Elofsson, U., von Scheele, B., Theorell, T., & Sondergaard, H. (2008). Physiological correlates of eye movement desensitization and reprocessing. *Journal of Anxiety Disorders, 22*(4), 622–34; Bossini, L., Tavanti, M., Calossi, S., Polizzotto, N., Vatti, G., Marino, D., & Castrogiovanni, P. (2011). EMDR treatment for posttraumatic stress disorder, with focus on hippocampal volumes: A pilot study. *The Journal of Neuropsychiatry and Clinical Neurosciences*; Bergmann, U. (2012). *Neurobiological foundations for EMDR practice.* Springer, NY; Pagani, M., Di Lorenzo, G., Verardo, A.R., Nicolais, G., Monaco, L., Lauretti, G., Russo, R., Niolu, C., Ammaniti, M., Fernandez, I., & Siracusano, A. (2012). Neurobiological correlates of EMDR monitoring—An EEG study. *PLoS One, 7*(9), e45753. https://doi.org/10.1371/journal.pone.0045753; Laugharne, J., Kullack, C., Lee, C.W., McGuire, T., Brockman, S., Drummond, P.D., & Starkstein, S.E. (2016). Amygdala volumetric change following psychotherapy for posttraumatic stress disorder. *Journal of Neuropsychiatry and Clinical Neurosciences, 28*(4), 312–318. https://doi.org/10.1176/appi.neuropsych.16010006

33. Kulkarni, B., Bentley, D., Elliott, R.M., Julyan, P.J., Boger, E., Watson, A., Boyle, Y., El-Deredy, W., & Jones, A.K. (2007). Arthritic pain is processed in brain areas concerned with emotions and fear. *Arthritis Rheum, 56*(4), 1345–1354. https://doi.org/10.1002/art.22460; Apkarian, A.V., Hashmi, J.A., Baliki, M.N. (2011). Pain and the brain: Specificity and plasticity of the brain in clinical chronic pain. *Pain.* https://journals.lww.com/

pain/Citation/2011/03001/Pain_and_the_brain__Specificity_and_plasticity_of.8.aspx; Tajerian, M., Hung, V., Nguyen, H., et al. (2018). The hippocampal extracellular matrix regulates pain and memory after injury. *Molecular Psychiatry*, *23*(12), 2302–2313. https://www.nature.com/articles/s41380-018-0209-z; Smallwood, R., Laird, A., Ramage, A., Parkinson, A., Lewis, J., Clauw, D., et al. (2013). Structural brain anomalies and chronic pain: A quantitative meta-analysis of gray matter volume. *The Journal of Pain*, *14*(7), 663–675.

34. Pagani, M., Di Lorenzo, G., Verardo, A.R., Nicolais, G., Monaco, L., Lauretti, G., Russo, R., Niolu, C., Ammaniti, M., Fernandez, I., & Siracusano, A. (2012). Neurobiological correlates of EMDR monitoring—An EEG study. *PLoS One*, *7*(9), e45753. https://doi.org/10.1371/journal.pone.0045753

35. Laugharne, J., Kullack, C., Lee, C.W., McGuire, T., Brockman, S., Drummond, P.D., & Starkstein, S.E. (2016). Amygdala volumetric change following psychotherapy for post-traumatic stress disorder. *Journal of Neuropsychiatry and Clinical Neurosciences*, *28*(4), 312–318. https://doi.org/10.1176/appi.neuropsych.16010006

36. Ghanbari Nia, N., Afrasiabifar, A., & Behnammoghadam, M. (2018, September 28). Comparing the effect of eye movement desensitization and reprocessing (EMDR) with guided imagery on pain severity in patients with rheumatoid arthritis. *Dovepress.* https://www.dovepress.com/comparing-the-effect-of-eye-movement-desensitization-and-reprocessing--peer-reviewed-fulltext-article-JPR

37. Mansour, A.R., et al. (2014). Chronic pain: The role of learning and brain plasticity. *Restorative Neurology and Neuroscience*, *32*(1), 129–39.29.

38. Amano, T., & Toichi, M. (2016). The role of alternating bilateral stimulation in establishing positive cognition in EMDR therapy: A multi-channel near-infrared spectroscopy study. *PLoS One*, *11*(10), e0162735. https://doi.org/10.1371/journal.pone.0162735

39. Elofsson, U., von Scheele, B., Theorell, T., & Sondergaard, H. (2008). Physiological correlates of eye movement desensitization and reprocessing. *Journal of Anxiety Disorders*, *22*(4), 622–34; Ghanbari Nia, N., Afrasiabifar, A., & Behnammoghadam, M. (2018, September 28). Comparing the effect of eye movement desensitization and reprocessing (EMDR) with guided imagery on pain severity in patients with rheumatoid arthritis. *Dovepress.* https://www.dovepress.com/comparing-the-effect-of-eye-movement-desensitization-and-reprocessing--peer-reviewed-fulltext-article-JPR

40. Baek, J., Lee, S., Cho, T., et al. (2019). Neural circuits underlying a psychotherapeutic regimen for fear disorders. *Nature.* https://www.nature.com/articles/s41586-019-0931-y

41. Grant, M. (2000). EMDR: A new treatment for trauma and chronic pain. *Complimentary Therapies in Nursing & Midwifery, 6*(2), 91–94. Harcourt; Grant, M, & Threlfo, C. (2002). EMDR in the treatment of chronic pain, *Journal of Clinical Psychology, 58*(12), 1505–1520.

42. Borsook, D., Moulton, E.A., Schmidt, K.F., & Becerra, L. (2007). Neuroimaging revolutionizes therapeutic approaches to chronic pain. *Molecular Pain, 3*, 1744–25. https://doi.org/10.1186/1744-8069-3-25; Borsook, D., Youssef, A.M., Simons, L.E., Elman, I., & Eccleston, C. (2018). When pain gets stuck: The evolution of pain chronification and treatment resistance. *Pain, 159*(12), 2421–2436. https://doi.org/10.1097/j.pain.0000000000001401; Siegel, D. (2020). *The developing mind* (3rd edition). Guilford Press.

43. Dworkin, M. (2005). *EMDR and the relational imperative.* Routledge, New York; Hase, M., & Brisch, K.H. (2022). The therapeutic relationship in EMDR therapy. *Frontiers in Psychology, 13.* https://doi.org/10.3389/fpsyg.2022.835470

44. Piedfort-Marin, O. (2018). Transference and countertransference in EMDR therapy. *Journal of EMDR Practice and Research, 12*(3), 158–172.

45. Hase, M., & Brisch, K.H. (2022). The therapeutic relationship in EMDR therapy. *Frontiers in Psychology, 13.* https://doi.org/10.3389/fpsyg.2022.835470

46. Schore, A.N. (2022). Right brain-to-right brain psychotherapy: Recent scientific and clinical advances. *Annals of General Psychiatry, 21*(1). https://doi.org/10.1186/s12991-022-00420-3

47. Taylor, A.G., Goehler, L.E., Galper, D.I., Innes, K.E., & Bourguignon, C. (2010). Top-down and bottom-up mechanisms in mind-body medicine: Development of an integrative framework for psychophysiological research. *Explore: The Journal of Science and Healing, 6*(1), 29–41. https://doi.org/10.1016/j.explore.2009.10.004.

48. LeDoux, J. (1998). *The emotional brain.* Simon & Schuster, US.

49. van der Kolk, B.A. (2015b). *The body keeps the score.* Penguin Press. p. 62.

50. Ulrich, L. (2009). The bottom-up protocol. In Marilyn Luber (Ed.), *Eye movement desensitization and reprocessing (EMDR): Scripted protocols.* Springer, NY, pp. 349–356; Levine, P. (2011). *Waking the tiger.* North Atlantic Books; D'Antoni, F., Matiz, A., Fabbro, F., & Crescentini, C. (2022). Psychotherapeutic techniques for distressing memories: A comparative study between EMDR, brainspotting, and body scan meditation. *International Journal of Environmental Research and Public Health, 19*(3), 1142. https://doi.org/10.3390/ijerph19031142; Macy, R.J., Jones, E., Graham, L.M., & Roach, L. (2018). *Sage Journals Home.* Sage Journals. https://journals.sagepub.com/doi/10.1177/1524838015620834

51. Spinazzola, J., & Wilson, K. (2019, March 1). The tip of the iceberg in adaptation to complex trauma. *Complex Trauma.* https://www.complextrauma.org/

52. van der Kolk. (2015c). *The body keeps the score.* Penguin Press. p. 206.

53. Porges, S.W. (2003). The polyvagal theory: Phylogenetic contributions to social behavior. *Physiology & Behavior, 79*(3), 503–513. https://doi.org/10.1016/s0031-9384(03)00156-2

54. Sanabria-Mazo, J., Colomer-Carbonell, A., Carmona-Cervelló, M., Feliu-Soler, A., Borràs, X., Grasa, M., Esteve, M., Maes, M., Edo, S., Sanz, A., & Luciano, J. (2022). Immune-inflammatory and hypothalamic-pituitary-adrenal axis biomarkers are altered in patients with non-specific low back pain: A systematic review. *Frontiers in Immunology;* Kolacz, J., & Porges, S.W. (2018). Chronic diffuse pain and functional gastrointestinal disorders after traumatic stress: Pathophysiology through a polyvagal perspective. *Frontiers in Medicine,* 5. https://doi.org/10.3389/fmed.2018.00145

55. Linnstaedt, S. (2018, August 27). Chronic pain after trauma may depend on what stress gene variation you carry. *The Conversation.* https://theconversation.com/chronic-pain-after-trauma-may-depend-on-what-stress-gene-variation-you-carry-102021

56. Linnstaedt, S. (2018, August 27). Chronic pain after trauma may depend on what stress gene variation you carry. *The Conversation.* https://theconversation.com/chronic-pain-after-trauma-may-depend-on-what-stress-gene-variation-you-carry-102021

57. Koenig, J., Loerbroks, A., Jarczok, M.N., Fischer, J.E., & Thayer, J.F. (2016). Chronic pain and heart rate variability in a cross-sectional occupational sample. *The Clinical Journal of Pain, 32*(3), 218–225. https://doi.org/10.1097/ajp.0000000000000242

58. Kolacz, J., & Porges, S.W. (2018b). Chronic diffuse pain and functional gastrointestinal disorders after traumatic stress: Pathophysiology through a polyvagal perspective. *Frontiers in Medicine, 5*. https://doi.org/10.3389/fmed.2018.00145

59. Yamada, K., Adams, H., Ellis, T., Clark, R., Sully, C., Larivière, C., & Sullivan, M. (2022). The temporal relation between pain and fatigue in individuals receiving treatment for chronic musculoskeletal pain. *BMC Musculoskeletal Disorders, 23*(1). https://doi.org/10.1186/s12891-022-05162-7

60. Porges, S.W. (2021). Cardiac vagal tone: A neurophysiological mechanism that evolved in mammals to dampen threat reactions and promote sociality. *World Psychiatry, 20*(2), 296–298. https://doi.org/10.1002/wps.20871

61. Woon, Fu L., & Hedges, Dawson W. (2008). Hippocampal and amygdala volumes in children and adults with childhood maltreatment-related posttraumatic stress disorder: A meta-analysis. *Hippocampus, 18*(8), 729–736.

62. Crook, R.J., Dickson, K., Hanlon, R.T., & Walters, E.T. (2014). Nociceptive sensitization reduces predation risk. *Current Biology, 24*(10), 1121–1125. https://doi.org/10.1016/j.cub.2014.03.043

Chapter Four

1. Shapiro, Francine (1989). Eye movement desensitization: A new treatment for post-traumatic stress disorder. *Journal of Behaviour Therapy & Experimental Psychiatry, 20*(3), pp. 211–217; Wilson, S.A., Becker, L.A., & Tinker, R.H. (1997). Fifteen-month follow-up of eye movement desensitization and reprocessing (EMDR) treatment for PTSD and psychological trauma. *Journal of Consulting and Clinical Psychology, 65*, 1047–1056.

2. Shapiro, Francine (2002). Appendix A: Evaluations of EMDR. In *EMDR as an integrative psychotherapy*. American Psychological Association, Washington; Tesarz, Jonas, Wicking, Manon, Bernardy, Kathron, & Seidler, Gunter H. (2019). EMDR's efficacy in the treatment of pain. *Journal of EMDR Practice and Research, 13*(4), 337–344; de Roos, C.J.A.M., Veenstra, A.C., den Holllander-Gijsman, M.E., van der Wee, N.J.A., de Jongh, A., Zitman, F.G., & van Rood, Y.R. (2006). Eye movement desensitization and reprocessing (EMDR) for chronic phantom limb pain (PLP): A preliminary study of 10 cases. *Pain* (In press); Schneider, J., Hofman, A., Rost, C., Shapiro, F. (2008). EMDR in the treatment of chronic phantom limb pain. *Pain Medicine, 9*(1), 76–82.

3. Matthijssen, S.J.M.A., Lee, C.W., de Roos, C., Barron, I.G., Jarero, I., Shapiro, E., Hurley, E.C., Schubert, S.J., Baptist, J., Amann, B.L., Moreno-Alcázar, A., Tesarz, J., & de Jongh, A. (2020). The current status of EMDR therapy, specific target areas, and goals for the future. *Journal of EMDR Practice and Research, 14*(4), 241–284. https://doi.org/10.1891/emdr-d-20-00039

4. Matthijssen, S.J.M.A., Lee, C.W., de Roos, C., Barron, I.G., Jarero, I., Shapiro, E., Hurley, E.C., Schubert, S.J., Baptist, J., Amann, B.L., Moreno-Alcázar, A., Tesarz, J., & de Jongh, A. (2020). The current status of EMDR therapy, specific target areas, and goals for the future. *Journal of EMDR Practice and Research, 14*(4), 241–284. https://doi.org/10.1891/emdr-d-20-00039

5. Nia, N.G., Afrasiabifar, A., & Behnammoghadam, M. (2018). Comparing the effect of eye movement desensitization and reprocessing (EMDR) with guided imagery on pain severity in patients with rheumatoid arthritis. *Journal of Pain Research, 11*, 2107–2113. https://doi.org/10.2147/jpr.s158981

6. Estergard, L. (2008). Eye movement desensitization and reprocessing in the treatment of chronic pain. *Walden University ProQuest Dissertations.* https://www.proquest.com/openview/2978cebada7cf8e19a1ddf4462e347ab/1.pdf?pq-origsite=gscholar&cbl=18750; Suárez, N.A., Pérez, J.M., Redolar-Ripoll, D., Hogg, B.M., Gardoki-Souto, I., Guerrero, F.G., Cabrera, S.J., Bernal, D.S., Amann, B.L., & Moreno-Alcázar, A. (2020). EMDR versus treatment-as-usual in patients with chronic non-malignant pain: A randomized controlled pilot study. *Journal of EMDR Practice and Research, 14*(4), 190–205. https://doi.org/10.1891/emdr-d-20-00004; Gerhardt, A., Leisner, S., Hartmann, M., Janke, S., Seidler, G.H., Eich, W., & Tesarz, J. (2016b). Eye movement desensitization and reprocessing vs. treatment-as-usual for non-specific chronic back pain patients with psychological trauma: A randomized controlled pilot study. *Frontiers in Psychiatry, 7.* https://doi.org/10.3389/fpsyt.2016.00201

7. Brennstuhl, M., Tarquinio, C., & Montel, S. (2014). Chronic pain and PTSD: Evolving views on their comorbidity. *Perspectives in Psychiatric Care, 51*(4), 295–304. https://doi.org/10.1111/ppc.12093

8. Rostaminejad, A., Behnammoghadam, M., Rostaminejad, M., Behnammoghadam, Z., & Bashti, S. (2017). Efficacy of eye movement desensitization and reprocessing on the phantom limb pain of patients with amputations within a 24-month follow-up.

International Journal of Rehabilitation Research, 40(3), 209–214. https://doi.org/10.1097/mrr.0000000000000227

9. Tesarz, J., Baumeister, D., Andersen, T.E., & Vaegter, H.B. (2020). Pain perception and processing in individuals with posttraumatic stress disorder: a systematic review with meta-analysis. *Pain Reports, 5*(5), p. e849. https://doi.org/10.1097/pr9.0000000000000849

10. Tesarz, J., Leisner, S., Gerhardt, A., Janke, S., Seidler, G.H., Eich, W., & Hartmann, M. (2013). Effects of eye movement desensitization and reprocessing (EMDR) treatment in chronic pain patients: A systematic review. *Pain Medicine, 15*(2), 247–263. https://doi.org/10.1111/pme.12303

11. Rostaminejad, A., Behnammoghadam, M., Rostaminejad, M., Behnammoghadam, Z., & Bashti, S. (2017). Efficacy of eye movement desensitization and reprocessing on the phantom limb pain of patients with amputations within a 24-month follow-up. *International Journal of Rehabilitation Research, 40*(3), 209–214. https://doi.org/10.1097/mrr.0000000000000227; Grant, M., & Threlfo, C. (2002b). EMDR in the treatment of chronic pain. *Journal of Clinical Psychology, 58*(12), 1505–1520. https://doi.org/10.1002/jclp.10101

12. Wilson, S.A., Becker, L.A., & Tinker, R.H. (1997). EMDR treatment of phantom limb pain. Conference report regarding EMDR treatment of six patients with phantom limb pain. *EMDR International Conference, 1997,* San Francisco USA.

13. Grant, M. (2014). Eye movement desensitization reprocessing treatment of chronic pain. *OA Musculoskeletal Medicine,* Aug, *17*(2), 17.

14. Apkarian, A.V., Hashmi, J.A., & Baliki, M.N. (2011). Pain and the brain: Specificity and plasticity of the brain in clinical chronic pain. *Pain, 152*(3), S49–S64. https://doi.org/10.1016/j.pain.2010.11.010

15. Kolacz, J., & Porges, S.W. (2018). Chronic diffuse pain and functional gastrointestinal disorders after traumatic stress: Pathophysiology through a polyvagal perspective. *Frontiers in Medicine, 5*. https://doi.org/10.3389/fmed.2018.00145

16. Froud, R., Patterson, S., Eldridge, S., Seale, C., Pincus, T., Rajendran, D., Fossum, C., & Underwood, M. (2014). A systematic review and meta-synthesis of the impact of low back pain on people's lives. *BMC Musculoskeletal Disorders, 15*(1). https://doi.org/10.1186/1471-2474-15-50

17. Hunter, M.E. (2009). *Understanding dissociative disorders: A guide for family physicians and health care professionals.* Crown House Publishing. p. 37. https://www.crownhouse-publishing.com/understanding-dissociative-disorders1

18. Kleiman, V., Clarke, H., & Katz, J. (2011). Sensitivity to pain traumatization: A higher-order factor underlying pain-related anxiety, pain catastrophizing and anxiety sensitivity among patients scheduled for major surgery. *Pain Research & Management, 16*(3), 169–177. https://doi.org/10.1155/2011/932590

19. Kleiman, V., Clarke, H., & Katz, J. (2011). Sensitivity to pain traumatization: A higher-order factor underlying pain-related anxiety, pain catastrophizing and anxiety sensitivity among patients scheduled for major surgery. *Pain Research & Management, 16*(3), 169–177. https://doi.org/10.1155/2011/932590

20. Tesarz, J., Leisner, S., Gerhardt, A., Janke, S., Seidler, G.H., Eich, W., & Hartmann, M. (2013). Effects of eye movement desensitization and reprocessing (EMDR) treatment in chronic pain patients: A systematic review. *Pain Medicine, 15*(2), 247–263. https://doi.org/10.1111/pme.12303

21. Koechlin, H., Coakley, R., Schechter, N.L., Werner, C., & Kossowsky, J. (2018). The role of emotion regulation in chronic pain: A systematic literature review. *Journal of Psychosomatic Research, 107,* 38–45. https://doi.org/10.1016/j.jpsychores.2018.02.002; Messman-Moore, T.L., & Bhuptani, P.H. (2017). A review of the long-term impact of child maltreatment on posttraumatic stress disorder and its comorbidities: An emotion dysregulation perspective. *Clinical Psychology: Science and Practice, 24*(2), 154–169. https://doi.org/10.1111/cpsp.12193; Ford, J.D., & Courtois, C.A. (2014). Complex PTSD, affect dysregulation, and borderline personality disorder. *Borderline Personality Disorder and Emotion Dysregulation, 1*(1), 9. https://doi.org/10.1186/2051-6673-1-9

22. Shalala, N., Tan, J., & Biberdzic, M. (2020). The mediating role of identity disturbance in the relationship between emotion dysregulation, executive function deficits, and maladaptive personality traits. *Personality and Individual Differences, 162,* 110004. https://doi.org/10.1016/j.paid.2020.110004; Nicola, M., Correia, H., Ditchburn, G., & Drummond, P.D. (2019). Invalidation of chronic pain: A thematic analysis of pain narratives. *Disability and Rehabilitation, 43*(6), 861–869. https://doi.org/10.1080/09638288.2019.1636888

23. Koechlin, H., Coakley, R., Schechter, N.L., Werner, C., & Kossowsky, J. (2018). The role of emotion regulation in chronic pain: A systematic literature review. *Journal of Psychosomatic Research*, *107*, 38–45. https://doi.org/10.1016/j.jpsychores.2018.02.002

24. Kolacz, J., & Porges, S.W. (2018). Chronic diffuse pain and functional gastrointestinal disorders after traumatic stress: Pathophysiology through a polyvagal perspective. *Frontiers in Medicine*, 5. https://doi.org/10.3389/fmed.2018.00145

25. Bean, D., Dryland, A., Rashid, U., & Tuck, N.L. (2022). The determinants and effects of chronic pain stigma: A mixed methods study and the development of a model. *The Journal of Pain*, *23*(10), 1749–1764. https://doi.org/10.1016/j.jpain.2022.05.006

26. Wu, D. (1982). Psychotherapy and emotion in traditional Chinese medicine. In *Springer eBooks* (pp. 285–301). https://doi.org/10.1007/978-94-010-9220-3_12

27. Patierno, C., Fava, G.A., & Carrozzino, D. (2023b). Illness denial in medical disorders: A systematic review. *Psychotherapy and Psychosomatics*, 1–16. https://doi.org/10.1159/000531260

28. Yvette, R. (2012). *Metaphysical anatomy*. Metaphysical Anatomy. https://metaphysicalanatomy.com/mat/index.php

29. Afrell, M., Biguet, G., & Rudebeck, C.E. (2007b). Living with a body in pain—between acceptance and denial. *Scandinavian Journal of Caring Sciences*, *21*(3), 291–296. https://doi.org/10.1111/j.1471-6712.2007.00475.x

30. van Middendorp, H., Lumley, M.A., Jacobs, J.W.G., van Doornen, L.J., Bijlsma, J.W.J., & Geenen, R. (2008). Emotions and emotional approach and avoidance strategies in fibromyalgia. *Journal of Psychosomatic Research*, *64*(2), 159–167. https://doi.org/10.1016/j.jpsychores.2007.08.009

31. Kolacz, J., & Porges, S.W. (2018). Chronic diffuse pain and functional gastrointestinal disorders after traumatic stress: Pathophysiology through a polyvagal perspective. *Frontiers in Medicine*, 5. https://doi.org/10.3389/fmed.2018.00145

32. Shaygan, M., Saranjam, E., Faraghi, A., & Mohebbi, Z. (2022). Migraine headaches: The predictive role of anger and emotional intelligence. *International Journal of Community Based Nursing and Midwifery*. *10*(1), 74–83. doi: 10.30476/IJCBNM.2021.90552.1706. PMID: 35005043; PMCID: PMC8724728.

33. van der Kolk, B.A., Fisher, D.J., Korn, D., & Levine, P.A. (2023). The assessment and treatment of complex PTSD. *ResearchGate.* https://www.researchgate.net/publication/265099248_The_Assessment_and_Treatment_of_Complex_PTSD

34. Vance, A. (2016b). *Elon Musk: How the billionaire CEO of SpaceX and Tesla is shaping our future.* Virgin Publishing.

35. Siegel, D.J. (2018). *Aware: The science and practice of presence.* TarcherPerigee. https://drdansiegel.com/book/aware/

Chapter Five

1. Naylor, B., Boag, S., & Gustin, S.M. (2017). New evidence for a pain personality? A critical review of the last 120 years of pain and personality. *Scandinavian Journal of Pain, 17*(1), 58–67. https://doi.org/10.1016/j.sjpain.2017.07.011

2. Saariaho, T., Saariaho, A., Karila, I., & Joukamaa, M. (2011). Early maladaptive schema factors, chronic pain and depressiveness: A study with 271 chronic pain patients and 331 control participants. *Clinical Psychology & Psychotherapy, 19*(3), 214–223. https://doi.org/10.1002/cpp.737

3. Hay, L. (1995). *You can heal your life* (30th anniversary edition). Hay House. https://books.google.com.eg/books/about/You_Can_Heal_Your_Life.html?id=piyr4LGA8-gC&redir_esc=y

4. Kabat-Zinn, J. (2013). *Full catastrophe living: How to cope with stress, pain and illness using mindfulness meditation* (revised). Piatkus. https://books.google.com.eg/books/about/Full_Catastrophe_Living.html?id=qkT8lQEACAAJ&redir_esc=y

5. Sarno, J.E. (1982). *Healing back pain: The mind-body connection* (1st edition). Wellness Central. https://www.goodreads.com/book/show/144873.Healing_Back_Pain

6. Dell, P.F. (2022). *Clarifying the etiology of the dissociative disorders* (p. 243). Routledge eBooks. https://doi.org/10.4324/9781003057314-18

7. Putnam, Frank (2016). *The way we are: How states of mind influence our identities, personality and potential for change.* International Psychoanalytic Books.

8. Peroutka, S.J. (2004). Migraine: a chronic sympathetic nervous system disorder. *Headache, 44*(1), 53–64. https://doi.org/10.1111/j.1526-4610.2004.04011.x

9. Hussain, F., Shapiro, P.A., & Muskin, P.R. (2013). Somatoform disorders and headache. In *Cambridge University Press eBooks* (pp. 149–163). https://doi.org/10.1017/cbo9781139206952.014

10. Spierings, E.L. (2017). A perspective on the comorbidities of chronic migraine. *Open Access Journal of Neurology & Neurosurgery, 6*(3). https://doi.org/10.19080/oajnn.2017.06.555688; Peterlin, B.L., Tietjen, G.E., Brandes, J.L., Rubin, S.M., Drexler, E., Lidicker, J., & Meng, S. (2009). Posttraumatic stress disorder in migraine. *Headache, 49*(4), 541–551. https://doi.org/10.1111/j.1526-4610.2009.01368.x

11. Maizels, M., & Burchette, R.J. (2004). Somatic symptoms in headache patients: The influence of headache diagnosis, frequency, and comorbidity. *Headache, 44*(10), 983–993. https://doi.org/10.1111/j.1526-4610.2004.04192.x

12. Saçmacı, H., Cengiz, G.F., & Aktürk, T. (2020). Impact of dissociative experiences in migraine and its close relationship with osmophobia. *Neurological Research, 42*(7), 529–536. https://doi.org/10.1080/01616412.2020.1753417

13. Peterlin, B.L., Tietjen, G.E., Brandes, J.L., Rubin, S.M., Drexler, E., Lidicker, J., & Meng, S. (2009). Posttraumatic stress disorder in migraine. *Headache, 49*(4), 541–551. https://doi.org/10.1111/j.1526-4610.2009.01368.x; Mays, I., Flynn, J., McGuire, B.E., & Egan, J. (2021). The role of attachment style, adverse childhood experiences and dissociation in migraine. *Journal of Trauma & Dissociation*, 1–34. https://doi.org/10.1080/15299732.2021.1989114

14. Schauer, M., & Elbert, T. (2010). Dissociation following traumatic stress. *Zeitschrift Für Psychologie Mit Zeitschrift Für Angewandte Psychologie, 218*(2), 109–127. https://doi.org/10.1027/0044-3409/a000018

15. Schalinski, I., Schauer, M., & Elbert, T. (2015). The shutdown dissociation scale (Shut-D). *European Journal of Psychotraumatology, 6*(1). https://doi.org/10.3402/ejpt.v6.25652

16. Marcus, S. (2008). Phase 1 of integrated EMDR an abortive treatment for migraine headaches. *Journal of EMDR Practice and Research, 2*(1), 15–25. https://doi.org/10.1891/1933-3196.2.1.15

17. Marcus, Steve (2023). Personal communication

18. de Roos, C.J.A.M., Veenstra, A.C., de Jongh, A.D., den Hollander-Gijsman, M.E., van der Wee, N.J.A., Zitman, F.G., & van Rood, Y.R. (2010). Treatment of chronic phantom limb pain using a trauma-focused psychological approach. *Pain Research & Management, 15*(2), 65–71.

19. McCracken, L. (2008). Psychological effects of chronic pain: An overview. In Peter J. Wilson, Paul J. Watson, et al. (Eds.), *Clinical pain management: Chronic pain*. CRC Press; Barbuto, John P., White, George L. Jr, Porucznik, Christina A., Holmes, Edward B., Chronic pain: Second, do no harm. *American Journal of Physical Medicine & Rehabilitation, 87*(1), 78–83, January 2008. doi: 10.1097/PHM.0b013e31815e87b1; Tedstone, J., & Tarrier, N. (2003). Posttraumatic stress disorder following medical illness and treatment. *Clinical Psychology Review, 23*, 409–448; Deatrich, K., Boyer, B. (2016). Post-traumatic stress disorder related to surgery: Prevalence and risk factors. In C.R. Martin et al. (Eds.), *Comprehensive guide to posttraumatic stress disorders* (pp. 351–366). Springer.

20. Kluft, R.P. (2022). Toward the effective treatment of dissociative symptoms and dissociative disorders, *Psychoanalytic Social Work,* doi: 6. 10.1080/15228878.2022.2095876

21. Bjick, S. (2001). Accessing the power in the patient with hypnosis and EMDR. Eye Movement Desensitization and Reprocessing. *American Journal of Clinical Hypnosis,* 2001 Jan–Apr, *43*(3–4), 203–16. doi: 10.1080/00029157.2001.10404277. PMID: 11269625; Fine, C.G., & Berkowitz, A.S. (2001). The wreathing protocol: The imbrication of hypnosis and EMDR in the treatment of dissociative identity disorder and other dissociative responses, *American Journal of Clinical Hypnosis, 43*(3–4), 275–290, doi: 10.1080/00029157.2001.10404282; Harford, P. M. (2010), The integrative use of EMDR and clinical hypnosis in the treatment of adults abused as children. *Journal of EMDR Practice and Research, 4*(2), 60–75. https://doi.org/10.1891/1933-3196.4.2.60; Ramondo, N., Gignac, G.E., Pestell, C.F., Byrne, S.M. (2021). Clinical hypnosis as an adjunct to cognitive behavior therapy: An updated meta-analysis. The *International Journal of Clinical and Experimental Hypnosis,* 2021 Apr–Jun, *69*(2), 169–202. doi: 10.1080/00207144.2021.1877549. Epub 2021 Mar 1. PMID: 33646087.

22. Nicosia, G.J. (1995). Eye movement desensitization and reprocessing is not hypnosis. Dissociation: Progress in the Dissociative Disorders, 8(1), 69.

23. Lawrence, M. (1998). EMDR as a special form of ego state psychotherapy: Part one. Dec 1998 *EMDRIA Newsletter.*

24. Phillips, M., & Frederick, C. (1995). *Healing the divided self.* WW Norton & Company. New York.

25. Hendrix, H., & Lakelly, H. (2005). *Receiving love: Transforming your relationship by letting yourself be loved.* Atria Books.

26. Duckworth, M.P., Iezzi, T., Archibald, Y., Haertlein, P., & Klinck, A. (2000). Dissociation and posttraumatic stress symptoms in patients with chronic pain. *International Journal of Rehabilitation and Health, 5*(2), 129–139; Goodwin, Jean, & Attias, Reina (1999). *Splintered reflections: Images of the body in trauma.* Basic Books. NY. USA.

27. Porges, S.W. (2009). The polyvagal theory: New insights into adaptive reactions of the autonomic nervous system. *Cleveland Clinic Journal of Medicine, 76*(Suppl 2), S86.

28. Siegel, Daniel (2010). *The mindful therapist.* WW Norton & Company. New York.

29. Ogden, P., & Fisher, J. (2015). *Sensorimotor psychotherapy: Interventions for trauma and attachment.* (Norton series on interpersonal neurobiology). WW Norton & Company.

30. Watkins, H.H. (1993). Ego-state therapy: An overview. *American Journal of Clinical Hypnosis, 35*(4), 232–240. https://doi.org/10.1080/00029157.1993.10403014

31. Badenoch, B. (2018). Safety is the treatment. In S.W. Porges & D. Dana (Eds.), *Clinical applications of the polyvagal theory: The emergence of polyvagal-informed therapies* (p. 75). WW Norton & Company. New York.

32. Rogers, C. (2003). *Client-centered therapy.* Constable Books.

33. Porges, S.W., Doussard-Roosevelt, J.A., & Maiti, A.K. (1994). Vagal tone and the physiological regulation of emotion. *Monographs of the Society for Research in Child Development, 240/59*(2–3), 167–186. doi:10.2307/1166144

34. Dohler, C. (2009). Wir haben uns immerzu in die augen geschaut und er hat sehr viel gelächelt [We looked into each other's eyes the whole time and he smiled a lot] (Interview with Margarethe Lutz). *Süddeutsche Zeitung Magazin*, Issue 13. Retrieved from http://sz-magazin.sueddeutsche.de/texte/anzeigen/28738/Er-hat-sehr-viel-gelaechelt [Google Scholar]

35. Watkins, H.H. (1993). Ego-state therapy: An overview. *American Journal of Clinical Hypnosis, 35*(4), 232–240. https://doi.org/10.1080/00029157.1993.10403014

36. Rosenthal, H. (2017). 12 things you didn't know about Milton H. Erickson and his daughter Betty. Psychotherapy.net. https://www.psychotherapy.net/blog/title/12-things-you-didn-t-know-about-milton-h.-erickson-and-his-daughter-betty-alice-erickson

37. Korn, D.L., & Leeds, A.M. (2002). Preliminary evidence of efficacy for EMDR resource development and installation in the stabilization phase of treatment of complex post-traumatic stress disorder. *Journal of Clinical Psychology*, *58*(12), 1465–1487.

38. Schmidt, S J. (2004). Developmental needs meeting strategy: A new treatment approach applied to dissociative identity disorder. *Journal of Trauma & Dissociation*, *5*(4), 55–78.

39. Schwarz, L., Corrigan, F., Hull, A., & Raju, R. (2017). The comprehensive resource model: Effective therapeutic techniques for the healing of complex trauma. Routledge/Taylor & Francis Group.

40. Ogden, P., & Fisher, J. (2015). *Sensorimotor psychotherapy: Interventions for trauma and attachment.* (Norton series on interpersonal neurobiology). WW Norton & Company.

41. Schneider, J., Hofmann, A., Rost, C., & Shapiro, F. (2008). EMDR in the treatment of chronic phantom limb pain. *Pain Medicine*, *9*(1), 76–82.

42. Phillips, M. (2019). It takes more than two to tango: Building secure attachment through hypnotic and ego-state relationships. *American Journal of Clinical Hypnosis*, *62*(1–2), 95–117.

43. Wade, T.C., & Wade, D.K. (2001). Integrative psychotherapy: Combining ego-state therapy, clinical hypnosis, and eye movement desensitization and reprocessing (EMDR) in a psychosocial developmental context. *American Journal of Clinical Hypnosis*, *43*(3–4), 233–245.

44. Lawrence, M. (1999). EMDR as a special form of ego state psychotherapy: Part two. *EMDRIA Newsletter.*

45. Schmidt, S.J. (1963). Internal conference room ego-state therapy and the resolution of double binds: Preparing clients for EMDR trauma processing. June, 1968, 1969.

Chapter Six

1. Watkins, H.H. (1993). Ego-state therapy: An overview. *American Journal of Clinical Hypnosis, 35*(4), 232–240. https://doi.org/10.1080/00029157.1993.10403014

2. Schore, A.N. (2022a). Attachment trauma and the developing right brain. In: *Routledge eBooks* (pp. 177–208). https://doi.org/10.4324/9781003057314-15

3. Amano, T., & Toichi, M. (2016b). The role of alternating bilateral stimulation in establishing positive cognition in EMDR therapy: A multi-channel near-infrared spectroscopy study. *PLoS One, 11*(10), e0162735. https://doi.org/10.1371/journal.pone.0162735

4. Brown, D.P., & Elliott, D.S. (2016). *Attachment disturbances in adults: Treatment for comprehensive repair.* WW Norton & Company. https://psycnet.apa.org/record/2016-40220-000

5. Siegel, D. (2004). *Parenting from the inside out: How a deeper understanding of your-self can help you raise children who thrive.* Tarcher-Perigree.

6. Schwartz, R. (2021b). *No bad parts: How the Internal Family Systems Model changes everything.* Sounds True.

7. Siegel, D. (2004). *Parenting from the inside out: How a deeper understanding of your-self can help you raise children who thrive.* Tarcher-Perigree.

8. Schmidt, S.J. (2009). *The Developmental Needs Meeting Strategy: An ego state therapy for healing adults with childhood trauma and attachment wounds.* DNMS Institute, LLC.

9. Siegel, D. (2004). *Parenting from the inside out: How a deeper understanding of your-self can help you raise children who thrive.* Tarcher-Perigree.

Chapter Eight

1. Halpin, S., Casson, A.J., Tang, N.K.Y., Jones, A., O'Connor, R.J., & Sivan, M. (2023). A feasibility study of pre-sleep audio and visual alpha brain entrainment for people with chronic pain and sleep disturbance. *Frontiers in Pain Research, 4.* https://doi.org/10.3389/fpain.2023.1096084; Zhou, W., Chonghuan, Y., Wang, H., Mao, Y., Zhang, W., Liu, A., Yang, C., Li, T., Hayashi, L., Zhao, W., Chen, L., Liu, Y., Tao, W., & Zhang, Z. (2022). Sound induces analgesia through corticothalamic circuits. *Science, 377*(6602), 198–204. https://doi.org/10.1126/science.abn4663

2. Jain, A., Bansal, R., Kumar, A., & Singh, K. (2015). A comparative study of visual and auditory reaction times on the basis of gender and physical activity levels of medical first year students. *International Journal of Applied & Basic Medical Research, 5*(2), 124. https://doi.org/10.4103/2229-516x.157168

3. Paulson, S., & Sandra, O. (2022). Personal communication; Boukezzi, S., Silva, C., Nazarian, B., Rousseau, P., Guedj, E., Valenzuela-Moguillansky, C., & Khalfa, S. (2017). Bilateral alternating auditory stimulations facilitate fear extinction and retrieval. *Frontiers in Psychology, 8.* https://doi.org/10.3389/fpsyg.2017.00990

4. Crook, R.J., Dickson, K., Hanlon, R.T., & Walters, E.T. (2014b). Nociceptive sensitization reduces predation risk. *Current Biology, 24*(10), 1121–1125. https://doi.org/10.1016/j.cub.2014.03.043

5. Grant, M. (2014). Eye movement desensitization reprocessing treatment of chronic pain. *OA Musculoskeletal Medicine, 2*(2), 17. https://www.researchgate.net/profile/Mark-Grant-8/publication/285068690_Pain_control_with_EMDR/links/5f9c747092851c14bcf637e9/Pain-control-with-EMDR.pdf

6. Grant, M. (2014a). The use of an app to manage carpal tunnel syndrome. *OA Behavioral Medicine, 20, 2*(1), 3. https://www.researchgate.net/publication/274254948_The_use_of_an_app_to_manage_carpal_tunnel_syndrome; Grant, M., Lau, R., & DiNardo, J. (2024). A randomized control trial regarding the efficacy of an app series based on EMDR for the effects of PTSD. (Manuscript in preparation.)

7. Grant, M. (2014). Eye movement desensitization reprocessing treatment of chronic pain. *OA Musculoskeletal Medicine,* Aug, *17*(2), 17.

8. Grant, M., Lau, R., & DiNardo, J. (2024). A randomized control trial regarding the efficacy of an app series based on EMDR for PTSD symptoms. (Manuscript in preparation.)

Chapter Nine

1. Leeds, Andrew (2007). Learning to feel good about positive emotions with the positive affect tolerance and integration protocol. *EMDRIA Annual Conference*, Dallas, USA.

2. Clark A. (2013). Whatever next? Predictive brains, situated agents, and the future of cognitive science. *Behavioral and Brain Sciences, 36*(3), 181–204. doi:10.1017/

S0140525X12000477; Cepelewicz, J. (2018). To make sense of the present, brains may predict the future. *Quanta Magazine*, July 2018.

3. Jerome, F. (1973). *Persuasion and healing* (revised edition). John Hopkins University Press, Baltimore, USA.

4. Colla, R., Williams, P., Oades, L.G., Camacho-Morles, J. (2022). "A new hope" for positive psychology: A dynamic systems reconceptualization of hope theory. *Frontiers in Psychology* (Sec. Positive Psychology), *13*, February 23, 2022. https://doi.org/10.3389/fpsyg.2022.809053

5. Chevetz, R.A. (2015). *Intensive psychotherapy for persistent dissociative processes* (p. vii). Norton.

6. Short, D., Erickson, B., Klein, R. (2005). *Hope and resiliency: Understanding the psychotherapeutic strategies of Milton H. Erickson.* Crown House Publishing.

Chapter Ten

1. Deatrich, K., Boyer, B. (2016). Post-traumatic stress disorder related to surgery: Prevalence and risk factors. In C.R. Martin et al. (Eds.), *Comprehensive guide to posttraumatic stress disorders* (pp. 351–366). Springer.

2. Nandhan, R., Kameswaran, M., Kameswaran, S. (2016). The evolution of hearing from fishes to Homo sapiens: A chronological review. *Scholars Academic Journal of Biosciences*, *4*(12), 1060–1069.

3. Paulsen, Sandra (2022). Personal communication; Richardson, P.S., Williams, S.R., Hepenstall, S., Gregory, L.J., McKie, S., & Corrigan, F.M. (2009). A single-case fMRI study: EMDR treatment of a patient with posttraumatic stress disorder. *Journal of EMDR Practice and Research*, *3*(1), 10–23. https://doi.org/10.1891/1933-3196.3.1.10

4. Grant, M. (2014a).The use of an app to manage carpal tunnel syndrome. *OA Behavioral Medicine*, *2*(2), p. 3; Grant, M. (2014b). Eye movement desensitization reprocessing treatment of chronic pain. *OA Musculoskeletal Medicine*, *2*(2), Article 17.

5. Grant, M. (2024). A randomized control trial regarding the efficacy of an app series based on EMDR for PTSD symptoms. In submission; Elofsson, U.O., von Scheele, B.,

Theorell, T., Sondergaard, H.P. (2007). Physiological correlates of eye movement desensitization and reprocessing. *Journal of Anxiety Disorders*, June 3, [Epub ahead of print].

6. Grant, M. (2014a).The use of an app to manage carpal tunnel syndrome. *OA Behavioral Medicine, 2*(2), p. 3. Grant, M. (2014b). Eye movement desensitization reprocessing treatment of chronic pain. *OA Musculoskeletal Medicine, 2*(2), Article 17.

7. Shapiro, Francine (1995). *Eye movement desensitization and reprocessing: Basic principles, protocols and procedures*. Guilford Press. New York.

8. Deatrich, K., Boyer, B. (2016). Post-traumatic stress disorder related to surgery: Prevalence and risk factors. In C.R. Martin et al. (Eds.), *Comprehensive guide to posttraumatic stress disorders* (pp. 351–366). Springer.

9. Nandhan, R., Kameswaran, M., Kameswaran, S. (2016). The evolution of hearing from fishes to Homo sapiens: A chronological review. *Scholars Academic Journal of Biosciences, 4*(12), 1060–1069.

10. Paulsen, Sandra (2022). Personal communication.

11. Richardson, P.S., Williams, S.R., Hepenstall, S., Gregory, L.J., McKie, S., & Corrigan, F.M. (2009). A single-case fMRI study: EMDR treatment of a patient with posttraumatic stress disorder. *Journal of EMDR Practice and Research, 3*(1), 10–23. https://doi.org/10.1891/1933-3196.3.1.10; Grant, M. (2014a). The use of an app to manage carpal tunnel syndrome. *OA Behavioral Medicine, 2*(2), p. 3; Grant, M. (2014b). Eye movement desensitization reprocessing treatment of chronic pain. *OA Musculoskeletal Medicine, 2*(2), Article 17; Grant, M. (2024). A randomized control trial regarding the efficacy of an app series based on EMDR for PTSD symptoms. In submission.

12. Elofsson, U.O., von Scheele, B., Theorell, T., Sondergaard, H.P. (2007). Physiological correlates of eye movement desensitization and reprocessing. *Journal of Anxiety Disorders*, June 3, [Epub ahead of print].

Chapter Eleven

1. Shapiro, F. (1995). *Eye movement desensitization and reprocessing: Basic protocols and procedures*. Guilford Press. pp. 244–271.

2. Tew, Marilyn (2023). *Interweaves—an explanation.* Downloaded from https://www.emdrgateway.com/videos on September 20, 2023.

3. Loewenstein, R.J. (1991). An office mental status examination for complex chronic dissociative symptoms and multiple personality disorder. *Psychiatric Clinics of North America.* 1991 Sep, *14*(3), 567–604. PMID: 1946025.

4. Kearney, B.E., Corrigan, F.M., Frewen, P.A., Nevill, S., Harricharan, S., Andrews, K., Jetly, R., McKinnon, M.C., & Lanius, R.A. (2023). A randomized controlled trial of Deep Brain Reorienting: A neuroscientifically guided treatment for post-traumatic stress disorder. *European Journal of Psychotraumatology,14*(2):2240691. doi:10.1080/20008066.2023.2240691. PMID: 37581275; PMCID: PMC10431732.

Chapter Twelve

1. Haley, Jay (1993). *Uncommon therapy*. WW Norton & Company. New York.

2. Spiegel, Herbert, & Spiegel, David (2004). *Trance and treatment: Clinical uses of hypnosis* (2nd edition). American Psychiatric Publishing. Washington DC.

3. Thompson, Trevor, Terhune, Devin Blair, Oram, Charlotte et al. (2019). The effectiveness of hypnosis for pain relief: A systematic review and meta-analysis of 85 experimental trials. *Neuroscience & Biobehavioral Reviews, 99.* doi: 10.1016/j.neubiorev.2019.02.013

4. Greenleaf, M. (2006). Mind styles and the hypnotic induction profile: measure and match to enhance medical treatment. *American Journal of Clinical Hypnosis*, Jul, *49*(1):41–58. doi: 10.1080/00029157.2006.10401551. PMID: 16889361.

5. Kluft, R.P. (1992). The use of hypnosis with dissociative disorders. *Psychiatric Medicine, 10*(4), 31–46. PMID: 1289960.

6. Harford, P.M. (2010). The integrative use of EMDR and clinical hypnosis in the treatment of adults abused as children. *Journal of EMDR Practice and Research, 4*(2), 60–75. https://doi.org/10.1891/1933-3196.4.2.60

7. Fine, C.A., & Berkowitz, A.S. (2001). The wreathing protocol: The imbrications of hypnosis and EMDR in the treatment of dissociative identity disorder and other dissociative responses. *American Journal of Clinical Hypnosis, 43*, 275–290.

8. Phillips, M. (2001). Potential contributions of hypnosis to ego-strengthening procedures in EMDR. *American Journal of Clinical Hypnosis, 43*, 247–262.

9. Dell, P.F. (2019). Reconsidering the autohypnotic model of the dissociative disorders. *Journal of Trauma & Dissociation,* Jan-Feb, *20*(1):48–78. doi: 10.1080/15299732.2018.1451806. Epub 2018 Mar 22. PMID: 29565750.

10. Sadler, Pamela, & Woody, Erik (2010). Dissociation in hypnosis: Theoretical frameworks and psychotherapeutic implications. In S.J. Lynn, J.W. Rhue & I. Kirsch (Eds.) *Handbook of Clinical Hypnosis*. APA. Washington DC.

11. Patterson, David R. (2010). *Clinical hypnosis for pain management.* American Psychological Association. Washington DC.

12. Ewin, Dabney (2019). Constant pain: I live with it. American Society of Clinical Hypnosis scientific meeting. San Antonio, USA.

Chapter Thirteen

1. Smith, T.J., Wilson, M.A., Karl, J.P., Orr, J.S., Smith, C., Cooper, A., Heaton, K.J., Young, A., & Montain, S.J. (2018). Impact of sleep restriction on local immune response and skin barrier restoration with and without "multinutrient" nutrition intervention. *Journal of Applied Physiology, 124*(1), 190–200. https://doi.org/10.1152/japplphysiol.00547.2017; Irwin, M.R., Olmstead, R.G., & Carroll, J. (2016). Sleep disturbance, sleep duration, and inflammation: A systematic review and meta-analysis of cohort studies and experimental sleep deprivation. *Biological Psychiatry, 80*(1), 40–52. https://doi.org/10.1016/j.biopsych.2015.05.014

2. Smith, T.J., Wilson, M.A., Karl, J.P., Orr, J.S., Smith, C., Cooper, A., Heaton, K.J., Young, A., & Montain, S.J. (2018). Impact of sleep restriction on local immune response and skin barrier restoration with and without "multinutrient" nutrition intervention. *Journal of Applied Physiology, 124*(1), 190–200. https://doi.org/10.1152/japplphysiol.00547.2017; Irwin, M.R., Olmstead, R.G., & Carroll, J. (2016). Sleep disturbance, sleep duration, and inflammation: A systematic review and meta-analysis of cohort studies and experimental sleep deprivation. *Biological Psychiatry, 80*(1), 40–52. https://doi.org/10.1016/j.biopsych.2015.05.014

3. Davies, K., Macfarlane, G.J., Nicholl, B.I., Dickens, C., Morriss, R., Ray, D., & McBeth, J. (2008). Restorative sleep predicts the resolution of chronic widespread pain: Results from the EPIFUND study. *Rheumatology, 47*(12), 1809–1813. https://doi.org/10.1093/rheumatology/ken389

4. Haack, M., & Mullington, J.M. (2005). Sustained sleep restriction reduces emotional and physical well-being. *Pain,* Dec 15, *119*(1–3), 56–64. Epub Nov 16.

5. Killgore, W.D., Kahn-Greene, E.T.T., Lipizzi, E.L., Newman, R.A., Kamimori, G.H., & Balkin, T.J. (2007). Sleep deprivation reduces perceived emotional intelligence and constructive thinking skills. *Sleep Medicine, August* [Epub ahead of print].

6. Older, S.A., Battafarano, D.F., Danning, C.L., et al. (2005). Delta wave sleep interruption and fibromyalgia symptoms in healthy subjects. [Abstract] *Journal of Musculoskeletal Pain, 3*(Suppl 1), 159.

7. Davis, Gail C. (2003). Improved sleep may reduce arthritis pain. *Holistic Nursing Practice,* May/June, 128–135.

8. Angoli-Israel, Sonia (2001). "Sleep is not tangible" or what the Hebrew tradition has to say about sleep. *Psychosomatic Medicine, 63,* 778–787.

9. Warburton, D.E., Nicol C.W., & Bredin, S.S. (2006). Health benefits of physical activity: The evidence. *CMAJ, 174*(6), 801–809.

10. Trivedi, M.H., Greer, T.L., Grannemann, B.D., Chambliss, H.O., Jordan, A.N. (2006). Exercise as an augmentation strategy for treatment of major depression. *Journal of Psychiatric Practice, 12*(4), 205–13.

11. Ratey, John (2008). *Spark: the revolutionary new science of exercise and the brain.* Little Brown & Co. NY. USA.

12. Blumenthal, James A., Babyak, Michael A., Doraiswamy, P. Murali et al. (2007). Exercise and pharmacotherapy in the treatment of major depressive disorder. *Psychosomatic Medicine 69,* 587–596.

13. Hayden, Jill, van Tulder, Maurits, Malmivaara, A.V., Koes, Bart W. (2005). Meta-analysis: Exercise for non-specific low back pain. *Annals of Internal Medicine, 142*(9), 765–775 (May 3, 2005).

14. Rhudy, J., Williams, A., McCabe, K., Rambo, P., & Russell J. (2006). Emotional modulation of spinal nociception and pain: The impact of predictable noxious stimulation. *Pain, 126*(1), 221–233.

15. Davidson, R.J. (2000). Affective style, psychopathology, and resilience: Brain mechanisms and plasticity. *American Psychologist, 55,* 1196–1214.

16. Siegel, Daniel (1999). *The developing mind.* Guilford Press. New York.

17. Siegel, Daniel (1999). *The developing mind.* Guilford Press. New York.

18. Rosen, Sidney (1982). My voice will go with you. *The teaching tales of Milton H. Erickson* (pp. 47–52). WW Norton & Co. New York.

19. Urry, Heather L., Nitschke, Jack B., Dolski, Isa., et al. (2004). Making a life worth living: Neural correlates of well-being. *Psychological Science, 15*(6), 367–372.

20. Michener, J.A. (2003). *Chesapeake* (p. 851). Dial Press Trade Paperback. Reprint edition.

Index

T

U

V